# The Nursing Process

# The Nursing Process
## Theory, Application, and Related Processes

**Norma Nolan Pinnell, R.N., B.S.N., M.S.N.**
Instructor, School of Nursing
Southern Illinois University at Edwardsville
Edwardsville, Illinois

**Mary de Meneses, R.N., M.A., M.S., Ed.D.**
Associate Professor, School of Nursing
Southern Illinois University at Edwardsville
Edwardsville, Illinois

 APPLETON-CENTURY-CROFTS/Norwalk, Connecticut

0-8385-7036-4

Notice: The author(s) and publisher of this volume have taken care that the information
and recommendations contained herein are accurate and compatible with the standards generally
accepted at the time of publication.

Copyright © 1986 by Appleton-Century-Crofts
A Publishing Division of Prentice-Hall

86 87 88 89 90 / 10 9 8 7 6 5 4 3 2 1

Prentice-Hall of Australia, Pty. Ltd., Sydney
Prentice-Hall Canada, Inc.
Prentice-Hall Hispanoamericana, S.A., Mexico
Prentice-Hall of India Private Limited, New Delhi
Prentice-Hall International (UK) Limited, London
Prentice-Hall of Japan, Inc., Tokyo
Prentice-Hall of Southeast Asia (Pte.) Ltd., Singapore
Whitehall Books Ltd., Wellington, New Zealand
Editora Prentice-Hall do Brasil Ltda., Rio de Janeiro

**Library of Congress Cataloging-in-Publication Data**
Pinnell, Norma Nolan.
    The nursing process.

Includes index.
1. Nursing.  I. de Meneses, Mary.  II. Title.
[DNLM: 1. Nursing Process. WY 100 P656n]
RT41.P58  1986     610.73     85-28804
ISBN 0-8385-7036-4

Design: M. Chandler Martylewski

PRINTED IN THE UNITED STATES OF AMERICA

To:

My husband Tom for his help, understanding, encouragement, and love.

*Norma*

My family, especially my sons Luis and Daniel.

*Mary*

# Contents

# Preface

Through the years societal needs and changes within the overall health care system have created a need for nurses to examine themselves and their role. Because of this introspection and reflection, nursing has gradually evolved from an intuitive, compassionate form of care to a scientific form. Today's professional nurses recognize the importance of theory-based care. They see as their goal the need to maximize the health of their clients by diagnosing potential and actual health concerns and by delivering care that maintains, restores, and promotes health. Effective use of the nursing process promotes achievement of this goal.

The purpose of this book is to increase the nurse's knowledge of all steps of the nursing process—assessing, diagnosing, planning, implementing, and evaluating. A comprehensive approach to the nursing process is made within the framework of the problem-solving process. The nursing process is viewed as a conceptual, intellectual, and dynamic process that can be used in any health care setting and applied to any client—individual, family, or community.

In addition to the nursing process, this book includes chapters on the related processes of research, teaching, decision making, and change. The content within these chapters is organized to present new material before its application to the nursing process is discussed. These processes are conceptualized as integral components of nursing action and as such are part of the nursing process.

We wish to take this opportunity to express appreciation to our families and friends who offered us their patience, understanding, and assistance during the development of this book. We wish to thank Barry Merkin who helped us during the early planning phase and David Gordon, Nursing Editor, Appleton-Century-Crofts, who helped us through the publishing process. We appreciate the efforts and contributions of the reviewers and wish to express our thanks to them. We also wish to thank our students (past and present) who produced a need in us to clarify our thinking about the nursing process.

# Development of Contemporary Nursing

To understand why the nursing process evolved into a problem-solving method, it is important to study the historical events of its origin and growth. The act of nursing can be traced from antiquity through the Dark Ages to the present. In this chapter, we will consider how nursing has responded to the needs of society, milestones in nursing education, significant studies and reports affecting nursing, and the transition in the scope of practice and focus of care.

Study of this chapter will help you to:

1. Discuss how nursing has responded to problems, issues, and needs of society.
2. Discuss the evolution of theory-based care.
3. Identify health trends affecting the nursing profession.
4. Describe the change in the scope of nursing practice.
5. Identify three studies that were important to the growth of the nursing profession.
6. Discuss the transition in health care focus.

## THE RESPONSE OF NURSING TO THE NEEDS OF SOCIETY

Nursing is affected by the changes, problems, and issues of society. Since early civilization, nursing has assumed the structure and functions that best met societal needs at that time.

### Early Christian Period

It was not until the early Christian period that nursing actually took root. Christ's teachings urged people to love and care for their neighbors. These teachings were implemented by church groups whose primary concern was the care of the sick, poor, aged, orphans, widows, slaves, and prisoners. Most active in such services were women.[7,9]

Women were classified into three groups: deaconesses, widows, and virgins. Virgins were more concerned with church duties than with the charitable work with the sick;

widows worked among the sick and poor but had less church work to perform. The deaconesses performed both secular as well as religious duties.[7]

The deaconesses in the Eastern churches were of particular importance. Many of these women had wealth and social position. Deaconesses were the early counterparts to the community health nurse of today. Phoebe was the first deaconess and perhaps the first visiting nurse. She carried the letters of St. Paul and cared for him. In the Epistle of Paul to the Romans, dated about 58 A.D., reference is made in Chapter 16, verses 1 and 2, to Phoebe and her work.[7]

Although the position of the deaconess originated in the Eastern Church, it spread to Rome, Italy, Gaul, and Ireland. In Rome, women holding similar positions were called Roman Matrons. Three Roman matrons who contributed significantly to nursing were Fabiola, St. Marcella, and St. Paula. Fabiola founded the first free hospital in Rome in 390 A.D. St. Marcella established the first monastery for women and taught her followers the care of the sick. In the broadest sense, she might be considered the first nurse educator. St. Paula (347 to 404 A.D.) devoted her fortune to the establishment of hospitals and roadside shelters for pilgrims traveling to Jerusalem. She built a hospital in Bethlehem and, with her community sisters, nursed the sick. Some historians credit her with being the first to teach nursing as an art rather than as a service.[6,7]

## Middle Ages

The Middle Ages constituted the period in European history between Antiquity and the Renaissance—476 to 1453 A.D. The first half of this period has been called the Dark Ages.

During the Dark Ages, the world was in a state of chaos: civilization deteriorated; the population decreased both in number and strength; crime increased; and impoverished people were tortured and imprisoned when they were unable to pay high taxes. Because of extreme moral decay, the Roman Empire faced destruction. Disorganized and persecuted communities turned to feudalism and monasticism in an attempt to survive.

**Feudalism** was a political and economic system whereby a person who held land under a feudal lord received protection in return for service and homage. Although feudalism afforded protection to many, it prevented the development of a strong central government and prevented progress because of constant warfare. The feudal system encouraged the growth of chivalry—which eventually led to the institution of knighthood.

**Monasticism**, on the other hand, offered the opportunity for men and women to live a Christian life while pursuing an occupational career of their choosing. The monasteries played a large role in the preservation of culture and learning as well as offering refuge to the persecuted, care to the sick, and education to the illiterate.

Monasticism provided the organizational structure needed to meet some of the changes, problems, and issues of that period. One form of monasticism still flourishing today is the order of Benedictines founded by St. Benedict (480 to 543 A.D.). St. Benedict was born of noble parents. He became disgusted at the moral decay that he found in Rome and, as a result, organized a monastic family. He eventually founded monasteries throughout Europe.

The care of the sick was an important part of the community life in all Benedictine monasteries. Monastery gardens were the source of plants, herbs, and minerals used for healing. St. Benedict established infirmaries within the monasteries for the care of sick members of the order and to help organize the care of pilgrims and wayfarers. The monasteries gave women the opportunity to pursue a career and satisfy their intellectual and spiritual needs. Because the nurses were part of a community of scholars in the monasteries, they were able to strengthen the scientific, artistic, and cultural components of nursing.[7]

The Crusades, which swept through Northern Europe during the late Middle Ages, lasted almost 200 years (1096 to 1291). Ideas, customs, values, and beliefs, as well as attitudes concerning health and illness, were spread between the East and West by the Crusades. In addition, the nomadic movements of individuals during this time produced major health problems. Leprosy, bubonic plague, syphilis, and mental illness were widespread.[7] Provisions for health care were not adequate to meet the mounting needs of society, and, once again, changes within the structure of nursing occurred. The Deaconess movement became almost extinct, and in its place, military, mendicant, secular, and religious orders of nurses evolved.

**Military nursing orders** drew large numbers of men into the field of nursing. The membership in these orders consisted of knights, monks, and serving brothers. The Knights Hospitallers was such a military order. The original purpose of this order was to bring the wounded from the battlefield to the hospitals and to care for them there. Eventually two other branches of the Knights were formed, one group to defend the pilgrims and the other to defend the wounded while they were being brought to the hospital. The effect of these early care providers was not lost completely through the years. The Knights, who were at times required to defend the hospital and its patients, wore a suit of armor under their habits. On the habit was a black mantle with a white Maltese cross. Years later when a badge was designed for the Nightingale School, this same cross was used. The idea of a badge representing a school of nursing was the forerunner of the nursing pin as we know it today.[4,7]

The **mendicant orders** of nursing came into existence as a direct response to the rapid spread of poverty and sickness. These orders were based on the practice of begging or accepting alms to provide the necessary food and supplies to care for the sick and poor. St. Francis of Assisi (1182 to 1226) and St. Dominic were the dominant leaders in this area and each founded three orders.[7,10]

**Secular orders** of nurses were composed of members who could terminate their vocation at any time and who were not bound to the vows of monastic life. Their work was similar to that of the monastic orders, but they lived in their own homes. The Order of Antonines (1095), the Order of the Holy Ghost (1180), and the Beguines of Flanders, Belgium (1184), were some of the prominent secular orders. The only nursing education offered was an apprenticeship.[4,7]

With the continued decline of the deaconesses, the **religious orders** grew stronger. The monastic orders comprised of monks and nuns controlled hospitals but were more concerned with patients' religious problems than with their illnesses. The Order of St. Benedict, previously described, was still in existence and quite active. The Alexian Brotherhood order, which came into being in 1348 as a secular order, was organized into a religious order in 1431. This order was among the pioneers of organized nursing in Europe.[7]

## Renaissance Period and Reformation

The Renaissance, a revival of classical art, literature, and learning, originated in Italy and spread through Europe. The approximate period for this revival was from the 14th to the 16th century. This new impetus to education affected most areas except nursing and medicine; a renaissance in these professions occurred later.

During the 16th century, the Reformation occurred. The Reformation was an attempt to reconstitute the life-style and teachings of Western Christendom. One of the unexpected results of the movement was the separation of the Protestant churches from the Roman Catholic Church. Although the Renaissance was a period of intellectual enlightenment and achievement, the Reformation itself caused the overall quality of health care to deteriorate.

Reformers, in an attempt to diminish the control and power of the Catholic Church, suppressed Catholic religious orders. This resulted in the closing of hundreds of hospitals. No one had anticipated the consequences of this action. The government and the Reformation leaders were unprepared to handle the large numbers of aged, sick, orphaned, and poor who were forced from monasteries and other religious shelters. These people had nowhere to go; many died on the streets from disease or starvation. Others were forced to serve as slaves or laborers for the wealthier citizens. Eventually, charitable institutions to care for the sick and poor were founded. Even in these institutions, however, the sick were expected to help in the care of the more seriously ill. Countries that remained primarily Catholic escaped some of the societal disorganization caused by the Reformation; England and France were two countries especially affected.[6,7]

With so much poverty and human abuse, social reform was inevitable. Unfortunately, most women did not profit by the reforms. The Reformation had changed the role of women drastically. Women were considered subordinate to men, and the Protestant church did not allow them much freedom. This attitude greatly affected nursing during this time. Nursing was no longer considered a respectable occupation; it existed without organization and without social standing. Eventually hospital care was delegated to women of low social status—prisoners, drunks, and prostitutes. Nurses were considered menial servants; they worked long strenuous hours for very low pay. This era has been called the Dark Age of Nursing and lasted from the end of the 17th century to the middle of the 19th century.[7]

## Nursing in America: 1700 to 1900

Nursing in America from the late 1600s until the mid-1850s was probably at the same stage of development as nursing in Europe at that time. As the growth of settlements in America continued, the need for nursing became urgent. Catholic orders organized themselves similarly to their prototypes in Europe and cared for the sick in their communities. In the Protestant settlements, less-organized efforts were apparent and the care of the sick usually fell on the shoulders of mothers whose care showed creativity and compassion.[7,11]

The need for organized nursing efforts was especially felt during the American Revolution (1775 to 1783). The Catholic orders were the only organized groups with any actual knowledge of nursing; they placed their facilities and nurses at the disposal of the army. In addition, wives, sisters, and mothers followed the army and tended to the sick and wounded.[7]

The 19th century was a period of political, geographical, economic, medical, and social expansion blended with inventions, discoveries, and creativity in every aspect of human endeavor. In the early 1800s, the actual care of the sick remained the responsibility of the women in the family. Although hospitals existed, they were unattractive, crowded, and inhabited by the poor. Almost the only acceptable hospital nursing was done by religious orders.[7]

At about midpoint of the 19th century, at the same time that Florence Nightingale was making her presence known in Europe, social reforms and demands for emancipation of women started in America. Efforts to improve the treatment of the mentally ill, poor, aged, and sick were made. Gradually, women received more freedom and were eventually readmitted into the field of medicine and accepted at institutes of higher learning.

Because the women had more freedom, they became involved in more activities and reform movements. Just prior to the onset of the Civil War, women in New York City formed the Women's Central Association for Relief. This organization worked to improve sanitary conditions and brought about the establishment of the United States Sanitary Commission. When the Civil War (1861 to 1865) started, the association worked to send nurses to war areas.[7]

It soon became apparent that the Women's Central Association for Relief was unable to supply the quantity of nurses needed. Dorothea Lynde Dix, who had become known because of her social reform movements for the mentally ill, was quickly appointed Superintendent of Female Nurses of the Union Army. She was given the responsibility and authority to recruit and equip a corps of army nurses. These two organized efforts to supply the Union Army with nurses proved insufficient; the number of wounded overwhelmed the number of trained nurses. Eventually, citizen volunteers were used.[11]

On the Confederate side, no director of nursing was appointed. Religious sisters and lay women provided the necessary nursing care. It is estimated that 1000 women performed nursing duties for the Southern armies compared to some 6000 women for the Northern armies. This wide variation in the number of women used as nurses was attributed to the attitude supported by Southerners that caring for men was unfit for ladies.[11]

One of the significant movements of the 19th century was the development of the Red Cross Society. For centuries there had been societies for helping the wounded in time of war. The Red Cross Society expanded the idea to an international basis and suggested teamwork between nations.

In October of 1863, an international conference was held in Geneva, Switzerland, where representatives of 16 nations agreed to a provisional program. This led to the formation of the International Red Cross Society. (The United States did not participate since it was in the midst of the Civil War.) In August of 1864, a formal diplomatic congress was held, and the Geneva Convention was signed. Under the Geneva agreement, each nation was to form a national committee or society whose function was to make preparation beforehand for war or disaster. The emblem of the society, the Red Cross, was also adopted at the 1864 congress.

The United States was the 32nd country to enter the Red Cross. Clara Barton, a nurse who served during the Civil War and who worked with the Red Cross in the Franco-Prussian War, worked tirelessly for the establishment of a Red Cross society in America. Because of her efforts, an American Association of the Red Cross was incorporated in 1881 in the District of Columbia. Final ratification of the Geneva Convention by the United States came in 1882.[7,11]

## Nursing in America: 1900 to 1945

Following the turn of the century, within the span of 45 years, nurses were confronted with three major events that required reorganization of the health care structure. The United States was involved in two major wars and a depression: World War I from 1914 to 1918; the Depression of the 1930s; World War II from 1939 to 1945.

As with earlier wars, the supply of nurses during World War I did not meet civilian and war zone needs. At the time that the United States declared war, there were about

400 army nurses. Jane Delano was appointed superintendent of the Army Nurse Corps and Chairman of the Red Cross Nursing Service. By coordinating the activities of these two organizations, she was able to supply about 20,000 nurses for duty with the Army and Navy during the war. Because of the increase in military nurses, the number of health care providers in civilian hospitals was depleted.[5,7,11]

During the war, nurses were assigned to camps, base hospitals, evacuation and mobile hospitals, and hospital trains. Although the conditions during the war were atrocious, nurses once again proved themselves able and brave in military situations. They were not always *wanted*, but they stood their ground and gave care to the sick and wounded wherever they were *needed*.

Prior to World War I the United States was a rural society; after the war the United States became an urban society. As a result of this change, new nursing roles developed. The visiting nurse and public health nurse continued to be active, but in addition, the nurse began to assume active roles in school nursing, midwifery, occupational health nursing, maternal and child nursing, cancer nursing, and tuberculosis nursing. Also during this postwar time, national nursing organizations were formed; practice acts and nurse registration were advocated.[5] Because of societal changes and needs, nurses were motivated to look at themselves and their role in society.

The Great Depression of the 1930s also affected nursing. People could not afford health care or private duty nurses. Unemployment of graduate nurses rose sharply. For once, the supply of nurses exceeded the demand, causing a lowering of income throughout all segments of nursing. Hospitals reduced service to three 8-hour shifts in an attempt to spread the work around and many nurses worked for room and board.[7,11]

As World War II accelerated, military personnel in the United States increased. Again the need for nurses increased. In an attempt to meet military nursing needs, the Bolton Bill, which created a Cadet Nurse Corps, was passed in July of 1942. Lucille Petry was appointed the chief nurse and director of the Cadet Nurse Program. Because of her efforts, acceleration of existing nursing education programs and establishment of special programs occurred. These program changes met the military nursing needs and maintained nursing service to the civilian population. Within the war zone, nurses from different countries worked side by side. Some 75,000 nurses served in World War II; after the war, some of these nurses received special recognition for their services.[5,7,11]

## Nursing in America: 1946 to 1985

During this 40-year period, several major factors influenced health care and dictated nursing's direction. Among these factors were: growth of knowledge, change in attitude toward health, change in health care personnel supply and distribution, decreased number and length of hospitalizations, changes in population growth and composition, continued emancipation of women, expanded role of the nurse, entry into practice issue, and the American Nurses' Association Social Policy Statement.

The growth of knowledge includes technological, scientific, and medical advances. Diagnoses are made more quickly and accurately. New drugs, equipment, and diagnostic and surgical procedures make treatment easier and more exact. Computer use has been introduced for billing, accounting, diagnosing, and data recording. Contagious diseases, such as smallpox, diphtheria, and typhoid fever, have almost been eliminated due to improved preventive measures.

With this growth of knowledge has come a new attitude toward health. No longer is health considered the absence of disease. It is viewed as a state of physical, psychological, and social well-being; the optimal functioning of an individual. The public has become more aware of the prevention of various diseases and more concerned with health promotion and maintenance measures. They view health care as a right, not just a privilege. In addition, emphasis is placed on the individual's responsibility for his or her own health.

When health and health care is viewed in this manner, changes may be needed within society and the health care structure. In the United States, Medicare and Medicaid are intended to provide financial access to this right for older citizens and others who are financially eligible. Industrial plants provide nurses and health services as well as insurance programs. School health programs have been developed and well-child clinics established.

Although these measures have increased the accessibility of health care, a problem does exist in providing adequate health care to the total population. This problem centers around the supply and distribution of health care personnel. Most health workers and health facilities are located in urban and suburban centers. Although rural health teams have been developed and more community hospitals and clinics have been established, the problem still exists. State, regional, and federal medical, health, and nursing organizations continue to seek possible solutions.

There has also been a decrease in the number and length of hospitalizations. The emphasis has shifted from hospital care to home care. Follow-up care is provided in clinics or by community health nurses. Extended-care facilities and outpatient clinics manage long-term chronic illnesses. Because of this shift in health care settings, many hospitals have been forced to close nursing units and reduce the number of employees. This, in turn, has caused nurses to seek employment away from the acute-care settings.

Changes in population growth and composition have occurred. Between 1900 and 1952, the nation's population doubled. After World War II, however, the family planning movement surfaced. More effective contraceptive techniques were introduced; more information was made available about birth control. The result of this activity was a zero population growth in 1973. With the decreased birth rate, there came an increased longevity—people are living longer. This increased longevity has changed the focus of health care delivery. Heart disease, cancer, and kidney disease now rank high as major causes of death. Chronic problems associated with the increased incidence of degenerative diseases are more frequent.

The continued emancipation of women has also influenced health care and given direction to nursing. Nursing, from its American beginning, was primarily composed of women, and, as such, has almost always been involved in women's rights movements. Advancement in nursing was frequently slowed because early female nursing leaders were unable to get appropriate and necessary legislative action.

Nursing has also felt the impact of the stereotyping of male–female roles, especially the physician–nurse relationship. The absence of autonomy for nurses is seen as one direct result of sex discrimination in nursing. As American women became more liberated, female nurses have moved closer to professional autonomy.[4,7,10,11]

The nurse's role continues to expand and to become more specialized. Two expanded roles that have had a major impact on the nursing profession are those of nurse practitioner and clinical specialist. Preparation for these roles varies. Originally, nurse practitioner programs could be entered regardless of previous educational preparation. These early certificate programs are gradually decreasing in number as new programs at a master's level increase. Practitioner programs prepare the nurse to function in a speciality area—pediatrics, medical–surgical, maternal–newborn, and so forth. Clinical specialist programs prepare nurses at the graduate (master's) level and require a baccalaureate degree in nursing for entrance into the program. These programs also prepare the nurse to function in a speciality, such as psychiatric–mental health nursing, maternal–child nursing, oncology nursing, adult medical–surgical nursing, and gerontology nursing.

Nurse practitioners function most frequently in ambulatory care and community health settings. They work under established medical protocols and serve well clients or those with stable chronic conditions. Most clinical specialists find positions in large hospital centers. They serve as role models because of their expertise in developing nursing care standards and protocols and using the nursing process. Clinical specialists also promote research and staff development within their designated settings.[3,5]

The entry-into-practice issue significantly influenced nursing during this period. This issue has caused the nursing profession to take a closer look at itself and to examine how it is meeting the needs of society.

The entry-into-practice issue surfaced in 1974 when the New York Nurses' Association adopted a resolution calling for the baccalaureate degree as the minimum preparation for entry into professional practice by 1985. The resolution did not become law, but it created much debate and consideration of similar legislation in other states.

At the American Nurses' Association (ANA) convention in 1978, the entry-into-practice issue was debated extensively. A resolution was passed which supported the 1985 date for requiring a baccalaureate degree in nursing as the minimum preparation for entry into professional practice.[3,5]

For this resolution to be implemented, issues of competency, titling, licensure, and the concept of grandfathering must be considered. At present, all graduates from associate degree, diploma, and baccalaureate programs write the same examination for licensure and are required to achieve the same minimum score. In addition, all individuals passing the examinations are titled registered nurses. Should different tests be required for each group or should different passing scores for each group be established? The grandfathering aspect is just as confusing. Grandfathering would allow all nurses licensed as registered nurses prior to a given date to continue to use the title of registered nurse. Would such action protect less well-prepared practitioners and thus weaken the profession?

Definite answers to this issue do not appear imminent. While debates and discussions continue, nurses proceed to deliver health care with the welfare of the client as their major concern. The issue, however, has precipitated other events. Large numbers of registered nurses have returned to school to acquire a baccalaureate degree. In addition, health agencies across the nation have increased their efforts to employ only nurses with a baccalaureate degree or to require their present staff to acquire a degree.

It is important to note that the 1980 ANA Social Policy Statement directly addressed nursing's social responsibility. The statement sees the 1980s as a decade of increasing regulations with regard to the quantity, costs, and quality of health care. Social and political priorities for action will continue to be based on society's values and needs.[2]

Educational changes paralleled those changes that occurred within nursing as a result of problems, issues, or needs of society. We will now look at some of the major developments within nursing education.

## MILESTONES IN NURSING EDUCATION

Historically, nursing and medicine had independent origins and existed for many centuries without much contact. Not until the evolution of medicine and surgery into highly complex bodies of knowledge were specially educated nurses needed. This brought nursing and medicine closer together, helped to expand the role of the nurse, and produced major changes within nursing education.

## Early Educational Efforts

During early civilization, education of the individuals who cared for the sick did not exist. Actual nursing skills developed from intuitive responses and from trial and error behavior. Individuals who showed themselves adept in caring for the sick were called upon in times of illness. Caring for the ill was not their primary function or responsibility, but they seemed to have inherent knowledge concerning the care of the sick.

Early attempts at formal education of health care providers can be traced to 400 A.D. when early deaconesses taught care of the sick to their followers. Much later, in the 17th century, attempts at teaching nurses in the community setting were made by the Sisters of Charity. However, it was not until the Florence Nightingale era that major attempts at developing formal educational programs occurred.[4,6,7]

## Florence Nightingale's Influence on Nursing Education

Miss Nightingale's activities in the Crimean War demonstrated the need for educated nurses. Her ability to use the scientific method of gathering data and her skills as a statistician exemplified this need.

Immediately after the war, Miss Nightingale devoted most of her time to writing. Her *Notes on Matters Affecting the Health, Efficiency and Hospital Administration of the British Army* and *Notes on Nursing: What It Is and What It Is Not* caused major changes within medicine and nursing. In the book, *Notes on Nursing*, Miss Nightingale stressed the importance of primary prevention. She emphasized that there were two major components of nursing—health nursing and sick nursing—and insisted that prevention was better than cure. Miss Nightingale also advocated a holistic client approach, maintaining that the whole person should be understood and treated. She believed that nursing encompassed a body of knowledge and a role separate from that of medicine. She envisioned the nurse functioning in a collaborative role with the physician. Her beliefs concerning nursing eventually led to the establishment of the Nightingale Training School for Nurses.

This school, which was established by the Nightingale Fund, opened in 1860 as a completely independent educational institution—not associated with any one particular hospital. Although Miss Nightingale did not actually teach in the school, she supervised all of the school's activities, including the selection of students, faculty, and the development of the curriculum.

With the establishment of her own school of nursing, Miss Nightingale was able to introduce her beliefs about nursing and nursing education more easily. She insisted that intelligent, competent women be recruited for the nursing program. She limited the enrollment in the 1-year program to about 30 students—selecting carefully from among the 1000 to 2000 applicants. She incorporated into the curriculum what she thought was the major role of the nurse—assessment and intervention based on a plan of care, followed by evaluation. She stressed the need to *learn* how to observe, what to observe, and how to ask questions. All of these important components currently are found in the assessment step in the nursing process.[7,8,12]

It is impossible to measure the impact that this one woman had on nursing. Her influence touched many facets of nursing: education, research, community nursing, hospital nursing, and the nursing process. Perhaps most significant is the fact that Florence Nightingale advanced nursing as a profession.

## Early Nursing Programs in America

In the United States, one of the first attempts at organizing a school of nursing occurred in 1839. The Nurse Society of Philadelphia started a school which awarded a certificate after a period of lectures, demonstrations, and experience at a hospital. The instructions were quite basic and elementary, with nurses being taught in the same classes as medical students. About 20 years later, in 1861, Women's Hospital in Philadelphia established a school. The program was designed to appeal to the higher class of young women. In this program, a diploma was given at the end of the 6-month course. Although more individuals became interested in training nurses, neither school produced large numbers of trained nurses.[11]

In 1837, three important schools appeared almost simultaneously: the Bellevue Hospital Training School in New York City, the Boston Training School, and the Connecticut Training School in New Haven. These schools were patterned after the ideas of Florence Nightingale and represented an important step in nursing education in America.[4,7,11]

Originally these schools were formed independently of hospital structures and were administered independently. In time this separation became more difficult to maintain. Because there was a close association between nursing schools and hospitals, it became easy for a school to be absorbed into the hospital's organizational structure. This incorporation of nursing schools into the hospital's structure made it easy for hospitals to look at the students as sources of free labor. This attitude deterred independent growth within nursing education and tied the development of nursing to the growth and development of hospitals.

Other changes in nursing education occurred during the 19th century. The length of programs within schools of nursing was gradually increased from 1 to 3 years. In addition to lengthening the programs, nurses were taught differently. They were taught the "why" behind their actions. For example, they were taught physiology and the pathology of disease processes so that they could understand why certain nursing therapies were successful. Nurses were no longer asked to administer drugs without knowing the drug's action. Courses that dealt with ethical and professional problems and social and behavioral sciences were added to the curriculum. Although earlier nursing leaders had spoken of the need to have "trained" nurses, this was one of the earliest indications that the profession was preparing "educated" nurses.

The medical profession and society soon began complaining that nurses were becoming "overtrained." This attitude did not alter the direction of nursing education but instead strengthened the convictions of the nursing leaders of that period. Eventually, toward the end of the 19th century, nursing recognized the need for some nurses to receive advanced education. It was felt that nurses who wanted to assume teaching and administrative positions needed experiences not offered in the basic educational programs. An education at a university level was considered essential for these nurses. However, the growth of baccalaureate programs was slow and it was not until the 1950s that significant progress was seen. The first school of nursing established in a university setting was at the University of Minnesota in 1909. The school actually resembled the diploma programs in existence at that time. No higher general education requirements existed, and education was predominantly by apprenticeship. It was not until 1919 that an undergraduate baccalaureate program was created at Minnesota.[9,13]

## Educational Changes: 1900 to 1965

In 1919, eight baccalaureate programs existed in the United States. Originally most baccalaureate programs were 5 years in length. Three years were spent completing a nursing school curriculum, and 2 additional years of liberal arts were required. Gradually baccalaureate nursing programs became located in 4-year colleges and universities. The majority of the nursing studies are taught at the upper division (junior and senior years). Nursing theory builds on the liberal arts and science courses taken by the student during the first 2 years of college. This type of educational program is a generic baccalaureate program.

The preparation of the nurse in community colleges was perhaps the most dramatic change in nursing education since its beginning. The first programs in nursing within the framework of community colleges followed the publication of Dr. Mildred Montag's doctoral thesis, *Education of Nursing Technicians*, in 1951. Montag's study proposed a new type of education consisting of 2 years in a community college. The curriculum would be an integrated one, half general education and half nursing. Graduates from these programs would be called nursing technicians and would provide bedside care. These nurses would not be prepared to assume administrative responsibilities. The first three programs modeled on the principle suggested in Montag's study were started in 1952. By 1965 there were over 130 programs.[9,11]

Prior to the close of 1965, two other events occurred that affected nursing education—the Nurse Training Act and the American Nurses' Association Position Paper. The Nurse Training Act of 1964 provided financial assistance to students, diploma, associate degree, and baccalaureate degree schools. The act was an attempt to help assure more and better schools of nursing, more carefully selected students, higher standards of teaching, and better health care. Because of these funds, institutions of higher education took a renewed interest in providing educational programs for nurses.

Another major influence on nursing education during this period was the ANA Position Paper (The American Nurses' Association's First Position on Education for Nursing). This statement was prepared by the ANA Committee on Education and was adopted by the ANA Board of Directors in September, 1965.

The paper took four important positions. They were:

1. The education for all those who are licensed to practice nursing should take place in institutions of higher education.
2. Minimum preparation for beginning professional nursing practice at the present time should be baccalaureate degree education in nursing.
3. Minimum preparation for beginning technical nursing practice at the present time should be associate degree education in nursing.
4. Education for assistants in the health service occupations should be short, intensive preservice programs in vocational institutions rather than on-the-job training programs.[1]

The position paper created quite a tumult in nursing. Many nurses misunderstood the paper's intent and considered it a threat. Students, faculty, and hospital administrators who were associated with diploma programs were especially upset and threatened by the content of the paper. They saw the omission of diploma school education from the paper as a move to eliminate diploma education. Although repeated attempts were made to clarify the content and intent of the document, the storm raged for over 15 years. Eventually, social and economic trends brought about many of the changes proposed by the position paper.[11]

During the 1930s and 1940s, there were a limited number of nurses with a master's degree in nursing. This was primarily due to the lack of availability of master's programs. Because of the shortage of master's programs in nursing, nurse educators were forced to seek master's degrees in education. In the 1950s and early 1960s, funding for master's programs in nursing was directed at nurses seeking preparation for teaching, supervisory, and administrative positions. Clinical programs at the master's levels did not develop until the late 1960s.[11]

Nursing research also evolved slowly during this time. Studies of nursing service, nursing education, and nurses were done with or by social scientists or medical researchers—nurses "assisted" with the research. Nursing leaders realized that nursing could not develop as a profession without clinical research that focused on nursing. Movements in that direction included the publication of *Nursing Research* in 1952 and the ANA's establishment of the American Nurses' Foundation in 1955. The Foundation conducts studies, surveys, and research; it also funds nurse researchers and publishes scientific reports.[11]

## Current Educational Patterns

There are three major educational routes that prepare graduates to write the National Council Licensure Examination (NCLEX): diploma programs, associate degree programs, and baccalaureate programs. In 1979, 23 percent of the new graduates were from generic baccalaureate programs, 47 percent from associate degree programs, and 23 percent from diploma programs.[14] In addition to these traditional forms of nursing programs, other educational formats, such as external degree and direct articulation programs, can be used by individuals seeking to become registered nurses.

External degree programs provide the opportunity for students to complete the requirements for a degree without the traditional college or university structure. Students may earn all of the credits needed for graduation by examination without ever attending a formal class. The New York Regents External Degree Program of the University of the State of New York was the first successful external degree program in nursing. In 1971, the New York Board of Regents authorized an external associate degree program in nursing, and in 1976, the Board of Regents authorized an external baccalaureate degree in nursing. The W. B. Kellogg Foundation funded the start of both programs.

These programs have general education and nursing requirements. Transfer credits from didactic courses completed at colleges and universities can be used or credits can be earned by examination. The performance area of the associate degree or baccalaureate degree can only be satisfied by taking the Regents External Degree Performance Examination.[9]

The direct articulation program is a method of moving from lower-level educational programs to higher-level ones. This type of program makes it possible for nurses to begin and end their education at specific points or to continue moving up the educational ladder. Direct articulation programs are most beneficial to associate degree and practical nurse graduates. For example, a student in an articulated practical nurse or associate degree program could stop after 1 year and take the licensing examination for practical nurses. If the student desires to complete another year, an associate degree in nursing would be earned, and the student would take the licensing examination for registered nurses.[9]

In recent years there has been an increase in the number of baccalaureate programs for registered nurses who graduate from diploma or associate degree programs. These programs vary in format, but in most cases they offer nurses an opportunity to build upon their prior educational preparation.

There has also been an increase in the number of nurses enrolled in master's programs and doctoral studies. The master's programs usually include specialization in areas such as community, maternal–newborn, mental health, or medical–surgical nursing. Twenty-three doctoral programs in nursing existed in 1981. In addition, 33 universities were considering or definitely planning a doctoral nursing program.[13] Doctorates earned in the existing programs vary; they include Doctor of Nursing Science (D.N.Sc.), Doctor of Nursing (D.N.), Doctor of Nursing Education (D.N.Ed.), and Doctor of Philosophy in Nursing (Ph.D.). Other types of doctorates are also available to nurses; for example, Doctor of Education (Ed.D.) or Doctor of Public Health (D.P.H.).

In addition to these forms of education, specialized educational programs have been developed to help prepare nurses for roles not included in their formal education. These programs take the form of certificate programs and continuing education offerings.

Current trends support the baccalaureate degree as the educational preparation needed by all professional nurses. Nurses recognize the need for establishing a base of knowledge that evolves from the profession of nursing—and is not just borrowed from other disciplines. Individuals involved in all facets of nursing—clinical practice, education, research, etc.—are striving to establish a scientific basis for their actions.

## SIGNIFICANT STUDIES AND REPORTS AFFECTING NURSING

Nursing service and nursing education might not have taken their present direction if studies had not been completed along the way. These studies were used to solve existing problems and to advance the profession. Some of the significant studies and reports affecting nursing will be described in the next section.

### Early Efforts to Evaluate Nursing Education: 1900 to 1960

The greatly increased demands for nurses in World War I forced many schools of nursing to relax their entrance requirements. Such a variation in educational standards developed that it was necessary to investigate and analyze the existing admission policies.

One study that was designed to evaluate nursing education was financed by the Rockefeller Foundation. The Committee for the Study of Nursing Education was formed in 1918 with its main purpose to study the educational requirements for public health nursing. References vary in their interpretation of the committee membership, but most reports agree that Professor C. E. A. Winslow of Yale University was the head of the committee with Josephine Goldmark doing most of the work. By 1920 it became apparent to the committee that public health nursing could not be investigated separately; the study was extended to cover the entire field of nursing education.

In 1923, the *Goldmark Report* was published in *Nursing and Nursing Education in the United States.* The report affirmed that: (1) widespread neglect of the field of public health existed; (2) many instructors in nursing schools were inadequately prepared; (3) courses were not standardized; (4) schools were deficient in technical facilities; and (5) problems existed when the head of the hospital was also head of the school of nursing. The findings of this study were not shared with the public. Some improvements were gradually seen—substandard schools closed, better-prepared instructors were hired, schools adopted acceptable educational curricula—but the full importance of the study was never understood by the profession.

Another attempt at improving the standards of nursing education was made by the National League of Nursing Education Committee on Curriculum. In 1917 it published *A Standard Curriculum for Schools of Nursing* that offered suggestions on how to improve courses being taught in nursing schools. In 1929, a revision was published, *A Curriculum for Schools of Nursing*, which covered the advancements made in nursing since the 1917 edition and incorporated the recommendations from the *Goldmark Report*. As an aftermath of these two publications, the initial committee studied existing teaching methods as to their suitability for use in nursing schools. *A Curriculum Guide for Schools of Nursing* was published in 1937 that stressed the role of the clinical instructor and the need for creative teaching methods.[7,11]

In 1944, the National Nursing Council, a large group of representatives from many health organizations, formed a committee (National Nursing Planning Committee) to study society's need for nursing. The committee was headed by a nonnurse, Dr. Esther Lucille Brown. In general, the areas to be studied were: the improvement of nursing services, the total program of nursing education, the distribution of nursing services, and the study of standards. The study was published in 1948 and is known as the *Brown Report*. The report recommended that the term *professional* be applied only to graduates from accredited professional schools. Other recommendations included: (1) schools of nursing should be nationally classified and accredited; (2) faculty standards should be established; (3) nursing courses in hospital schools should be shortened; (4) state and regional planning for nursing service and nursing education should be started; and (5) public and private financial support for nursing education was needed.

On the whole, the report made nurses, doctors, hospital administrators, and the public look at nursing and nursing education more thoroughly. A later study in 1970 found that many of the recommendations were still unfulfilled and still valid.[4,7,9,11]

At the 1950 convention, the ANA membership requested a study of all phases of nursing care. The ANA Program of Studies of Nursing Functions launched a 5-year research plan to determine the functions and relationships of all types of institutional nursing personnel, to determine what proportion of nursing care could be provided by each group, and to develop techniques to improve care and to use personnel more economically and effectively. The preliminary report, *Nurses Invest in Patient Care*, was released in 1956.[7]

## Significant Studies of the 1960s to the 1980s

Another study of nursing service and nursing education was conducted in the 1960s. The National Commission for the Study of Nursing and Nursing Education was an independent group established by the American Nurses' Association and the National League for Nursing (NLN). The commission, which received financial support from both the Avalon Foundation and the Kellogg Foundation, was fully formed by January, 1968, with Jerome Lysaught, a nonnurse, as project director.

Basically the study focused on supply and demand for nurses, nursing roles and function, nursing education, and nursing careers. Current practices and patterns were analyzed and future needs were assessed. The final report, entitled *An Abstract for Action*, was published in the mid-1970s and is referred to as the *Lysaught Report*.

Four major recommendations resulted from the study:

1.  Increase research into the practice of nursing and the education of nurses.
2.  Improve educational systems and curricula based on the results of that research.
3.  Clarify roles and practice associated with other health professions to ensure the delivery of optimum care.

4. Increase financial support for nurses and for nursing to ensure adequate career opportunities that will attract and retain the number of individuals required for quality health care.[7,11]

Initially the report was received with mixed reactions and controversy. Eventually all of the major nursing organizations, the American Medical Association, the American Hospital Association, and other health groups either published statements of support or endorsed in principle the recommendations. The ANA, NLN, and the Kellogg Foundation gave additional money to the commission to assist with the implementation of the recommendations. In 1973, the status of the implementation effort was reported in *From Abstract into Action.*[7,9,11]

It is difficult to evaluate accurately the effect of the National Commission report on nursing and health care. Many of the changes that occurred after the report may have evolved on their own. An evaluation survey conducted by Lysaught in 1977 showed minimal progress toward implementation of some of the major recommendations of the study. Because some of these recommendations had first appeared in the Brown Report, 29 years had passed without implementation.

In 1980 the National Commission on Nursing was formed. This commission, which was composed of representatives from nursing, hospital management, business, government, education, and medicine, was to study nursing-related problems in the health care system, especially the apparent shortage of nurses. The American Hospital Association, Hospital Research and Educational Trust, and American Hospital Supply Corporation sponsored the study group.

Some aspects that the group examined were: forces influencing the nurse's work environment; the relationship among nursing education, nursing practice, and professional interaction; and the professional characteristics of nurses in relation to organizational structures of health care agencies. An initial report was published in September of 1981, and final recommendations were published in 1983. The findings were not unexpected. They included: (1) physicians and health care administrators do not understand the role of the nurse in the health care system; (2) traditional and outdated images are preventing the acceptance of the nurse's current role; (3) nursing lacks a clear understanding of its role; (4) individuals and professional groups have not agreed about the educational preparation for the nurse or the professional goals for nursing; and (5) many diverse associations represent nurses.[6,9] These problems and concerns have existed for some time; the commission did not offer a plan for resolving them.

The Institute of Medicine Committee on Nursing and Nursing Education also conducted a study in the early 1980s. This 2-year study was mandated by the 1979 Nurse Training Amendments and was funded by the Department of Health and Human Services. The purpose of the study was to determine: if and why the attrition rate of nurses from the work force had increased; whether federal funds should continue for nursing education; and what measures might improve the usefulness of nursing resources. The results of the study were released in January of 1983. The group found that the nursing shortage of the 1960s and 1970s had largely disappeared. They recommended that future federal financial support be directed at graduate education and that support of "generalist nurses" be discontinued.[7,9]

It is correct to say that these studies and reports had an impact on nursing and nursing education. On the other hand, it is alarming to realize how many recommendations are never implemented but instead appear in subsequent studies. Does this point to a weakness within the profession of nursing? Why is the nursing profession slow to implement changes which are meant to strengthen the profession?

## SUMMARY

Nursing evolved in response to society's needs, and the scope of practice varied according to the needs at that time. At first, nursing was task oriented and concerned with only the physical needs of the individual. Gradually nursing became aware of the whole individual, taking a holistic approach. In addition, the scope of practice widened to include the family and community.

The focus of nursing care has also changed because of changes within society and nursing. Nursing care originally was given in the home. Later nursing care was primarily delivered within the structure of health care facilities. The pendulum has now swung the other way as more and more health care is given within the home and community structure.

Early health care providers showed an interest and concern for maintaining the health of the individual. Somewhere in the development of nursing, this concern was momentarily pushed aside as nurses became absorbed with restorative care in acute-care settings. Nurses now recognize that health care has three facets—maintenance of health, restoration from illness or injury, and prevention of disease.

The educational patterns within nursing have changed to meet the needs of the profession. At present, a baccalaureate degree in nursing is considered minimum preparation for entry into professional practice. The aim of baccalaureate education is to develop nurses who can give high-quality, theory-based care. Because of the emphasis on theory, nursing has gradually evolved from intuitive and compassionate nursing care to scientific and humanistic nursing care.

The remaining chapters in the book will add to your current knowledge and help you to organize and use your knowledge in an effective manner.

## STUDY GUIDE

1. Identify and describe one study that was important to the growth of the nursing profession.
2. How did societal needs affect the profession after World War I? since 1950?
3. What is meant by the expanded role of the nurse? How does a nurse in an expanded role differ from the generalist nurse?
4. Compare and contrast the three traditional formats within nursing education: diploma, associate degree, and baccalaureate degree.
5. What impact did Florence Nightingale have on nursing education?

## REFERENCES

1. American Nurses' Association's First Position on Education for Nursing. *American Journal of Nursing*, 1965, *65*(12), 107.
2. American Nurses' Association. *Nursing: A social policy statement*. Kansas City, Mo.: American Nurses' Association, 1980.

3. Bullough, B., Bullough, V., & Soukup, M. C. (Eds). *Nursing issues and nursing strategies for the eighties.* New York: Springer-Verlag, 1983.
4. DeLoughery, G. *History and trends of professional nursing.* St. Louis, Mo.: C.V. Mosby, 1977.
5. DeYoung, L. *Dynamics of nursing* (5th ed.). St. Louis, Mo.: C.V. Mosby, 1985.
6. DeYoung, L. *The foundations of nursing.* St. Louis, Mo.: C.V. Mosby, 1976.
7. Dolan, J. *Nursing in society: A historical perspective* (14th ed.). Philadelphia: Saunders, 1978.
8. Dreves, K. D. Nurses in American history: Vassar training camp for nurses. *American Journal of Nursing,* November 1975, *75*(11), 2000–2003.
9. Ellis, J. R., & Hartley, C. L. *Nursing in today's world: Challenges, issues, and trends.* Philadelphia: Lippincott, 1984.
10. Griffin, G. J., & Griffin, J. K. *History and trends of professional nursing* (7th ed.). St. Louis, Mo.: C.V. Mosby, 1973.
11. Kelly, L. Y. *Dimensions of professional nursing* (4th ed.). New York: Macmillan, 1981.
12. Nightingale, F. *Notes on nursing: What it is and what it is not.* New York: Dover Publications, 1969.
13. Vaughn, J. C. Educational preparation for nursing: 1981. *Nursing & Health Care,* October 1982, *3*(10), 448.
14. Vaughn, J. C., & Johnson, W. L. Educational preparation for nursing—1978. *Nursing Outlook,* September 1979, *27,* 608–614.

## BIBLIOGRAPHY

Aiken, L. (Ed). *Nursing in the 1980s: Crises, opportunities, challenges.* Philadelphia: Lippincott, 1982.

Austin, A. L. Nurses in American history: Wartime volunteers—1861–1865. *American Journal of Nursing,* May 1975, *75*(5), 816–818.

Bixler, G. K., & Bixler, R. The professional status of nursing. *American Journal of Nursing,* September 1945, *45*(9), 730–735.

Bullough, B. Nurses in American history. *American Journal of Nursing,* January 1976, *76*(1), 118–120.

Carnegie, M. E. Nursing in the warzones: Black nurses at the front. *American Journal of Nursing,* October 1984, *84*(10), 1250–1252, 1254.

Chaska, N. L. (Ed.). *The nursing profession: A time to speak.* New York: Mc-Graw Hill, 1983.

Christy, T. Entry into practice: A recurring issue in nursing history. *American Journal of Nursing,* March 1980, *80*(3), 485–488.

Christy, T. Portrait of a leader: Isabel Hampton Robb. *Nursing Outlook,* 1969, *17*(3), 26–29.

Christy, T. Portrait of a leader: Isabel Maitland Stewart. *Nursing Outlook,* 1969, *17*(10), 44–48.

Christy, T. Portrait of a leader: Lavina Lloyd Dock. *Nursing Outlook,* 1969, *17*(6), 72–75.

Elmore, J. A. Nurses in American history: Black nurses—their service and their struggles. *American Journal of Nursing,* March 1976, *76*(3), 435–437.

Fitzpatrick, M. L. Nurses in American history: Nursing and the great depression. *American Journal of Nursing,* December 1975, *75*(12), 2188–2190.

Goodnow, M. *Nursing history* (7th ed.). Philadelphia: Saunders, 1944.

Hawkins, J. B. W., & Higgins, L. P. *Nursing and the American health care delivery system.* New York: Tiresias Press, 1982.

Huxley, E. *Florence Nightingale.* New York: G.P. Putnam's Sons, 1975.

Kalisch, B., & Kalisch, P. Heroine out of focus: Media images of Florence Nightingale—Part I: Popular biographies and stage productions. *Nursing & Health Care,* April 1983, *4*(4), 181–187.

Kalisch, B., & Kalisch, P. Nurses in American history: The cadet nurse corps in World War II. *American Journal of Nursing,* February 1976, *76*(2), 240–242.

Marks, G., & Beatty, W. K. *Women in white.* New York: Charles Scribner's Sons, 1972.

McCloskey, J. C., & Grace, H. K., (Eds). *Current issues in nursing.* Oxford: Blackwell Scientific Publications, 1981.

Palmer, I. S. Florence Nightingale and international origins of modern nursing. *Image,* June 1981, *13*(2), 28–31.

Pletsch, P. Mary Breckinridge: A pioneer who made her mark. *American Journal of Nursing,* December 1981, *81*(12), 2188–2190.

Selavan, I. C. Nurses in American history: The revolution. *American Journal of Nursing,* April 1975, *75*(4), 592–594.

Shannon, M. L. Nurses in American history: Our first four licensure laws. *American Journal of Nursing,* August 1975, *75*(8), 1327–1329.

Smith, J. *The idea of health: Implications for the nursing professional.* New York: Teachers College Press, 1981.

# 2

# The Problem-solving Process

Problem solving is a learned behavior. It is an essential skill for any nurse regardless of the clinical setting. In this chapter, we will discuss the process of problem solving and distinguish the characteristics of effective from ineffective problem solvers. The scientific method of problem solving will be discussed as well as several modified scientific methods. The nursing process will be introduced as a problem-solving process which helps nurses to apply their knowledge and skills in an efficient manner.

Study of this chapter will help you to:

1. Define problem solving.
2. Identify four problem-oriented behaviors that are important in effective problem solving.
3. Distinguish the characteristics of effective from ineffective problem solvers.
4. Explain the steps of the scientific method of problem solving.
5. Explore the barriers to effective problem solving.
6. Define the nursing process.
7. Discuss the historical evolution of the nursing process.
8. State the steps in the nursing process.
9. Describe the nursing process as a problem-solving process.
10. Discuss the benefits of using the nursing process as a method of resolving clinical problems.
11. Identify three limitations of the nursing process.

## OVERVIEW OF PROBLEM SOLVING

In order to use the problem-solving process, you must start with a clear understanding of the terms *problem* and *problem solving*. A **problem** is generally defined as any question in need of a solution or an answer. If you promised your best friend you would pick her up from the airport, but your car would not start . . . you have a problem. The question in need of solution may be, "How can I get my car started?"or "How will I pick my friend up from the airport?"

Two types of problems have been identified—restructuring problems and straightforward problems. Problems that can only be solved if the solver changes his or her initial perception of the problem are called **restructuring problems**. **Straightforward problems** do not require a change in perception.[3,8,21,26] These two types of problems will be explored in greater detail later in the chapter.

The process used to resolve or answer the question or achieve a solution is called **problem solving**. Ray,[26] drawing upon the work of Duncker,[8] divided the problem-solving task into the following three parts: "a) the given situation, b) the desired situation, and c) the method of proceeding from the one to the other" (p. 135).

It is easy to identify these parts in any situation where a solution or answer to a question is needed. For example, consider the individual who is wanting a new car. Perhaps the individual's present car is no longer reliable and is requiring frequent, expensive repairs (given situation). The individual wants to buy a new car but doesn't want the monthly payments any higher than $156.00 (desired situation). To accomplish the desired situation, the person must look for a car that will meet budgetary restraints, provide a down payment large enough to reduce the monthly payments to the desired level, or spread the payments over a long period of time to reduce the monthly amounts. Regardless of the method chosen, the individual can move from the given situation to the desired situation.

## Problem-oriented Behavior

In the discussion of problem solving, there are four problem-oriented behaviors that are important—goal-setting, information-seeking, mastery, and help-seeking (Fig. 2–1).

Setting goals, gathering needed information, seeking help, or gaining a sense of mastery of a particular subject area are unfamiliar behaviors for some people. These individuals may be spontaneous in their thoughts and unplanned in their actions. Their behavior may produce results that are incomplete, disorganized, or finished late. Other people are problem oriented in their behavior. They plan the activities that they wish

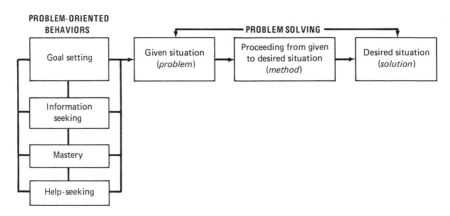

**Figure 2–1.** Problem-oriented behaviors.

to accomplish. If they want to carry out an activity but lack the knowledge and skill, they read about the task or ask others for help.

*Goal-setting.* A goal can be defined as a broad statement of what is to be accomplished. It is an overall statement of what is desired—the outcome, end state, or point to be achieved. In order to solve a problem effectively, goals are necessary. By setting goals, you are making a judgment concerning the desired outcome of a particular situation. Goal-setting is achieved by gathering information about the problem from the given situation, from past experiences, and from your knowledge base.

Even though you may solve problems without identifying goals, there are benefits to be derived from goal-setting. First, you have accomplished what you set out to do. Second, goal-setting is efficient; this practice is an organized way of achieving in an expedient period of time. Lastly, persons who routinely set goals tend to experience less stress because they know what to expect; they control their own activities. (Refer to Chapter 6 for discussion of goal-setting as it relates to the nursing process.)

*Information-seeking.* Questioning and examining are methods that are used to seek information. The assessment interview, nursing health history, wellness assessment, and physical assessment discussed in Chapter 4 are information-seeking tools.

To be proficient in seeking information about a given situation, one must be able to recall from memory information one has learned. Information is more likely to be remembered if three conditions exist—the information is relevant, organized, and associated with previously acquired information.

To have relevance, information must be meaningful and directed toward an identified goal. Meaningfulness of new material will make a memory storage system more responsive to cues. A cue is a perceived signal for action that produces a conditioned response. To retrieve information from long-term memory (LTM), cues are needed to trigger its release. This means that almost any information can be retrieved with a correct cue. If organized logically, meaningful material enables you to encode information so you can retrieve it. The more information you acquire, the more cues you can use and the richer the association between old and new information. In addition, if you are highly familiar with the material, it will be more easily remembered.

Now that we have identified the importance of memory to the problem-oriented behavior of information-seeking, we will examine the concept of memory in more detail.

Until recently, memory was thought of as a type of library where one's experiences were cataloged neatly in files. Memory is now viewed as an entire system comprising different storage areas. A model of memory (Fig. 2–2) can help you understand the memory system.

For learning to occur, physical stimuli such as light, heat, pressure, or sound must be communicated to the sensory system through the senses—hearing, sight, touch, smell, and feeling. The sensory system sends the information to short-term memory where the information is rehearsed (enhanced associations). By enhanced associations, we mean that methods are used to make the information more meaningful and associated with what is already known. "Show and tell" is a method of making the information more interesting and meaningful, and, therefore, less likely to be forgotten. With "show and tell," the sense of hearing is used as well as the sense of sight. This combination of senses enhances association among data. If one does not rehearse or pay attention for a period of time, the information is forgotten. If the information is rehearsed, it

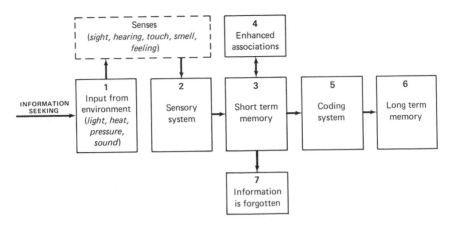

**Figure 2–2.** Information-processing model of memory. *(Adapted from Gage, N. L. and Berliner, D. C. Educational Psychology, (3rd ed.). Boston: Houghton Mifflin, 1984, pp. 168–208, with permission.)*

is sent directly to the coding system. From the coding system, information goes into LTM. If the information is not coded, it is forgotten.

The structure and capacity of the two main memory systems—short-term memory (STM) and LTM—impose limitations on what you learn and remember. The STM is your working memory[12,16]—the active part of your mind that processes all that comes in from the environment. If you look at Figure 2–2, you will note that once the information is processed in the STM you either forget it or the information is stored in your LTM for later use.

Short-term memory has a very short duration and information remains there only about 15 to 20 seconds. Information can, however, remain longer if rehearsed. When new information enters STM, previous information is lost. An example of how this works is when you ask the telephone operator for a number. You say it over and over to yourself so you will not forget it. Before you are able to dial the number, however, someone interrupts you and the number is forgotten. In addition to a short duration, the STM has a limited capacity. This is why telephone numbers and zip codes are usually no longer than seven digits. When longer numbers are used, they are broken into units by hyphens or parentheses (314–32–6872).

Short-term memory also responds better to relevant, organized information. For example, if your grocery list is short with only about five items on it, you probably could remember to purchase everything without referring to the list. Even with a longer list you would be able to remember more of the items if they were organized according to whether the items were vegetables, fruits, or meats. Other means of organization may be by the lanes in which the foods are located or by associating foods with letters of the alphabet (F: fish, fruit).

How does this apply to problem solving? The problem solver is confronted with a large amount of unorganized information to process. If the data are not organized as they enter STM, the problem solver is unable to process the information and it may be forgotten. Forgetting information may cause decreased efficiency, important omissions, and improper resolutions of a problem.

The **long-term memory** contains two types of memory systems—episodic memory and semantic memory.[16] **Episodic memory** stores significant peak experiences in your life. This type of memory system is also referred to as declarative or "fact" memory.[12] The year you graduated from high school will be stored in episodic memory. By contrast, **semantic memory** retains information such as rules and principles and is also called procedural or "skill" memory.[12] It involves learning repetitious activities and requires no conscious thought. The rule of spelling—"*i* before *e* except after *c*"—is an example of semantic memory. Information in episodic memory has a greater tendency to become distorted or unretrievable as new information comes into the system. Semantic memory changes less frequently because the information is organized.

Long-term memory is dependent upon knowledge base, cues, and retrieval system. By becoming open to all possible learning experiences, your knowledge base will become stronger and more expansive. This added knowledge will be stored in LTM and will serve as cues for future incoming information.

*Mastery.* **Mastery** can be defined as a full command of knowledge on a particular subject. The solving of problems requires mastery of specific content. The type of information you seek, the sources of information you use, and the way in which you interpret the information **influence** mastery. At the same time, these same factors are **influenced** by mastery. For example, if you lack knowledge about certain content areas, you may not know that a problem even exists. Or if you use inadequate or inappropriate resources, you will have insufficient knowledge to solve a problem.

*Help-seeking.* To facilitate problem solving, you may need to seek help. There will be times when you lack the necessary knowledge and skills to solve problems on your own. This is not uncommon. You should feel free to acknowledge your limitations and seek assistance. In addition to human resources, it may be helpful to refer to media and other nonhuman sources.

We have identified and discussed four problem-oriented behaviors. With these prerequisite behaviors in mind, let us look at some characteristics of effective problem solvers.

## Characteristics of Problem Solvers

Researchers[5,33] have studied the difference between effective and ineffective problem solvers (Table 2–1). Ineffective problem solvers were found to be passive in their thinking, mentally careless, and superficial in solving problems. They often rushed through a problem. Because they either failed to comprehend what was required or spent too little time considering the question, wrong answers were selected. Their answers were selected on the basis of a few clues, such as a feeling, an impression, or a guess.

By contrast, effective problem solvers made an active attack on problems. They often employed a lengthy, sequential analysis in arriving at an answer when a question was initially unclear. They started with what they understood, drew on information that they possessed, and went through a chain of steps that finally brought them to a solution.

Other strategies used by effective problem solvers are inductive thinking, deductive thinking, and synthesis.

**TABLE 2–1. GUIDELINES FOR EFFECTIVE PROBLEM SOLVERS[5,33]**

1. *Maintain a Positive Attitude*—Effective problem solvers strongly believe that problems can be solved through careful, persistent analysis. Ineffective problem solvers, by contrast, frequently express the opinion that either you know the answer to a problem or you don't know it, and if you don't know it, you might as well give up or guess. Ineffective problem solvers lack both confidence and experience in dealing with problems through gradual (sometimes lengthy) analysis.
2. *Have a Concern for Accuracy*—effective problem solvers take great care to understand the facts and relationships in a problem fully and accurately. They are compulsive in checking whether their understanding of a problem is correct and complete. By contrast, ineffective problem solvers lack an intense concern about understanding. For example, effective problem solvers may reread a problem several times until they are sure they understand it. Ineffective problem solvers may miss a problem because they do not know exactly what it states.
3. *Break the Problem into Parts*—Effective problem solvers have learned that analyzing complex problems and ideas consists of breaking the ideas into smaller steps. They have learned to attack a problem by starting at a point where they can make some sense of it, and then proceed from there. By contrast, ineffective problem solvers have not learned the approach of breaking a complex problem into subproblems—dealing first with one step and then another.
4. *Avoid Guessing*—Ineffective problem solvers tend to jump to conclusions and guess answers without going through all the steps needed to make sure that the answers are accurate. Sometimes they make intuitive judgments in the middle of a problem without checking to see whether the judgments are correct. At other times they work a problem part of the way, but then give up on reasoning and guess at an answer. Effective problem solvers tend to work problems from beginning to end in small, careful steps. The tendency for ineffective problem solvers to make more errors—to work too hastily and sometimes skip steps—can be traced to these characteristics.
5. *Be Active in Problem Solving*—Effective problem solvers tend to be more active than ineffective problem solvers when dealing with problems. Put simply, they do more things as they try to understand and answer difficult questions. For example, effective problem solvers may try to create a mental picture of the ideas in order to "see" the situation better, or they may try to pin the situation down in terms of familiar experiences and concrete examples. Effective problem solvers may ask themselves questions about a problem, answer the questions, and "talk to themselves" as they clarify their thoughts. All in all, effective problem solvers are active in many ways that improve their accuracy and help them get a clearer understanding of ideas and problems.
6. *Possess Knowledge of Content Area*—In order for the process of problem solving to be carried out with expediency, efficiency, and positive results, the process is reliant upon facts. Factual knowledge of a content area is essential. Without background knowledge you will not recognize facts that are necessary to complete the steps of problem solving.

*Inductive Thinking.* With **induction** you gather isolated pieces of unassociated information. Then you evaluate all the data that you have collected and arrive at a conclusion that can be supported by theoretical knowledge. For example, often a woman who experiences tiredness, nausea in the morning, emotional sensitivity, and a late menses will conclude that she is pregnant even before confirmation by a physician.

*Deductive Thinking.* When you use the **deductive method,** the move is from the conclusion or generalization (confirmation of pregnancy) to the specific data (tiredness, nausea in the morning, and so forth). In other words, the problem is first identified and then the woman becomes aware of the physical cues. (Refer to Chapters 5 and 9 to learn more about inductive and deductive thinking.)

*Synthesis.* The linking of data to a specific problem requires the ability to synthesize the material and bring it together into meaningful relationships. **Synthesis** refers to the ability to tie together concepts, data, methods, and ideas from one source with those available from other sources. These other sources can be courses, books, journals, newspapers, and life experiences.

Synthesis is a complex process. The ability to synthesize information makes new information more understandable and meaningful. Suppose you were asked to discuss a lengthy Russian novel which describes 25 characters and 3 wars; it may be next to impossible to recall all the details. But what if you have a degree in Russian history, spent the last two summers in Russia, and recently saw a movie based on the film? Your experiences allow you to make associations and meaningful relationships among the various sources of data.

Now that we have explored the characteristics that distinguish effective problem solvers from ineffective problem solvers, let us examine the relationship between cognitive style and problem solving.

## Relationship of Cognitive Style and Problem Solving

Each of us has an identifiable cognitive style, or characteristic way of thinking, that is exhibited in our activities. Numerous cognitive learning styles have been researched. Two of these styles relate to problem solving—cerebral specialization and field perception.

*Cerebral Specialization.* **Left/right cerebral specialization** denotes a person's tendency to rely more on one hemisphere of the brain than on the other when processing information.[23,25,28] The left hemisphere is the language processing, sequential, if–then (hypothetical) part of the brain. This hemisphere mediates input in a "sorting out" way, processing information systematically to find the best solution. People who process information with the left hemisphere are more analytical, objective, and logical in their thinking. They tend to solve problems in an orderly, systematic manner.

The right hemisphere is the global view, the visual–spatial part of the brain. The right side of the brain functions on multiple-image inputs, experiences, emotions, and a wide assortment of mental operations in a way that encourages invention.[27] People who process information with the right hemisphere are more intuitive, subjective, and creative in their thinking. They solve problems using their emotions and personal experiences. The differences in intellectual characteristics of individuals with left/right cerebral specialization are summarized in Table 2–2.

**TABLE 2–2. COMPARISON OF INTELLECTUAL CHARACTERISTICS OF INDIVIDUALS WITH LEFT/RIGHT CEREBRAL SPECIALIZATION**[28,30,32]

| Left Hemisphere | Right Hemisphere |
| --- | --- |
| 1. Perceives data analytically | 1. Perceives data globally |
| 2. Responds to verbal commands | 2. Responds to visual commands |
| 3. Solves one problem at a time in sequential order | 3. Solves several problems simultaneously |
| 4. Processes information objectively | 4. Processes information subjectively |
| 5. Memory enhanced by systematic and controlled presentation | 5. Memory enhanced by use of creativity |
| 6. Solves problems by use of logic (inductive thinking) | 6. Solves problems by use of intuition |
| 7. Possesses a hypothetical orientation to problem solving | 7. Possesses a heightened spatial orientation to problem solving |
| 8. Processes data systematically in a reductive (sorting out) way | 8. Processes data by means of multiple-image inputs, experiences, and emotions that encourage invention |

Does this mean that if you tend to rely more on the right hemisphere to process information you will not be objective or use logic to solve problems? Hemispheres are thought to act interdependently to facilitate the activity of one another.[20,35] The left and right hemispheres may complement each other in perceiving, analyzing, and remembering information. It is more accurate to say that one particular hemisphere is dominant in a given function than it is to imply that one particular hemisphere is dominant for all functions.

*Field Perception.* Field-dependence/field independence is probably the most thoroughly researched cognitive style. The label of **field-dependence/field-independence** reflects a person's tendency toward perceiving events in one mode versus another. There is evidence that the preferred mode of thinking is quite stable and not drastically modified after adolescence.

**Field-dependence** refers to the tendency to accept a background as it is. In other words, these people adhere to the existing structure without any attempt to restructure. In field-dependence, events are experienced globally in an undifferentiated fashion. People who are field-dependent are extrinsically motivated and prefer guidance by others. They are more successful at structured tasks.

**Field-independence** refers to the tendency to mentally separate embedded figures from contextual backgrounds. This analytic ability can be illustrated by activities found in children's books. The child is instructed: circle all animals hidden in the picture. People who are field-independent seem to rely on their own perceptions to structure what they observe. This predisposing characteristic enables them to break up the contextual background to identify distinct yet hidden parts. This ability helps field-independent people to organize what they observe as well as to impose a structure from their own creation.[37,38] People who are field-independent are intrinsically motivated and require minimal guidance. They are guided by ideas and principles and are effective in analyzing situations. The differences in intellectual tasks of field-independence and field-dependence are summarized in Table 2–3.

**TABLE 2–3. COMPARISON OF INTELLECTUAL TASKS OF INDIVIDUALS WITH FIELD-INDEPENDENCE/DEPENDENCE[10,18,38]**

| Field-independence | Field-dependence |
|---|---|
| 1. Approaches environment in analytical terms | 1. Approaches environment in global terms |
| 2. Favors learning that requires separation of elements from the background | 2. Favors learning tasks with a global view |
| 3. Differentiates objects from embedding contexts | 3. Experiences events in an undifferentiated fashion |
| 4. Is competent at tasks requiring analysis | 4. Succeeds at tasks which refer to an already existing structure |
| 5. Is insensitive to social cues | 5. Is more proficient in social situations |
| 6. Is inner-directed; will make discovery without assistance | 6. Prefers to be directed by others; needs extensive guidance |
| 7. Tends to be more interested in things as opposed to persons | 7. Spends time looking at faces of those with whom they interact |
| 8. Has a well-developed sense of own identity | 8. Lacks a well-developed sense of own identity |
| 9. Prefers solitary, impersonal situations | 9. Prefers situations that require interpersonal contact |
| 10. Is concerned with ideas and abstract principles | 10. Is interested in interpersonal relationships |

There are some important similarities among field perception, hemispheric special-ization, and problem solving. Field-independent people, those dominated by the left hemisphere, and effective problem solvers are classified as analytic. Researchers[28,29] claim that people with these modes of thinking deal sequentially with one problem at a time. They are characterized as being more adept in working independently and mak-ing discoveries on their own.[32] Field-dependent people and right hemispheric dominated people use a holistic or global approach to problem solving. In these modes, people can deal with many problems at the same time. They require more guidance and structure, and prefer working with others.[31,38] Field-dependent, right hemisphere dominant people perform less well at solving problems that require isolating essential elements from the contextual background in which they are presented and in using them in different con-texts. People who are field-independent and dominated by the left hemisphere are more successful when the problem's solution requires that an embedded context be over-come.[14,25]

Now that we have explored the relationship between cognitive style and problem solving, it is time to discuss the problem-solving process itself.

## THE PROBLEM-SOLVING PROCESS

Problem solving is often undifferentiated from decision making. (Decision making is discussed in Chapter 11.) As stated earlier, problem solving is the method used to arrive at a solution (Fig. 2–3).

A problem can be straightforward or require restructuring of the original situation. A straightforward problem is one in which there is a definite answer, such as a mathe-matical problem: $2 + 2 = 4$. Restructuring problems require that one's initial perceptions be altered. For example, in determining the answer to the question (1)"For what career shall I prepare?" there is no given answer. It takes critical thinking (2) (i.e., inductive thinking, deductive thinking, and synthesis) and the ability to distinguish between rel-evant and irrelevant data. In the choice of a career, you would need to think of what

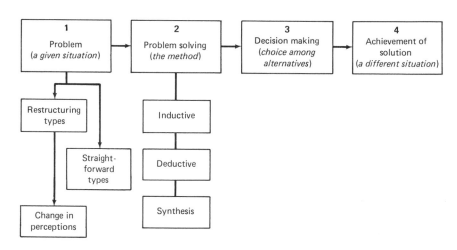

**Figure 2–3.** Depiction of problem solving as a method.

your aptitude and interests were as well as the requirements of various careers. This necessitates sifting through much data about yourself and career options to come up with data that are relevant to the original question of choosing a career. Decision making (3) is the choice one makes among alternatives generated by the problem-solving method. In this third step, you must choose among the potential careers that you would be capable of undertaking. Depending on your attitudes, values, beliefs, and interests, one option is more appealing, and you make your choice of a career. The last step (4) requires making a commitment concerning the alternative one will use to achieve the solution to the problem. In the example of choosing a career, commitment may be in the form of selecting the proper prerequisite courses to enable you to prepare for this choice.

## Methods of Problem Solving

There are several problem-solving methods. The choice of which method to use depends upon the complexity of the problem and the experience, skill, and knowledge of the problem solver. Some methods used to solve problems are unlearned, trial and error, intuitive, and scientific. Descriptions of these methods of problem solving are listed in Table 2–4.

An example of unlearned problem solving is one's reaction to touching an object that is hot. The reflex action is to withdraw contact immediately to prevent a burn injury. An individual does not have to be taught this action; it is innate. You may use trial and error problem solving when you select fruit or vegetables. You pick up each piece, feel it for ripeness, examine it for bruises, and you may even smell it. Each piece is scrutinized, and those that do not measure up to your standards are replaced. Intuitive problem solving is used when you sense the need to act in a certain way, but have no data on which to substantiate your action. Children are sensitive to the proper time to ask their parents for a special privilege. They may base their timing on past successes and failures; they remember the way their parents reacted and the explanations given at that time. On the basis of their experiences, they select the timing that correlates with past successes. The scientific method is probably most familiar to you and will be discussed in the next section.

Modifications of the scientific method exist. These methods of problem solving reflect changes that have resulted from the generation of new knowledge. Many of the modifications have been devised to meet the needs of specific disciplines. For example, Elstein and others devised a medical inquiry model to instruct medical students in problem solving. This model was used specifically to prepare students to make accurate medical diagnoses.[9] Newell and Simon based their theory of problem solving on the concepts of information processing and computer programming.[22] As the theoretical base in nurs-

TABLE 2–4. METHODS OF PROBLEM SOLVING

| Methods | Explanation of Methods |
| --- | --- |
| Unlearned | Reactions to problems that are not acquired by training or study but occur as the result of reflexes. |
| Trial and error | Testing and rejecting of solutions to problems without forethought and without recording the outcome.[7,15] |
| Intuitive | Subjective reactions based on feelings, emotions, attitudes, values, and beliefs without the benefit of theory. |
| Scientific | Reliable method using both inductive and deductive reasoning to arrive at logical conclusions. |

ing expanded, the profession needed an orderly method for resolving client problems. This led to the development of the nursing process.

In order to have a basis for understanding the modified scientific method—nursing process—you must understand the scientific method from which it evolved.

## Scientific Method of Problem Solving

Six steps are present in the scientific method of problem solving.[17] The first step is **understanding the problem**. In this step, it is important to recognize, define, and limit the problem. Generally, a problem is recognized when one is aware that a discrepancy exists between what is observed and what is expected. At times, you may experience frustration or realize that there is a barrier that prevents you from attaining a particular goal. Defining the problem means that you have pinpointed or isolated what is causing the frustration or barrier. When you limit a problem, you establish the boundaries that surround or "rope off" matters needing investigation.

The second step is **data collection**. Once the boundaries have been established, you must observe each piece of isolated information and decide if that information is relevant. Irrelevant data are discarded. In deciding relevancy of data, it is important to determine if a pattern exists among the isolated bits of data or if the event is unlikely to recur.

**Formulation of hypotheses** is the third step. Greater detail will be given to the discussion of hypotheses in the chapter on research. However, we will discuss briefly hypotheses as they relate to this chapter. **Hypotheses** are defined as tentative propositions suggested as explanations of abstract phenomena. These tentative propositions are possible solutions—alternatives—to the problem. During this step, it is important to generate as many possible answers to the problem as possible. The more tentative explanations you have to select from, the more substantial the solution to the problem.

The fourth step is **preparing a plan** for testing hypotheses. Depending on the nature of the problem and the problem solver's experience and knowledge base, the plan may be simple or complex. It is important to specify your intended actions. Any plan of action is more likely to succeed if it is recorded. A written plan decreases the possibility of omitting an important action.

**Testing the hypothesis** is the fifth step. This step involves the implementation of the plan. The testing period may vary in length. No plan is valuable unless it can be implemented successfully. When the actions you specified in the plan are enacted, you are testing their usefulness and can more realistically evaluate their effectiveness.

The sixth step is **interpretation and evaluation** of the results of the implemented plan. During this step, a decision is made as to whether the plan was effective in resolving the problem. The evaluation may be done on a daily basis or periodically to see how well the proposed actions are solving your problem.

Perhaps an example of how the scientific method works will clarify this important method. Let us imagine that you have been working part-time at various jobs for the past several years. Soon you will graduate from college and will apply for your first full-time position. On past evaluations there were very general comments about how you had some problems relating to others, but nothing specific. You wish to be successful in securing a full-time position. What should you do? The first step would be to clearly ask yourself, "What is the problem I have, based on past experiences and interactions with others?" You may need to list the specific comments made to enable you to state the precise problems. Your sister called you "stuck up." Your best friend said you were "sometimes a real snob." A fellow worker once told you that "you think you're better than anyone else." The statement of the problem may be: I convey a sense of superiority to others through my verbal and nonverbal messages. The next step in solving your problem would be to collect data and to determine patterns of behavior that recur. You discover that it is not so much what you say, but how you say it and how you appear when you speak. You therefore decide to focus your attention on the nonverbal messages and the tone of your message while communicating with others. The next step is to think of all the possible solutions to your communication problem with peers: "I need to be relaxed when I speak with others; I need to be sensitive to the way in which I am perceived by others; I need to find out why I must feel superior to others." The next step is to prepare a detailed plan of how you will improve communication with others. Since a plan is more effective when it is written, you decide to write your plan in a notebook. The next step is to test separately each item of your plan while speaking with others. The last step is to evaluate how effective your plan was. You choose to try each item in your plan one at a time and evaluate that action before trying the next item. You may ask a trusted friend who has known you for a number of years to monitor your progress. You may look for signs of improved interaction—a smile, a desire to spend more time with you.

Will following these steps allow you to solve problems? The answer is yes and no. Even though you follow the steps, several barriers may prevent you from successful resolution.

## Barriers to Problem Solving

There are several barriers to effective problem solving. Among these barriers are:

1. Failure to specify goals. Even though one may have knowledge of the problem-solving process, failure to specify goals may result in fragmentation of the plan of action.
2. Failure to follow each step of the problem-solving process systematically and completely. Possible causes for this barrier are a knowledge deficit and lack of time.
3. Collection of insufficient information. This barrier may be attributed to insufficient time, lack of initiative, failure to identify the scope of the problem, or insufficient knowledge base.
4. Failure to validate initial impression of the problem. This action overlooks the importance of considering multiple sources of data to substantitate the initial impression of the problem. Failure to recognize inconsistencies between the initial impression and validated data will result in ineffective problem solving.
5. Inadvertent alteration of data. Because of lack of sleep, anxiety, illness, and so forth, one may unintentionally perceive data incorrectly. Values, beliefs, and attitudes that conflict with the data can cause unconscious altering. It is also possible to make errors when communicating data.
6. Failure to generate all relevant alternatives before acting. This action limits the scope of your plan and prevents the evaluation of potential consequences.
7. Failure to consider probable consequences of actions. This action may overlook the most efficient, beneficial, safe solution.
8. Lack of positive reinforcement for problem-solving behavior. Problem-solving behavior may not be rewarded or practiced because it is an intellectual skill rather than a psychomotor skill and may require time for deliberation.

Knowledge of these barriers to successful problem solving increases our awareness of the importance of following a systematic format in solving problems. Now that you understand what is involved in problem solving, let us apply this method to the nursing process.

## THE NURSING PROCESS: A PROBLEM-SOLVING METHOD

Nursing, unlike other health care disciplines, has an organized structure that helps nurses to efficiently apply their intellectual, psychomotor, and interpersonal skills. This structure is the nursing process.

We can easily understand the term *nursing process* if we consider the definitions for the terms *nursing* and *process*. **Nursing** is the act of diagnosing and managing human responses[1] to potential or actual changes in health status. Care is provided to maintain the client's health, restore the client's health status and well-being, and prevent illness or injury to the client. The term **process** denotes the act of continuously moving forward, proceeding from one point to another on the way to a goal. Process is a method used to produce, accomplish, or attain a specific result. Based on these definitions, **nursing process** can be defined as an organized, systematic method of examining the client's health status, identifying the client's needs, and determining appropriate solutions to meet these needs. The nursing process uses the steps of assessing, diagnosing, planning, implementing, and evaluating.

How are the two processes of problem solving and nursing process comparable? You will recall that problem solving is the process used to resolve or answer proposed questions or achieve a solution to a problem. Client needs that are identified in the assessing and diagnosing steps of the nursing process are the "questions" in need of a solution or an answer. The remaining steps—planning, implementing, and evaluating—are used to develop an appropriate plan that will resolve or answer the questions. Thus, the nursing process is a problem-solving method.

### Historical Evolution of the Nursing Process

The actual term *nursing process* did not appear in nursing literature until the mid-1960s. Limited mention of the term, however, appeared during the 1950s. For example, Hall and Alfano (1964) discussed their ideas about nursing with a group of nurses in New Jersey. Their basic assumption was—"Nursing is a process."[11] One of the reasons that Hall and Alfano referred to nursing as a process was because it was dynamic and capable of changing as health problems changed. Hall and Alfano saw teaching as the means of enacting the nursing process.

During this same time period, Orlando (1961) also used the term nursing process. In her text *The Dynamic Nurse–Patient Relationship,* published at the beginning of the 1960s, Orlando identified three aspects of the nursing experience—client behavior, nurse's action, and nurse's reaction. Nursing process was the interaction among these three elements.[24]

Another author who broadly spoke of specific functions of the nurse was Wiedenbach (1964). She identified the purpose of nursing as supplying clients with assistance in meeting their needs. She classified the functions of the nurse as recognizing the client's need for help, administering to the client's needs, and evaluating whether the help given was adequate in meeting the client's needs. Although the terminology differs, these functions are the forerunners of the current steps in the nursing process.[34]

Besides those who contributed to the definition and the steps of the nursing process, Henderson (1966) strongly influenced the thinking of nurses. The nature of nursing was the topic of her writings, which were included in a nursing textbook and influenced thinking in the 1950s and early 1960s. She advocated a strong knowledge base in the biologic sciences as well as in the social sciences. Man was viewed as a whole, complete, and independent being. Nursing was seen as a complement to the client—supplying what was needed to carry out activities and prescribed treatment. The nursing process was equated with the nursing activity. Henderson's broad framework enabled nurses to assess, plan, implement, and evaluate care with clients at any point on the health continuum.[13]

Toward the latter 1960s, nursing leaders were more specific as to the purpose of nursing and the components of the nursing process. Yura and Walsh (1967) wrote that the nursing process was a series of actions that were intended to fulfill the purposes of nursing. They identified four components: assessing, planning, implementing, and evaluating. The process was depicted as a mutual interaction between client and nurse.[39]

During the 1970s most nurse educators taught the nursing process as a four-step process. Also, nurses were acquiring more sophistication in using the nursing process.

Carnevali (1973) viewed the nursing process as an organized means to determine the client's need for assistance, the type of assistance needed, and the effectiveness of the assistance once it was given. She broke the nursing process into two broad phases— a diagnostic phase (assessment and analysis of the problem) and a management phase (planning, intervention, and evaluation). She felt that one should not diagnose a need for coping with activities and demands of daily living unless information was collected concerning four areas—activities of daily living, demands of daily living, internal resources, and external resources.[6]

As nursing diagnosis gradually evolved into an accepted function of professional nurses, it was incorporated into either the assessing or planning step of the nursing process. It was not until the 1980s that diagnosing was considered as a separate step in the process (Table 2–5).

## Benefits and Limitations of the Nursing Process

Although the nursing process stresses a dominant and independent function of the profession, there are benefits and limitations to its use. Some of the benefits of the nursing process are that it:

1. Provides an open approach to problem solving. No two persons solve the same problem in the same way. And yet, several may arrive at the correct solution.
2. Makes possible a variety of strategies to solve problems. The nursing process does not adhere to any one particular method of solving problems. This open approach provides a flexible format. If a specific theoretical framework is used, the method is limited rather than open.
3. Provides for continuous feedback during the planning and implementing steps of the nursing process. The feedback leads to rejecting or restructuring of the hypotheses.
4. Allows nurses the advantage of generating hypotheses before planning care.
5. Enables nurses to generate and remember a greater number of hypotheses at a particular time, which forms the basis for encouraging care planning.
6. Translates a conceptual and cognitive way of thinking into client-centered, action-oriented nursing interventions.

**TABLE 2–5. COMPONENTS OF THE NURSING PROCESS**

| | Yura and Torres (1967)[39] | Bailey and Claus (1975)[2] | Mayers (1978)[19] | Bircher (1984)[4] | Pinnell and de Meneses (1986) |
|---|---|---|---|---|---|
| Step 1 | Assessing | Defining overall needs, purposes, and goals | Gathering data | Assessment | Assessing |
| Step 2 | Planning | Defining the problem | Identifying problems | Knowledge | Diagnosing |
| Step 3 | Implementing | Weighing the constraints versus the capabilities and resources | Defining expected outcomes | Nursing diagnosis | Planning |
| Step 4 | Evaluating | Specifying an approach to solving the problem | Prescribing best solutions | Planning | Implementing |
| Step 5 | | Stating decision objectives and performance criteria | Evaluating at periodic and endpoint intervals | Implementation | Evaluating |
| Step 6 | | Generating alternative solutions | | Evaluation | |
| Step 7 | | Analyzing options | | | |
| Step 8 | | Choosing best options | | | |
| Step 9 | | Controlling and implementing decisions | | | |
| Step 10 | | Evaluating effectiveness of action | | | |

7. Enables nurses to use the problem-solving process to resolve personal and professional problems.

The limitations of the nursing process are that the process:

1. Lacks specific details to guide nurses in effective problem-solving methods. The use of a theoretical framework would give direction.
2. Requires a certain amount of knowledge and skill in order to be used effectively.
3. Becomes time-consuming and burdensome to nurses who work in short-staffed units or in environments with critically ill clients.

Although there are some limitations, we believe that the nursing process is an important model for promoting professional status.

## Overview of the Nursing Process

We previously identified five steps in the nursing process—assessing, diagnosing, planning, implementing, and evaluating (Fig. 2–4). The assessing step can be accomplished by four procedures—conducting an assessment interview, collecting a nursing health history, conducting a wellness assessment, and performing a physical assessment. For a family or community client, a separate family and community assessment are needed.

The diagnosing step is made up of the following substeps: analysis of data, derivation of conclusions, assignment of diagnostic labels, determination of sustaining factors, and formulation of a diagnostic statement.

During the planning step, six operations are involved: establishing priorities, determining prognosis, establishing goals, formulating behavioral objectives, identifying nursing interventions, and formulating a plan of care. In the implementing step, two activities are necessary—organization of interventions and performance of interventions.

The final step in the nursing process is evaluating. This step consists of determining outcome criteria, collecting data about the current situation, comparing data to the outcome criteria, summarizing inferences regarding evaluation outcomes, and taking appropriate action(s) based on evaluation outcomes. (Fig. 2–5).

This particular model of the nursing process has several attributes. Many of these qualities result from the fact that the nursing process is an open system. If you examine Figures 2–4 and 2–5 carefully, you will become aware of the following:

1. The process is circular in nature. By this we mean that each step is arranged in a sequential order that is continuous and repetitive until the client no longer needs nursing assistance.
2. This model is an open system which is characterized by a large network composed of a number of smaller units. Each of these smaller units works together to create a functioning larger network.

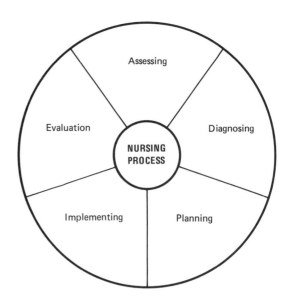

**Figure 2–4.** Overview of the nursing process.

APPLICATION TO AN INDIVIDUAL CLIENT

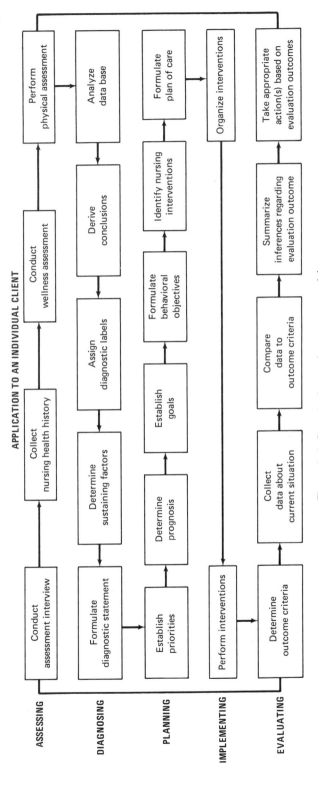

**Figure 2–5.** Steps in the nursing process model.

ASSESSING

DIAGNOSING

PLANNING

IMPLEMENTING

EVALUATING

**TABLE 2–6. COMPARISON OF SCIENTIFIC METHOD AND NURSING PROCESS**

| | Scientific Method | Nursing Process |
|---|---|---|
| Assessing | Recognizing a general problem area; broadly defining and describing the problem | a. Recognizing a client's need for help in certain general problem areas<br>b. Reviewing background information about the client<br>c. Developing "impressions" concerning client's problems |
| | Collecting data from all relevant sources | Developing data base<br>a. Nursing history<br>b. Physical examination<br>c. Review of laboratory test findings<br>d. Review of diagnostic studies<br>e. Consultation<br>f. Review of the literature |
| Diagnosing | Formulating an hypothesis | a. Analyzing and interpreting the data; making inferences<br>b. Defining the client's problems and stating the impact of these problems upon the client's life situation (nursing diagnosis) |
| Planning | Preparing a plan for testing the hypothesis | a. Setting priorities<br>b. Determining prognosis<br>c. Stating client's goals and behavioral objectives<br>d. Determine outcome criteria<br>e. Planning nursing interventions<br>f. Writing nursing orders |
| Implementing | Testing the hypothesis | a. Initiating the plan of care<br>b. Writing and recording results of nursing actions<br>c. Administering and supervising nursing care<br>d. Teaching the client<br>e. Referrals |
| Evaluating | Interpreting test results and evaluating the hypothesis | a. Establishing standards or criteria for evaluation of plan of care and client's progress<br>b. Reviewing client's progress recorded in chart and comparing with care plan<br>c. Evaluating nursing management and interventions and determining if goals are being achieved |
| | Modifying the plan of action based upon further data collection | Modifying the plan of care |

3. This process is dynamic and continually changing. The separate units are constantly interacting with one another and yet contribute to the functioning of the whole system.
4. This model is appropriate for use with individual clients, families, or communities. It is also applicable in the various levels of health care delivery—primary, secondary, and tertiary.
5. This model has utility. It can be used to maintain the client's health, to restore the client's health status, or to prevent the effects of stressors upon health.

Now that we have discussed the nursing process in general terms, we are ready to examine how the nursing process compares with the scientific method.

## Comparison of the Nursing Process with the Scientific Method

The purpose of this chapter has been to introduce you to the nursing process as a problem-solving approach. Remember when we talk about problem solving that we are not restricting discussion to problems as defined by theorists.[8,26] We see problem solving as an intellectual function used to resolve the needs of clients, families, and communities.

Depicted in Table 2–6 is a comparison of the elements of the scientific method and the nursing process. Some of the attributes of these related processes are the following:

1. Once the cycle is completed in each of these processes, it begins again. If the second cycle also relates to the same problem area as the first cycle, the difference is in the nature and amount of information available.
2. Both cognitive processes are capable of being learned. They are not static processes—they are dynamic. If one masters these processes one has the potential of being an effective problem solver.
3. Both cognitive processes are open systems. There is an input of information, a throughput, and an output. These cognitive processes are open to new information and create a change in existing information.
4. These cognitive processes rely on a knowledge base. The stronger one's knowledge base, the more effective one's ability to solve problems.

This broad comparison of the characteristics of the nursing process to the scientific method will prepare you to examine each step of the nursing process in greater depth in later chapters.

## SUMMARY

Problem solving is a dynamic process that is used to resolve or answer questions or achieve a solution to a problem. Four behaviors that are important to effective problem solving are goal-setting, information-seeking, mastery, and help-seeking. In addition, characteristics that distinguish effective from ineffective problem solvers are a positive attitude, concern for accuracy, systematic analytic techniques, active use of imagery, and possession of a strong knowledge base—theoretical and experiential.

The scientific method, a structured form of problem solving, is the basis for the nursing process. The nursing process which consists of five steps—assessing, diagnosing, planning, implementing, and evaluating—is more flexible and adaptable than the scientific method. The nursing process provides an organized, systematic method of examing the client's health status, identifying the client's needs, and determining appropriate solutions to meet these needs.

## STUDY GUIDE

1. Identify three characteristics of effective problem solvers that you possess. Identify three ineffective behaviors that you possess.
2. Compare the nursing process to scientific problem solving.
3. Discuss the barriers that interfere with your problem-solving abilities.
4. Outline a plan to follow that would correct these barriers to problem solving.
5. List five attitudes (positive or negative) that you have concerning use of the nursing process.

## REFERENCES

1. American Nurses' Association. *Nursing: A social policy statement.* Kansas City, Mo.: American Nurses' Association, 1980.
2. Bailey, J. T., & Claus, K. E. *Decision making in nursing.* St. Louis, Mo.: C.V. Mosby, 1975.
3. Berry, P. C. *An exploration of the interrelations among some non-intellectual predictors of achievement in problem solving* (Tech. Rep. 4, prepared under Contract Nonr 609, NR 150–166, for Office of Naval Research). New Haven, Conn.: Department of Industrial Administration and Department of Psychology, Yale University, December 1958.
4. Bircher, A. National conference on nursing diagnosis: St. Louis University, St. Louis, Mo., April 1984.
5. Bloom, B., & Broder, L. *Problem-solving processes of college students.* Chicago: University of Chicago Press, 1950.
6. Carnevali, D. L. *Conceptualizing: Storage of knowledge for diagnosis and management.* In P. Mitchell & A. Loustau (Eds.), *Concepts Basic to Nursing.* New York: McGraw-Hill, 1973.
7. Davis, G. A. Current status of research and theory in human problem solving. *Psychological Bulletin,* 1966, *66,* 36–4.
8. Duncker, K. On problem solving. *Psychological Monographs,* 1945, *58,* (5, Whole No. 270).
9. Elstein, A., Shulman, L., & Sprafka, S. *Medical problem solving: An analysis of clinical reasoning.* Cambridge: Harvard University Press, 1978.
10. Farr, R. S. Personality variables and problem solving performance: An investigation of the relationships between field-dependence—independence, sex-role identification, problem difficulty and problem solving performance." (Doctoral dissertation, New York University, 1968). *Dissertation Abstracts,* 1969, *29,* 2561A-2562A. (University Microfilms No. 69-3168).
11. Hall, L., & Alfano, G. Myocardial infarction: Incapacitation or rehabilitation. *American Journal of Nursing,* 1964 *64,* 20–25.
12. Haney, D. Q. Unraveling the mysteries of memory. St. Louis, Mo.: *Post-Dispatch,* September 3, 1984, 3E, 8E.
13. Henderson, V. *The nature of nursing.* New York: Macmillan, 1966.
14. Karp, S. A., Silberman, L., & Winters, S. Psychological differentiation and socioeconomic status. *Perceptual and Motor Skills,* 1969, *28,* 55–60.
15. Kieffer, J. Nursing diagnosis can make a critical difference. *Nursing Life,* May/June 1984, 18–21.
16. Klatzky, R. L. *Human memory: Structures and processes.* San Francisco: W. H. Freeman & Company Publishers, 1975.
17. Kleinmuntz, B. (Ed.). *Problem-solving: Research, method, and theory.* New York: Wiley, 1966.
18. Loeff, R. G. *Embedding and distracting field contents as related to the field-dependence dimension.* Unpublished master's thesis, Brooklyn College, 1961.
19. Mayers, M. A. *A systematic approach to the nursing care plan.* New York: Appleton-Century-Crofts, 1978.
20. Messick, S. Personality consistencies in cognition and creativity. In S. Messick and Associates (Ed.), *Individuality in learning.* San Francisco: Jossey-Bass, 1976.

21. Nakamura, C. Y. Conformity and problem solving. *Journal of Abnormal and Social Psychology,* 1958, *56,* 315–320.
22. Newell, A., & Simon, H. A. *Human problem solving.* Englewood Cliffs, N. J.: Prentice-Hall, 1972.
23. Olson, M. D. Cerebral lateralization in science. *Gifted Child Quarterly,* 1979, *23,* 142–150.
24. Orlando, I. J. *The dynamic nurse-patient relationship.* New York: Lakeside, 1961.
25. Orstein, R., & Galen, D. Lateral specialization of cognitive mode II: EEG frequency analysis. *Psychophysiology,* September 1974, *11,* 568–578.
26. Ray, W. S. Complex tasks for use in human problem-solving research. *Psychological Bulletin,* 1955, *52,*134–149.
27. Reynolds, C. R., & Torrance, E. P. Perceived changes in styles of learning and thinking (hemisphericity) through direct and indirect training. *Journal of Creative Behavior,* 1979, *12,* 247–252.
28. Sperry, R. W. Left-brain, right-brain. *Saturday Review,* August 9, 1975, pp. 30–33.
29. Torrance, E. P. *Encouraging creativity in the classroom.* Dubuque, Iowa: William C. Brown, 1970.
30. Torrance, E. P., & Mourad, S. Role of hemisphericity in performance on selected measures of creativity. *Gifted Child Quarterly,* 1979, *23,* 44–45.
31. Torrance, E. P., Reynolds, C., Ball, O., & Reigel, T. *Technical manual for your style of learning and thinking.* Athens, Ga.: University of Georgia, 1978.
32. Wheatley, G., Mitchell, R., Franklane, R., & Craft, R. Hemisphere specialization and cognitive development: Implications for mathematics education. *Journal for Research in Mathematics Education,* January 1978, *99,* 20–30.
33. Whimbey, A., & Lochhead, J. *Problem solving and comprehension: A short course in analytical reasoning.* Philadelphia: Franklin Institute Press, 1978.
34. Wiedenbach, E. *Clinical nursing: A helping art.* New York: Springer, 1964.
35. Witkin, H. Individual differences in ease of perception of embedded figures. *Journal of Personality,* 1950, *19,* 1–15.
36. Witkin, H., & Berry, J. *Psychological differentiation in cross cultural perspective.* Princeton, N.J.: Educational Testing Service, 1975.
37. Witkin, H., Dyke, R., Faterson, H., et al. *Psychological differentiation.* New York: Wiley, 1962.
38. Witkin, H., & Moore, C. *Cognitive style and the teaching-learning process.* Paper presented at the American Educational Research Association Meeting, Chicago, April 15, 1974.
39. Yura, H., & Torres, G. *The nursing process.* New York: Appleton-Century-Crofts, 1967.

## BIBLIOGRAPHY

Buffery, A. W. H., & Gray, J. A. Sex differences in the development of spatial and linguistic skills. In F. Ounsted & D. C. Taylor (Eds.), *Gender differences: Their ontogeny and significance.* London: Churchill, 1972.
Carnevali, D. L. *Nursing care planning, diagnosis and management.* (3rd ed.). Philadelphia: Lippincott, 1983.
Carnevali, D. L., Mitchell, P. H., Woods, N. F., & Tanner, C. A. *Diagnostic reasoning in nursing.* Philadelphia: Lippincott, 1984.
Ceronsky, C. Family staff conferences open communication, resolve problems. *Hospital Progress,* August 1983, *65*(8), 58–59.
Cochran, R. B. Don't let tactics trip you up . . . plays commonly used to block the resolution of problems. *American Journal of Nursing,* May 1983, *83*(5), 844.
Cohen, B., Berent, S., & Silverman, A. Field-independence and lateralization function in the human brain. *Archives of General Psychiatry,* February 1973, *28,* 165–168.

Cronenwett, L.R. Helping and nursing models. *Nursing Research,* November–December 1983, *32*(6), 342–346.

de Chesnay, M. Problem solving in nursing. *Image,* Winter 1983, *15*(1), 8–11.

de Chesnay, M. The creation and dissolution of paradoxes in nursing practice. *Topics in Clinical Nursing,* October 1983, *5*(3), 71–80.

Elstein, A. Clinical judgment: Psychological research and medical practice. *Science,* 1976, *194,* 698–700.

Fair, E. W. Short cuts to problem solving. *Supervisor Nurse,* April 1981, *12*(4), 62–63.

Frederickson, K., & Mayer, G. G. Problem-solving skills: What effect has education? *American Journal of Nursing,* July 1977, *77* (7), 1167–1169.

Gage, N. L., & Berliner, D. C. *Educational psychology* (2nd ed.). Chicago: Rand McNally, 1979, p. 305.

Hogarth, R. M. Process tracing in clinical judgment. *Behavioral Science,* 1974, *19,* 298–313.

Holzemer, W. L., Schleutermann, J. A., Farrand, L. L., & Miller, A. G. A validation study: Simulations as a measure of nurse practitioners' problem-solving skills. *Nursing Research,* May–June 1981, *30*(3), 139–144.

Jackson, D. N., Messick, S., & Meyers, C. T. Evaluation of group and individual forms of embedded figures measures of field-independence. *Education and Psychological Measurement,* 1964, *24,*177–192.

Jacobs, A. *Critical requirements for safe/effective nursing practice.* Kansas City, Mo.: American Nurses Association, 1978.

Johnson, M., & Davis, M. L. *Problem solving in nursing practice.* Dubuque, Iowa: William C. Brown Co., 1978.

Kaltsounis, B. Validity evidence on *Your Style of Learning and Thinking. Perceptual and Motor Skills,* 1979, *48,* 177–178.

Karp, S. A. Field-dependence and overcoming embeddedness. *Journal of Consulting Psychology,* 1963, *27,* 294–302.

Kassirer, J., & Gorry, G. A. Clinical problem-solving behavior. *Annals of Internal Medicine,* August 1978, *89,* 245–255.

Khatena, J., & Torrance, E. P. *Norms technical manual: Thinking creatively with sounds and words.* Lexington, Mass.: Personnel Press/Ginn, 1973.

Kleinmuntz, B. The processing of clinical information by man and machine. In B. Kleinmuntz (Ed.), *Formal representation of human judgment.* New York: Wiley, 1968.

Kogan, N. Sex differences in creativity and cognitive styles. In S. Messick & Associates (Eds.), *Individuality in learning.* San Francisco: Jossey-Bass, 1976.

Lenberg, C. *The clinical performance examination.* New York: Appleton-Century-Crofts, 1979.

Ludwig, L. Environments for learning. In M. Marty (Ed.), *Responding to new missions.* San Francisco: Jossey-Bass, 1978, pp. 45–54.

McCarthy, M. M. The nursing process: Application of current thinking in clinical problem solving. *Journal of Advanced Nursing,* May 1981, *6*(3), 173–177.

Newell, A. Heuristic programming: Ill-structured problems. In J. Aronofsky (Ed.), *Progress in operations research* (Vol. 3). New York: Wiley, 1969, pp. 360–414.

Orr, J. A. Nursing and the process of scientific inquiry. *Journal of Advanced Nursing,* November 1979, *4*(6), 603–610.

Page, G. Written simulation in nursing. *Journal of Nursing Education,* April 1978, *17,* 28–32.

Parnes, S. J., Noller, R. B., & Biondi, A. M. *Guide to creative action.* New York: Scribners, 1977.

Samples, R. Educating both sides of the human mind. *Science Teacher,* 1975, *42,* 21–23.

Style, A. Intuition and problem solving. *Journal of Royal College of General Practice,* February 1979, *199,* 71–74.

Suchman, J. R. A model for the analysis of inquiry. In H. J. Klausmeier, & C. W. Harris (Eds.), *Analysis of concept learning.* New York: Academic Press, 1966, p. 178.

Templeton, D. E. Analogizing: Its growth and development. *Journal of Aesthetic Education,* 1973, *7*(3), 21–33.

Torrance, E. P. Broadening concepts of giftedness in the '70's. In S. Kirk, & F. Lord (Eds.), *Educational resources and perspectives*. Boston: Houghton-Mifflin, 1974.

Torrance, E. P. Sociodrama as a creative problem-solving approach to studying the future. *Journal of Creative Behavior,* 1975, *9*, 182–195.

Torrance, E. P. *The Torrence test of creative thinking: Norms-technical manual*. Lexington, Mass.: Personnel Press/Ginn, 1974.

Torrance, E. P. Your style of learning and thinking. *The Gifted Child Quarterly*, Winter 1977, *21*, 563–585.

Vissing, Y., et al. Visualization techniques for health care workers. *Journal of Psychological Nursing Mental Health Service,* January 1984, *22*(1), 29–32.

Witkin, H. Cognitive styles in the educational setting. *New York University Education Quarterly,* Spring 1977, *8*, 14–20.

Witkin, H. *Educational implications of cognitive style*. Paper presented at the University Deans Meeting of the Council of Graduate Schools, Phoenix, Arizona, December 4, 1974.

Yura, H., & Walsh, M. *The nursing process: Assessing, planning, implementing, evaluating*. New York: Appleton-Century-Crofts, 1978.

# 3

# Theory: Relevance to Processes within Nursing

Professional nursing practice is a combination of valuing and believing, knowing, and doing. As a profession develops, all three areas change—values and beliefs are redefined, knowledge is expanded, and skills are perfected. The acquisition and organization of knowledge into meaningful patterns enriches professional practice. The quality of care is directly related to each nurse's knowledge base, which increases as nurses draw upon the expanding body of theory.

In this chapter we will discuss theory as it relates to processes inherent in the practice of nursing. Major interdisciplinary theories as well as nursing theories will be examined for their relevance to nursing practice. Process concept definition will be described and illustrated in relation to the nursing process. A relationship also will be made between theory and other important processes that will be discussed in this book.

Study of this chapter will help you to:

1. Relate the role of theory development to the emergence of nursing as a profession.
2. Explain how theories are developed.
3. Explain how theories from other disciplines are used in nursing practice.
4. Describe how nurses can apply selected nursing theories to the nursing process.
5. Develop process concept definitions to make the nursing process operational.
6. Describe the advantages of using a theoretical framework to guide nursing practice.
7. Use theoretical frameworks when applying other processes important to nursing—problem solving, research, teaching, decision making, and change.

## GENERAL THEORY DEVELOPMENT

A **theory** can be defined as a systematic set of interrelated concepts, definitions, and deductions that describe, explain, or predict interrelationships.[7,15,20] A theory is capable of being tested and thereby is supported by scientific research. (Refer to Chapter 9 which discusses the research process.)

A theory begins with an idea that occurs within your mind. Even though the idea may be abstract, it is still rooted in reality and has the potential for influencing your thoughts and behavior. This idea generally comes about as a result of observations you make of unrelated events. You begin to make sense of the bits and pieces of separate information that you have observed and to formulate ideas. In theory development these ideas are called concepts. By means of problem solving, several ideas or concepts are brought together to form a meaningful statement of relationships. A theory has been developed when this relationship is articulated.

The very term itself, *theory development*, indicates that theories are dynamic. They are vital and give meaning to the discipline they represent. The term **development** implies an increase, growth, or evolution. And when something grows, it also changes. The change may be subtle as in a child who, as he grows, increases in size but his form remains the same. Or the change can be dramatic, like a butterfly who changes from a caterpillar; the altered form is nothing like the original form. Similarly, theories change as they are developed. They alter as a result of deductive and inductive reasoning. Research may clarify, reformulate, verify, or nullify existing theory, or it may initiate new theory.

## Components of Theory

According to the definition stated earlier, there are three parts to a theory: definitions, concepts, and deductions. An understanding of these components is essential.

*Definitions.* Theories, like disciplines, have a language of their own. Theorists may coin or develop new words, redefine words in current use, or use uncommon words. This makes your task of understanding a theory more difficult and challenging. To increase your understanding of a particular theory, you need to look at how the theorist defines words or terms used within the theory. **Definitions** are operationally defined words or phrases that are expressed in observable and measurable terms. In other words, definitions will tell you how the theorist is using the word.

The coined words which are developed or invented by the theorist are the least familiar to us. These words are developed as a shorter way of saying something. Osmosis is much simpler to say than diffusion of fluid through a semipermeable membrane until there is equal concentration of fluid on either side of the membrane. Another example can be seen in the word **reciprocy** which was coined by Rogers. The word **reciprocity** can be found in the dictionary and means a mutual or cooperative interchange of favors or privileges. Reciprocy makes use of only the core element—recip-. Rogers' meaning is somewhat different although it retains much of the core meaning. She defines **reciprocy** as a "function of the mutual interaction between the human field and the environmental field."[22]

Common terms or words may be defined differently by theorists. For example, efficiency and effectiveness are synonymous. But to some theorists, **efficiency** is defined as work satisfaction or loyalty, and **effectiveness** as an organization's achievement of its goals. Some words are used by several disciplines. Problems occur when the words need to have a slightly different meaning for each discipline. **Homeostasis** is one such word. In biology, it means the process by which a system regulates itself around a stable state. The term is used to note the ingestion of food (the input) which is used by the catabolic and the anabolic processes of the body for tissue breakdown and restoration to preserve a steady state (homeostasis). When the word "homeostasis" is used in organizational theory, however, information is seen as the energy or food that the system needs to assist it in maintaining its steady state. Obviously, it becomes necessary to change the meaning somewhat for the word "homeostasis" to be useful in organizational theory.

Uncommon terms are also used by theorists. The definitions of the words may be the same or different from the dictionary definitions. An example is the term **ideographic**. If you were to look this word up in a dictionary, it would be defined in terms of a close study of an individual case. A theorist may use this word to refer to something personal—having to do with the person, the personality, and the person's needs.

*Concept.* When you are learning about a particular subject, you gain an impression by using your senses. The mental images you form by generalizing from these impressions are concepts. **Concepts** are abstract ideas of universal significance that give meaning to our sense perceptions and permit generalizations. They are stored in our memory to be recalled and used at a later time in new and different situations. Concepts can be translated into principles and laws.

When you were a young child, you gradually acquired concepts of various things— bed, chair, table, large, and small. These abstractions were whatever you thought they were. Some of these concepts represented physical properties of objects, while others were more abstract and were used in relation to something else (for example, large and small). If you never learned concepts, you would have to describe what you were referring to each time you wanted to talk about the subject, person, or event.

Some concepts are used to describe and characterize properties and relations of a class of things, persons, or objects. These words, such as environment, stress, and culture, provide the means for organizing our ideas. They bring order to our disconnected observations and related experiences.

Models are used to depict concepts. **Models** are patterns or word descriptions that depict the theory or concept in shortened form. You are probably familiar with the use of models. Many toys are models—soldiers, ships, automobiles, and doll houses. Models are used extensively in education, business, and industry because of their usefulness. Models depict tangible structures and systems; for example, a model of a heart can help us to learn complex skills.

Conceptual models have been very important in the development of theories because they provide the means of sorting and categorizing observations and research findings. A **conceptual model** can be defined as a group of concepts that are interrelated. A conceptual model differs from a theory in that it does not describe the interrelationships among the concepts nor does it explain how or why events occur. The various conceptual models view the events from different perspectives and thereby enhance understanding. Models should not be thought of as mutually inclusive or exhaustive in their depiction of a concept or theory. They are merely a means of depicting concepts and relationships of a theory.

There are certain advantages in using models. Most obvious is the advantage of economy of language. Another advantage is the potential for increased understanding that results from simplifying an otherwise complex theory. On the other hand, these advantages may also represent a disadvantage. The simplicity by which a theory is depicted in a model may be too limiting and too basic to serve the purpose of the theory. We have come to accept that certain phenomena are very complex and require several different frameworks to clarify and enhance understanding.

*Deductions.* The third component of a theory is deductions. **Deductions** are conclusions that are reached by logically proceeding from a clarification of definitions to acceptable concepts to deductions. The deductions can be tested through research.

Now that we have explored the components of theory, we will discuss the purposes and functions of theory and levels of theory development.

## Purposes of Theory

Theories are the capstone of all scientific work because understanding, which is the goal of science, is expressed in theoretical formulations. Theory development serves several purposes of science: It provides a typology or method of organizing and categorizing things, predicts future events, explains past events, provides a sense of understanding about the cause of events, and offers the potential for control of events.[7,19,20]

**Typology** is a study of systematic classifications. Providing typologies is the easiest purpose of science to fulfill. Concepts can be used as the organizing and classifying framework. For example, if the concept is energy, types of energy can be categorized according to their identifying characteristics. The typology should result in the concept's exhaustiveness. By this, we mean that there should not be any aspect of the concept that cannot be fitted into the classification system. There should not be any doubt as to where each "thing" belongs in the classification system. Typologies should be consistent with the other interrelated concepts included in the theory.

The second and third purposes of science, **prediction** and **explanation of past and present events**, are the same except from the perspective of time. It is important for theories to be stated correctly. If correctly stated, they can be used to predict future events and to explain past scientific events.

The most difficult purpose of science is to **provide a sense of understanding**. In order to understand a phenomenon, there must be a link between the changes occurring in one concept and the changes occurring in other concepts. An example is the ripening (concept of aging) of a banana after it has been left in a warm (concept of temperature) place over a period of time (concept of time). To understand the phenomenon of ripening, one must make a link between the dark areas of a ripening banana and the rise in room temperature and the passage of time.

The fifth purpose of science, the **ability to control events,** is not necessary for acceptance of theory as scientific knowledge because it is impossible to control all events. An example is the solar system. There is no way we can control this phenomenon, and yet there is a theory that can predict and explain what occurs within the solar system.

## Functions of Theory

A theory has several functions. Functions differ from purposes. A **purpose** is the result intended or desired, while a **function** is an action that contributes to an even larger action.

There are four major functions of theory.[5,20] Theory:

1. Guides research
2. Explains ideas
3. Summarizes existing knowledge
4. Predicts future trends

These functions, particularly the last three, are interrelated and can be used as criteria for evaluating a theory.

***Theory Guides Research.*** Theory can be thought of as the launch pad for research. It is the foundation on which research is built and justifies the choice of the research focus. Theory provides a particular way of looking at a phenomena. For example, there are many ways to view learning. It may be viewed from a development perspective (or framework) or it may be seen from the perspective of "play is a child's work." In each of these cases, we are observing the same set of phenomena, but we are looking at learning from a different frame of reference.

***Theory Explains Ideas.*** It offers an explanation of certain aspects of the world and gives reasons for the phenomena under observation. Explanations involve the "why" and "how" of phenomena.

***Theory Summarizes Existing Knowledge.*** A theory pulls together known phenomena. In other words, a theory will make a general statement about a group of phenomena. For example, "a substance will float if its density is less than that of water." This general statement accounts for a whole group of phenomena—wood floats, oil floats, paraffin floats, stones sink, metals sink; however, teakwood sinks and pumice stone floats. A useful theory pulls together known facts, summarizing aspects that are known. In doing this, it also assists in explaining the known world.

***Theory Predicts Future Trends.*** Essentially, a theory will say, "Given this, then that." For example, in stimulus–response theory, you will read that a stimulus will evoke a response. In other words, given a stimulus, then there will be a response.
    Theory development proceeds from forming one's basic assumptions about a phenomenon, to describing the observations made regarding the phenomenon, to developing lower (awareness) level concepts and intermediate level concepts, and arriving at a theory[7,20] (Fig. 3–1).

## Levels of Theory Development
The lowest level of theory development is that of awareness, wherein you readily form impressions and are responsive and sensitive. Because of this heightened sensitivity, you are more alert to certain facts, concepts, and phenomena. At this level, the formulated concept is a way of looking at something of which you are more aware.
    An intermediate level concept weaves together several lower level concepts into more complex concepts. In doing this, the intermediate level concept has more force and connotes greater meaning than a lower level concept.

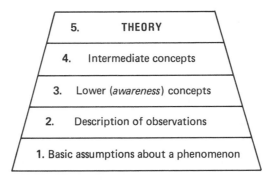

**Figure 3–1.** Five levels of theory development.

The highest level is theory, which is something apart from the lower and intermediate concepts. The lower and intermediate concepts are important to the development of the theory and are a part of it.

In the lower levels of theory development, observations are very important. This fact makes the lower levels more concrete and less abstract. At the higher levels of development, there is more abstractness because you are dealing with the concepts themselves—not merely observations.

When theory development proceeds from a concept to making observations, deductive reasoning is used. The reverse is true when theory development begins with observations and evolves to a theory. In this case, inductive reasoning is used to derive the theory from the observed phenomena.

Theories within these levels describe and explain phenomena. Some theories describe by identifying major concepts and the relationship among these concepts, but they do not attempt to explain why these concepts exist or how the concepts relate to each other. Theories that describe represent the lower levels of theory development and are important because they determine what the subject focus will be for a given theory.

The higher levels of theory development explain phenomena. In an attempt to state how and why the given concepts of a theory relate to each other, theories that explain may deal with cause and effect, associations, and the rules regulating interactions among theory constituents.

An example that illustrates these two types of theories may help to differentiate between their function. In a descriptive theory, the concepts of communication and lifestyle may be isolated as parts of the "family" phenomenon that a theorist thinks are important for understanding the goals of the family. In descriptive theory, the concepts and their relationships are merely named and defined, but the theory does not give an account of why the concepts act as they do. An explanatory theory expands upon the concepts and their relationship that have been isolated during the descriptive phase. For example, when one person interacts with another person in a passive and uncaring manner, animosity inevitably occurs; when one person interacts with another in an active and attentive manner, rapport inevitably occurs.

## MAJOR INTERDISCIPLINARY THEORIES

Two theories from disciplines other than nursing will be examined—role theory and systems theory. These two theories will be described briefly for the purpose of increasing your understanding of theory development.

### Role Theory

A **role** is the expectations that other individuals hold toward a person who falls into a particular category by virtue of that person's position in a social system. Role may also arise directly from within a person. Your perception of your role may be reflected in social behavior that you think is appropriate in terms of the demands and expectations of others. You develop your behavior patterns so that you can cope with internal and external pressures.

In some instances, one must deal with the role prescribed by others. Often the demands and expectations of some groups are inconsistent with those of other groups. For example, persons from the community may expect a mother to stay at home caring for her children, while professional peers may expect her to continue working and coordinate child-care efforts. To add to these contradictions, the mother must deal with cultural and traditional expectations and standards related to her other roles—those of wife, daughter, and consumer. If she is in a leadership position, she may be expected to be assertive and even outspoken. As a wife, she may be expected to be sedate and cooperative.

These incongruencies are called **role dilemmas**. Role dilemmas arise when you experience conflicting demands from your position, thus causing pressure. These demands may arise from pressure from others or from within oneself. These dilemmas present problems regardless of the source of pressure. For example, a mother whose child is ill must make the choice of going to work or staying home with the child.

Other role conflicts arise as a result of assuming several roles. Each role requires performing certain functions and tasks. When one is fulfilling and performing more than one role at the same time, the demands of the role or one's idea of how the roles should be performed may conflict. An example would be if the mother has a child in the school where she is also the principal. (Other terms besides role dilemma are used to describe this conflict. They include: role strain, role stress, role imbalance, role incongruity, and role ambiguity.)

Several theories have been proposed to explain the phenomenon of role. In each of these theories, there is a definition, a set of functions that describe that role, and a description of the way in which the concepts within the theory relate to each other. Concepts from each of these frameworks imply certain identifiable characteristics. These characteristics link together to form statements that explain the relationship between the concepts of role. For example, Kramer,[12] Oda,[16] and Baker[2] described and explained one aspect of role—the role development of nurses. Even though all three authors were describing and explaining the same phenomenon—role development—they did it from a different perspective. Each author spoke of role development occurring in phases. Kramer's phases were honeymoon, shock or rejection, recovery, and resolution. Oda's phases were role identification, role transition, and role confirmation. Baker identified the phases of role development as orientation, frustration, implementation, and reassessment. Each author also described the characteristics of the phases they depicted in the development of a role.

## General Systems Theory

Another theory that is from a discipline other than nursing is general systems theory.

A **system** is defined as an aggregate of discrete component parts that are interdependent and interrelated.[26] The interaction of these separate parts describes and constitutes the whole (called a **system**). In other words, a whole system is not only the sum of its parts, but also their relationship.

Systems have goals, process, and content. **Goals** refer to the ultimate purpose of the system—to attain and maintain optimum functioning. **Process** refers to the functions or series of sequential events over time by which the discrete parts work together. **Content** refers to the sum of the discrete parts that are organized to accomplish a particular goal.

A basic systems model is depicted in Figure 3–2. The input side of the figure includes some of the internal and external inputs that are significant in the functioning of the system. For example, if you think of a human as a system, the internal input may be the individual's personality, experience, and knowledge. The external input may consist of the person's position in a profession, the support from family and friends, and the expectations of society.

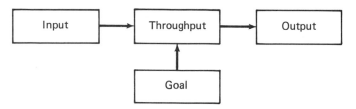

**Figure 3–2.** General systems model.

The output of the system is composed of the effects of the input. Using a human as an example, output may be personal growth, professional activities, maturation, and particular role behaviors. The process, as defined earlier, refers to the series of sequential events over time that enable the discrete parts of the system to work together. The goal directs all activities.

As another example of how the general systems theory operates, you can think of your school (a system). The school is comprised of smaller units—departments of chemistry, history, and so forth (subsystems). The internal input would be the faculty, staff, and the resources available, such as the library. The external input would be the expectations of the community and the support of parents. The output may be special awards, achievements of alumni, and admission of graduates to prestigious schools. The process would be the means that enabled the school to reach the goal of providing superior education to its students.

Now that we have discussed general theory development and examined two interdisciplinary theories, we will explore the development of nursing theories.

## DEVELOPMENT OF NURSING THEORIES

Nursing theories gave nursing its unique body of knowledge and played a major role in developing nursing into a profession. Stevens[25] defined **nursing theory** as a theory that attempts to describe or explain the phenomenon called nursing. If you will recall, earlier in this chapter theory was defined as a systematic set of interrelated concepts, definitions, and deductions that describe, explain, or predict the interrelationships.[7,15,20]

Currently, conceptual models and nursing theoretical frameworks describe the relationships that exist among the nurse, client, health, and environment. Nurses use these conceptual models and theoretical frameworks to guide their practice, particularly to interpret data about clients' health statuses and to plan effective interventions.

### Historical Perspectives

Early nursing leaders attempted to isolate specific concepts to explain the discipline of nursing. The central concepts—person, environment, health, and nursing—appeared in articles written by various nursing scholars as early as the 1950s. They were not identified as parts of a framework for nursing until Walker's writing (Fig. 3–3) in 1971. Walker categorized all the events occurring within nursing into "four subsets: 1) persons providing care, 2) persons with health problems receiving care, 3) the environment in which care is given, and 4) an end-state, well being."[27]

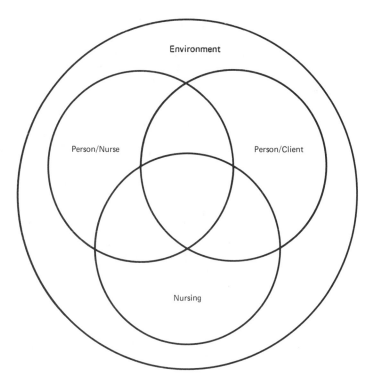

**Figure 3–3.** The central concepts of nursing.

In examining Figure 3–3 we see the concepts of person. The persons who are of prime importance in studying the phenomenon of nursing are the client and the nurse. The nurse is the provider of care; the client is the recipient of care. Environment is another important concept of nursing. This concept encompasses any setting where care of a client is provided by the nurse. The setting may be in a hospital, a community clinic, a school, or an industry. The concept of nursing is very broad. It incorporates not only the end-state of well-being that Walker spoke of,[27] but it includes the nursing process, professional standards, and other components that enable the nurse to bring the client to a state of health. Also depicted in Figure 3–3 is the continual interaction among the concepts of person (nurse and client), environment, and nursing. If one component is affected, all components will react to the change.

Different emphases in nursing theory can be seen within the literature. During the 1950s, emphasis was placed upon the social, interpersonal, and health aspects of nursing. Theorists described realities within nursing as they perceived them. They were influenced not only by their philosophical and educational backgrounds, but also by theories from other disciplines. Some of these theories, such as adaptation and interaction, helped our profession focus on concepts and problems specific to nursing.

Dorothy Johnson (1959)[10] presented her conceptual model for practice at Vanderbilt University. Johnson's behavioral systems model for nursing was based on sound theoretical knowledge. She felt that nursing was a needed service for clients who were under stress as a result of their basic needs being unmet. Clients had certain problems that needed assessment, nursing judgment, and action. Once stability was achieved, effort was made to maintain the client's health.

In 1960, Faye Abdellah's nursing-centered theory[1] identified 21 nursing problems that were later converted into statements of goals in an effort to promote comprehensive nursing care that was client-centered. The focus of the profession during this decade was to serve individuals and their families, and in so doing to provide service to society. Abdellah's three main concepts were health, nursing problems, and problem solving. She defined nursing in terms of the use of the problem-solving approach with 21 prime nursing problems related to the health needs of individuals. Abdellah viewed problem solving as the means of moving the client from a nursing problem toward the outcome of health. Abdellah never directly defined health; however, she implied that health was a dynamic state of human functioning whereby clients adapt to internal and external stresses in order to attain the maximum potential for daily living. She spoke of client health needs as problems that were either overt (an apparent condition) or covert (a concealed condition). To provide quality professional nursing care the nurse must be able to identify and solve these overt and covert nursing problems. Abdellah defined problem solving in terms of a process that involved identifying the problem, selecting relevant data, formulating hypotheses, testing these hypotheses through data collection, and when necessary revising hypotheses on the basis of conclusions obtained from the data. Many of these steps parallel the steps in the nursing process that will be presented in later chapters of this book.

In 1961, Ida Jean Orlando[18] described the practices that were basic to nursing—observation, reporting, recording, and actions carried out with or for the client. According to Orlando, the nursing process was unique because the nurse used all the senses, perceptions of client behavior, thoughts, feelings, and client actions. Orlando focused on those concepts she felt were unique to nursing. She spoke of the process involved in interacting with ill clients to meet an immediate need. The interaction was described as a dynamic one because of constant changes in the situation. These concepts of uniqueness, process, interaction, individual, immediate need, and dynamics provided the basis for her theory. Orlando's theory viewed the uniqueness of nursing from the perspective of a process—not a function. The nurse was defined in terms of the process of interaction with clients rather than by the activities enacted. From this viewpoint, nurses assessed client's needs, determined appropriate actions to meet these needs, and saw that the actions were implemented. Of prime importance was the effectiveness of the nurse–client relationship which culminated in resolution of the client's need. The interaction involved the client's behavior, the nurse's reaction, and the nursing actions designed to meet the client's needs. Again, similarities between aspects of Orlando's concept of process and the nursing process that will be discussed in later chapters can be seen.

Another early nursing theorist who defined the roles of both the nurse and the recipients of care was Ernestine Wiedenbach (1964).[28] Wiedenbach delineated the four components of nursing as: philosophy, purpose, practice, and art; and the four components of the art of helping as: identification, ministration, validation, and coordination. She also developed a model for clinical teaching, which she termed a "prescription." Wiedenbach viewed nursing as nurturing and caring for another in a motherly manner and therefore did not restrict the act of nursing to professional nurses. She defined nursing as a helping service that one rendered with compassion, skill, and understanding to people who needed care, advice, and confidence in the area of health. The nurse's central purpose (commitment) determined the quality of care given to clients. This commitment was based on the nurse's philosophy. Nurses, according to Wiedenbach's theory, subscribed to certain values and expressed these values in their attitudes and activities while working with clients. Wiedenbach emphasized the need for respect of others. Once nurses identified their own philosophy and recognized that clients had autonomy and individuality, they had the capacity to develop a prescription (plan of care). The prescription evolved from the nurse's philosophy and was affected by the reality of the situation. Wiedenbach defined the nursing process as an internal personalized mechanism that was influenced by the nurse's cultural background, knowledge base, wisdom, and sensitivity. Wiedenbach identified seven levels of awareness: sensation, perception, assumption, realization, insight, design, and decision. The nursing process began when a situation acted as a stimulus to alert the nurse. This alert led the nurse to interpret the first three levels, which were subjective, involuntary, and intuitive rather than objective, voluntary, and cognitive. The nurse then progressed from intuition to cognition, which included the next four levels. Although this model has many significant differences from the nursing process model that will be discussed in this book, there is some degree of similarity.

Lydia E. Hall (1964)[21,25] applied her nursing theory to nursing practice in the Loeb Center for Nursing and Rehabilitation of Montefiore Hospital and Medical Center in the Bronx. Hall, who based her conceptual model on the theories of Harry Sullivan, John Dewey, Hans Selye, and Carl Rogers, viewed nursing as having three aspects—core (based on the social sciences; therapeutic use of self), care (based on the natural and biologic sciences; intimate body-care aspects), and cure (based on the pathologic and therapeutic sciences; seeing client and family through the medical care). Hall's concept of care depicted the nurturing aspect of nursing. Unlike Wiedenbach's concept, care was represented as being exclusive to nursing, but Hall also incorporated the mothering concept (care and comfort of a person). When the nurse cared, knowledge of the natural and biologic sciences was applied. This background provided the strong theoretical base for nursing actions. The core of client care involved the therapeutic use of self. Hall did not see this concept as being exclusive to nursing—other members of the health team used self therapeutically. The nurse helped clients by developing an interpersonal relationship with them. The concept of cure was also shared with members of the health team. The nurse assisted the client through medical, surgical, and rehabilitative activities by being an active client advocate. In the care component, there was a positive tone (the nurse as a source of comfort), whereas in the cure component, the tone was negative (the nurse as a source of discomfort). All three concepts were interrelated. Hall's theory influenced nurses' approach to the phases of the nursing process. According to Hall, data collection (assessment phase) was for the benefit of the client rather than the nurse. Data collection was made to increase the client's self-awareness. The statement of the client's need or problem (nursing diagnosis) was based on the interpretation of the assessment data and the conclusions, which were influenced by how nurses envisioned their role. In Hall's opinion, the client decided what was of highest priority and what goals were desirable (planning). Hall viewed the core as being involved in planning. The actual institution of the plan of care (implementation) was the actual giving of nursing care. Assessing the client's progress toward the health goals (evaluation) was deciding whether the client was successful in reaching established goals. Aspects of each of Hall's concepts are applicable to each phase of the nursing process.

In 1965, Myra Estrin Levine[14] described her theory of nursing in a paper presented at a regional American Nurses' Association conference. Levine used a deductive approach to develop her theory by synthesizing existing theories from the sciences and humanities. She emphasized the individualization of client care based upon principles. (Levine's theory will be discussed in greater depth later in this chapter.)

Virginia Henderson's (1966)[9] major contribution to nursing theory was a succinct definition of nursing and the introduction of the terms *basic nursing care* and *independent nursing practice*. Henderson's conceptualization of nursing, which was based on theories of interpersonal relationships, provided the basis for the later development of Orem's concept of self-care.

Historically, the year 1968 was a landmark in the development of conceptual models for nursing practice. In addition, there was a great increase in the number of studies published on the nursing process. Dickoff and James (1968),[4] whose paper was published in *Nursing Research*, also provided a guide for evaluating nursing theories.

During the 1970s, there were mandates from the National League for Nursing that resulted in schools of nursing developing their curricula from specific conceptual frameworks. This action brought about efforts to integrate social, interpersonal, and health concepts and values into nursing practice and education. Nursing gradually evolved from a task-oriented service to a goal-oriented profession. The need to clarify the nature of nursing brought about theory development in nursing. Nurses came to realize that facts without theories held little meaning.

Initially, there was a search for one universal theory that the profession could adopt to explain all the various facets of the discipline. In time, the usefulness of one all-encompassing theory was questioned, and later this idea was abandoned. Rogers, King, Orem, and Roy were instrumental in developing varying frameworks to describe and explain nursing.

Martha Rogers proposed a theoretical basis of nursing in her book, which was published in 1970.[22] Human beings were conceptualized as unified wholes and open systems—thinking beings with pattern and organization. Rogers viewed life as a "unidirectional evolutional" process that moved along a space–time continuum. The goal of nursing was maintenance and promotion of human health. (Rogers' theory will be discussed in greater depth later in this chapter.)

In 1971, Imogene King's book on a nursing theory was published.[11] She defined the terms *people, environment, health,* and *nursing.* The focus of her conceptual framework was people—they functioned in social systems through interpersonal relationships, and their perceptions influenced both life and health. (King's theory will be examined in greater depth later in this chapter.)

The evolution of Dorothea Orem's theoretical model was described in the first edition of her book, which was published in 1971.[17] However, her model actually dated back to 1958. Orem's model built upon and elaborated on the earlier works of Henderson, Frederick and Northam, and Wiedenbach—all of whom viewed people as self-care agents. (Orem's theory will be discussed later in this chapter.)

The Roy Adaptation Model surfaced for the first time in 1964, and was used as the conceptual framework for a baccalaureate curriculum in 1968.[23] However, it was not widely adopted until 1974. The Roy model was based upon the following assumptions about people: they were biopsychosocial beings in constant interaction with the environment and they used innate and acquired mechanisms for coping. (Roy's theory will be discussed later in this chapter.)

In 1975, the Nursing Theories Conference Group was formed, and a text evolved from this group that described the theories of 12 nurses who were identified for their contributions to nursing. These people included Florence Nightingale, Lydia Hall, Virginia Henderson, Hildegard Peplau, Dorothea Orem, Faye Abdellah, Ida Jean Orlando, Ernestine Wiedenbach, Myra Levine, Martha Rogers, Imogene King, and Sister Callista Roy.[15]

Before we discuss some of the contemporary nursing theorists and their conceptual frameworks, we will identify the characteristics of a nursing theory and the steps in nursing theory development.

## Characteristics of Nursing Theory

Some of the identifiable characteristics of a nursing theory are its scope, complexity, terminology, implicit values, usefulness, testability, and ability to generate information.[5,6,8,20]

*Scope.* The scope of a nursing theory should be sufficient to cover a number of generalizations and provide a framework for organizing observations about a variety of phenomena within nursing. The scope should include both biologic and behavioral phenomena of the client. This characteristic relates to a goal of science—to describe and summarize a phenomenon from existing knowledge. A theory that has scope pulls together known phenomena. If a theory has scope, it will contain general statements about a group of phenomena.

*Complexity.* A theory should have complexity, either treating a number of variables or relationships or treating the complexity of a single variable. Even though a theory may have many intricate concepts that are interrelated it should meet another goal of science—the goal of parsimony. The concepts and relationships should be stated in the simplest of terms.

*Terminology.* A theory should develop a cogent terminology that can be applied to observed phenomena. As has been pointed out, well-defined terms may also be conceptualizations. The terminology of theories should describe clearly the relationship or connection between phenomena. The terms should spell out the how and why of phenomena. In addition, the terminology of theories should relate facts systematically and should be logical in its semantics and syntax.

*Implicit Values.* In a theory implicit values are made explicit. They are identified and used. For example, a theory of behavior implies that there are normal or desired behaviors but they are rarely made explicit. These implicit values predict outcomes.

*Usefulness.* A theory should be useful for clinical practice. A theory should explain and contribute to the understanding of nursing phenomena in a logical, meaningful, and testable manner. If a theory is useful, it will offer reasons for the observed phenomena. A theory must provide an explanation to be understood.

*Testability.* A theory should generate hypotheses that can be tested. To be testable, a theory must have operationally defined concepts. To ensure testability, concepts must be measurable and accurately reflect the theoretical concepts. A theory can be found to be false or can be confirmed. A theory is tested through empirical research, which will be discussed in Chapter 9.

***Generate Information.*** A theory should generate information. This information may result from hypotheses that have been developed. These hypotheses, in turn, may identify variables that were not thought of before. A theory guides nursing research and practice. It also provides the basis for research and practice. By generating information, a theory provides a way of looking at phenomena.

## Steps of Theory Development in Nursing

When a nursing theory is developed, the theorist proceeds through various steps. These steps are identified in Figure 3–4. In the first step, certain persons, places, and events (phenomena) relating to nursing are systematically observed. The phenomena are then defined, described, and explained (step 2) before they are applied to practice (step 3). In the practice setting, the theory is tested by use of empirical research (step 4). On the basis of research, the theory is modified (step 5), and a unique body of knowledge results (step 6).

In developing a theory, it is important to define what is meant by each concept. A major difficulty in defining concepts is that many of the concepts used in a nursing theory are directly related only to sensory experience—there is no concrete thing that can be observed. These concepts can be only defined in terms of their relationship to other concepts. A theory in its entirety rests upon an empirical base.

Now that we have identified several characteristics of a theory and have listed the steps of theory development, we will examine several contemporary nurse theorists and compare their theories of nursing.

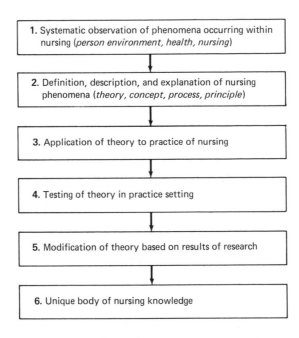

**Figure 3–4.** Steps of theory development in nursing.

## Contemporary Nurse Theorists

The subject matter of the different nursing theories varies according to the theorist. However, most of the theories focus upon the client, the nurse, or health. Some of the theories are client-centered, while others are nurse-centered, and still others are health-centered.

*Myra Estrin Levine.*[13] According to Levine, holistic nursing care is dependent upon recognizing the total responses of the client arising from the client's internal environment as well as the interaction occurring with the external environment. Nurses actively participate in the client's environment—to support the client's adaptation while the client is in a state of ill health. Nurses intervene by interposing their skills and knowledge into the events that affect clients. Nursing actions are founded on scientific knowledge but, more importantly, on recognition of the client's holistic response. The client's response indicates the nature of the adaptation taking place. The nurse's ability to read the messages (assessment) provides the basis for decision making by the nurse who acts in behalf of the client. Nursing actions are designed to foster successful adaptation. When nursing interventions favorably influence adaptation, the nurse is therapeutic; when interventions are unable to change the course of adaptation, the nurse is supportive. Levine views nursing principles as conservation principles—principles aimed at maintaining a proper balance between active nursing actions and the client's ability to participate. Levine's four conservation principles are based on the postulate of the unity and integrity of the client. In accordance with Levine's principles, nursing interventions are based on the client's energy, structural integrity, personal integrity, and social integrity. Depicted in Table 3–1 are descriptions of the central concepts of Levine's theory of nursing. Many aspects of this theory correlate with the steps in the nursing process that will be discussed later.

*Martha Rogers.*[22] Rogers' original theory, which was later refined, developed three principles of homeodynamics. Her first principle of helicy describes the nature and direction of human and environmental change. This change is continuously innovative, probabilistic, and is characterized by increasing diversity of the human and environmental fields. The pattern and organization of these fields emerge out of the continuous, mutual, simultaneous interaction between the person and the environment. Her second principle of resonancy is that the person and the environment are identified by wave pattern and organization. This pattern and organization manifest continuous change. The principle of complementarity refers to the continuous, mutual, simultaneous interaction process between the person and the environment. Rogers' theory focuses on the concept of "unitary man" and how man is continually changing. She views nursing's role as maintaining and promoting the health of man. To accomplish this role, major changes in attitudes and nursing action are required.

Rogers' conceptualization of the nursing process is similar to that of other theorists. In the assessment phase, the client is seen in the context of the client's environmental field at a specific point in time. Individual differences in the sequential patterning of the developmental process are identified in order to formulate nursing diagnoses and short- and long-term goals. Intervention by the nurse is directed toward repatterning the client and the environment so the client can develop a total human potential. Descriptions of the central concepts of Rogers' theory of nursing are shown in Table 3–1.

TABLE 3–1. CONCEPTS OF NURSING THEORIES

| Theory of Nursing | Man | Nursing | Health | Environment |
|---|---|---|---|---|
| Levine | Holistic<br>Dependent on relationships with others<br>Client adapts to environmental factors<br>Client actively participates in care | Involves human interactions<br>Involves integrated process by which clients adapt to factors of internal and external environment<br>Supports and promotes adjustment of client by supportive and therapeutic interventions | Maintenance and promotion of client's unity and integrity so client can adapt to environmental factors | The major focus of of this theory applies a conservation principle to maintain and promote a balance of integrity and unity of the client<br>1. Energy<br>2. Structural integrity<br>3. Personal integrity<br>4. Social integrity |
| Rogers | Man is the major focus of this theory<br>Man's wholeness is reflected in pattern and organization<br>Man is an open system continually interacting with his environment<br>Man has capacity for abstraction and imagery, language, and thought sensation and emotion | An art and a science<br>Continuous, mutual, and simultaneous interaction<br>Regulation of type and amount of input | Maintenance and promotion of health; prevention of illness, and care and rehabilitation of the sick and disabled | Strongly emphasized importance of environment and environmental factors<br>An energy field that encompasses everything outside man<br>Identified by pattern and organization |
| King | The major focus of this theory<br>A reacting being<br>A time-oriented being<br>A social being<br>Constantly interacts with others and environment through social systems | Assisting man to meet basic needs throughout life cycle<br>Through interpersonal relationships. Perceptions influence interactions and health | A dynamic and continuous adaption to external and internal stresses in the environment. Achieved through use of resources to reach maximum potential | Man's perception directly influences response to environment<br>Environmental changes and demands result in continual changes in biopsychosocial areas |
| Orem | An integrated whole within the community<br>Performs universal self-care to maintain health and well-being | Major focus of this theory<br>Assisting clients in meeting their self-care needs<br>Three approaches to nursing care: | Maintenance and promotion of structural integrity, functioning, and development | Together; man and environment form an integrated whole or system<br>Physical, biological, and social environment |

**TABLE 3–1. (cont.)**

| Theory of Nursing | Man | Nursing | Health | Environment |
|---|---|---|---|---|
| | Functions biologically, symbolically, and socially | 1. Supportive—educative<br>2. Partly compensatory<br>3. Wholly compensatory | | |
| Roy | Man interacts and adapts to the environment<br>Biopsychosocial beings interacting with a dynamic environment<br>Client may be a person, family, group, community, or society<br>An adaptive system | Assisting client in adapting in 4 modes:<br>1. Basic physiologic needs<br>2. Self-concept<br>3. Role mastery or function<br>4. Interdependence<br>Client's adaptation is promoted by changing stimuli (focal, contextual, | High-level wellness and by promoting adaptation<br>Energy is freed from inadequate coping attempts | Adaptation occurs when man interacts with the environment<br>Inputs from environment:<br>Focal stimuli—physical, physiologic, or psychosocial<br><br>Contextual stimuli—physical, physiologic, or psychosocial<br>Residual stimuli—attitudes, beliefs, experience, traits<br>Cognator and regulation subsystems are used to adapt to changing environments. |

***Imogene King.***[11] The person, who is viewed as a reacting, time-oriented, and social being, is the central focus of King's theoretical framework. In addition to these three premises, an individual possesses certain characteristics. A person has the capacity to perceive, think, feel, choose, set goals, select the means to achieve the goals, and make decisions. From King's perspective, a person functions in social systems through interpersonal relationships. Nurses work with three levels of social systems—individual, group, and society. The individual level is related to the concept of perception. The group level is associated with interpersonal relationships, and the society level focuses on the concept of health. The goal of interpersonal relationships is health. Health affects the client's life cycle in a dynamic way. In order to facilitate adaptation to internal and external stressors to achieve good health, one makes optimal use of resources. King defines nursing in terms of action, reaction, interaction, and transaction. All are aimed at helping clients to meet their basic needs and to assist them in coping with the problems inherent in wellness and illness. King combines the concepts to support nursing as a process. The nursing process, therefore, consists of action, reaction, interaction, and transaction. During assessment, the nurse acts, reacts, and interacts with clients. The nurse uses perception in deciding pertinent data. The client's health status is the focus of the assessment phase. The nursing diagnosis is based on the nurse's analysis of the client's health, social system, perceptions, and interpersonal relationships. In the planning and implementation phases, transaction is achieved. Planning involves setting mutual goals to move the client toward health. Evaluation involves all the concepts. Table 3–1 describes King's concepts.

***Dorothea Orem.***[17] Orem's theory attempts to explain why nursing exists as a health service in society and to explain the end product that is created by nurses in practice. Orem feels that nursing science mastered by nurses is a major component of the nurse's knowledge base and is antecedent to nursing practice. There are three components to Orem's general theory of nursing—the theory of self-care, the theory of deficits for engagement in self-care, and the theory that nursing systems are the end products created and made by nurses. Orem views the client as an integrated whole with the community. The client performs universal self-care (mental and physical basic needs or activities of daily living) to maintain health and well-being. When the client is unable to meet therapeutic self-care needs (supportive, remedial, or curative activities that are initiated to maintain health and well-being), nursing steps in to assist the client. Orem depicts the nursing process in three steps—1) assessment, 2) planning and implementation, and 3) evaluation. These steps, which are composed of many parts, have a sequential relationship. Assessment must be in progress prior to or concurrent with planning and implementation and evaluation. Orem views the nursing process as both an intellectual and a practical activity. Assessment and planning are identified as intellectual in nature. The nurse considers the client, the client's background, and the client's life-style as they affect the performance of self-care. The nurse also designs a system that effectively contributes to achieving health through therapeutic self-care. Orem formulates three types of nursing systems to meet client needs. The three systems are: wholly compensatory, partly compensatory, and supportive–educative. In the wholly compensatory system, the client has no active role in performing self-care. The nurse acts in behalf of the client. In the partly compensatory system, both the client and the nurse perform care activities. In the supportive–educative system, the client is assisted in care activities through support, guidance, and teaching. The practical aspect of the nursing process, according to Orem, encompasses implementation and evaluation. This phase is described as the initiation, conduction, and control of nursing actions. A description of the concepts of Orem's theory is given in Table 3–1.

***Sister Callista Roy.***[23] Roy's adaptation model contains three elements: the client, the goal, and the nursing intervention. She focuses on the interrelationship between the client and the environment. Adaptive subsystems and modes of adaptation are used to organize the nursing assessment of the client, to determine goal setting, and to formulate nursing interventions. Roy uses four modes of adaptation: physiologic needs, self-concept, role function, and interdependence relations. The goal of nursing is to help people adapt, using the four adaptive modes. The framework or environment within which nursing occurs is any setting and any time. Wellness and illness exist on a continuum from highest-level wellness to death. Roy views humans as biopsychosocial beings who must be understood by the nurse as holistic. According to Roy, a human is in constant interaction with the environment and copes with environmental change through adaptation. The process of adaptation occurs when the client responds to internal and external change. Roy defines health as a state of human functioning whereby the client continually adapts to change. The client's adaptation level is determined by focal, contextual, and residual stimuli. Changes in the environment are the focal stimuli. The contextual stimuli consist of the client's internal and external world that affects the client. Residual stimuli are relevant characteristics of the client. The four adaptive modes enable the client to adapt to change. The physiologic needs mode is activated when the client experiences need excesses or deficits. The self-concept mode refers to the psychologic integrity of the client, which is an unmet need. Roy recognizes two aspects of the role function mode—holding a position in society and interacting with a person who also holds a position in society. Social integrity is dependent on the role function mode and the independence mode. Through independence, the client's life becomes meaningful. Roy states that regulation and cognator effectiveness are required. When either or both of these mechanisms fail, maladaptation is suspected. Roy's concepts and their descriptions are given in Table 3–1.

## PROCESS CONCEPT DEFINITION

Learning to develop concept definitions[3] will assist you in understanding how theorists arrive at the concepts within their theories. Process concept definitions will also increase your understanding of some of the more abstract biopsychosocial concepts in nursing.

If you recall, concepts are tripartite relationships between an *idea*, a *pattern* of a number of attributes, and a name which serves as a *label* for the entire group. Concepts provide a structure for collecting, ordering, and analyzing your assessment data so you can more fully prescribe individual nursing interventions for your client. A very simple example is bird. The name of the concept is the word "BIRD." The idea of the concept is the pattern of the following recurring attributes: a moving thing with two legs, feathers, and a beak, that peeps loudly, flies in the sky, builds nests, lays eggs, eats worms, and so forth. The concept (bird) is mental shorthand that summarizes characteristics (moving thing with two legs, etc.) into a single idea. A memorizable word (bird) provides us with a single cue for a complex pattern.

### Steps in Process Concept Definition

A **process concept definition** comprises statements of all observable behaviors. These statements are general so that all possible variations of each characteristic can be included (for example, feathers is general, but all different colors of feathers would be too specific to include in a process concept definition). If the concept describes stages, phases, or changes that occur, then you would state the phases in the order in which they emerge. (An example are the stages of grieving clients go through as they approach death.)

To develop a process definition of a concept, you would follow these steps:

*Step 1: Identify the Main Problem.* The first step in developing your process definition of a concept is to observe your client. From your assessment data, try to determine the term that best describes what your client's problem is.

A. Observe your client to assess the primary concern.
B. Select a term (concept) that most accurately describes, explains, or seems important relative to this primary concern.

For example, Mrs. Smith has been admitted to your unit, and her nursing care plan calls for emotional support and encouragement of constructive expression of emotions. You may wonder, what are emotions all about? How are emotions supported? How are they expressed constructively? If you are not sure how to answer these questions, then it would be beneficial to process-define "emotion."

***Step 2: Collect Information.***  Once you have identified the concept, you shift your attention away from the clinical situation and to the literature resources available to you. The meaning of the concept which describes and explains the clinical situation would be explored.

A. Search literature for all possible definitions, discussions, and explanations of the concept.
B. In addition to your own definition of the concept and one or more from dictionary references, review the literature of other disciplines. You should select those definitions and statements that best illustrate or explain the concept.

***Step 3: Analyze the Information.***  Once you have gathered the information, it is time to sort it and to organize it.

A. In analyzing the information, you should:
   1. Review all the definitions and statements you have collected in regard to the concept. What does it really say? Are there several authors who say the same thing but use different words?
   2. List all the suggested behaviors that are connected to the concept: Those that are objective (what you observe) and those that are subjective (what the client states).
   3. Sort the behaviors in the order that they emerge. You may need to use inference as well as observation.
   4. Consider your past clinical experiences to fill in the gaps in process-defining the concept.
B. Before going to Step 4, decide whether the information you have collected is relevant and adequate, or whether you need to discard some of the collected statements and definitions. You may have to return to Step 1 before proceeding to Step 4.

***Step 4: Develop the Process Concept Definition.***  After you review the results of the first three steps, you are ready to write the emerging phases of the concept. The phases should be written in the sequence of their emergence. They should also be written in general terms so they may be applicable to a number of clients.

A. Write a short, concise statement of the central idea of the concept.
B. List the sequence of emerging phases of behaviors.

***Step 5: Validate the Process Concept Definition.***  The process concept and the sequence of emerging phases should be checked with someone else—someone whom you consider an expert in the field.

***Step 6: Determine the Applicability of the Process Concept Definition.***  It may be helpful to identify nursing situations in which the process concept definition may deepen your understanding.

*Step 7: Identify Meaningful Nursing Interventions.* After you have developed each phase of the process concept, you are ready to formulate appropriate nursing interventions.

A. Focus on all areas of care that apply to the client: life sustaining, remedial, personal, restorative, preventive, and health-promoting care.
B. Ask yourself these questions: What are the specific actions you can take to assist a client in that phase? What are the nursing actions necessary in helping the client to move into the next phase? (For example, a grieving client can be assisted in reaching the phase of acceptance.) What are the nursing actions necessary to prevent the client from reaching the next phase, if that phase is detrimental to the client's health and welfare? (For example, an emotionally distraught person experiencing high levels of anxiety could go to the next phase of disorganized behavior and exhibit uncontrolled panic and rage. What are the nursing actions that are likely to prevent this development? What are the nursing actions that are likely to precipitate it?)

*Step 8: Summarize Conclusions.* For future reference, write a short concise statement of the crux of the whole function. State one or more general principles which you will be able to recall easily and use to guide your nursing practice. For example, when heightened levels of tension and anxiety rise beyond the limits of tolerance in the client, the person loses control and organization of behavior, and panic or rage ensue.

**TABLE 3–2. STEPS 1 AND 2 OF PROCESS CONCEPT DEFINITION OF LONELINESS**

*Step 1—Process Concept: Loneliness*
*Step 2*—1. Experiences a need
    2. Desires personal contact or interaction with another human being
    3. Experiences lack of close relationship and meaningful communication
       a. Intense feeling of loss, confusion, numbness
       b. Feelings of loss of control and meaninglessness occur
       c. Loss of inner feelings, removal from world, no outside perception possible
       d. Alone; separated

| *Existential* | *Anxious* |
|---|---|
| 4. Maintenance of truthful self-identity<br>  a. Differentiation of self<br>  b. Perception of self as isolated, solitary individual | 4. Lack of intrinsic sense of worth<br>  a. Separation of self as feeling and knowing person<br>  b. Superficial social interaction |
| 5. Strength through isolation<br>  a. Search for fulfillment of inner nature | 5. Lack of fulfillment of human intimacy<br>  a. Inability to do anything while alone |
| 6. Self-awareness emerges<br>  a. Development of deeper sensitivities<br>  b. Bond or relatedness with self, others and nature develops | 6. Inability to love with negation of being<br>  a. Lack of affect, experiences restlessness and emptiness |
| 7. Expansion of individuality<br>  a. Development of new values<br>  b. Perception of new patterns for old ways and habits | 7. Alienation of self<br>  a. Stifling emergence of self<br>  b. Breach between what one is and what one pretends to be |

**TABLE 3–3. PROCESS CONCEPT DEFINITION FOR ALTERED COMMUNICATION PATTERN OF INDIVIDUAL, FAMILY, COMMUNITY**

| Nursing Process | Individual | Family | Community |
|---|---|---|---|
| Assessment (use of process concept definition) | Lack of awareness of one's own feelings<br>Incongruent verbal and nonverbal messages<br>Inability to empathize with others<br>Threatening and judgmental messages | Inability to express feelings or emotions<br>Lack of sharing ideas<br>Insensitivity in verbal messages<br>Devaluing the remarks of others | Lack of public health information by media (radio, TV, papers)<br>Minimal interaction between community leaders and residents in health planning<br>Deficit of health programs for community residents<br>Absence of forum where residents may express own opinions and concerns<br>Lack of community meeting places |
| Nursing diagnosis | Altered communication pattern related to shyness and depression | Altered communication pattern within family unit related to fear, lack of family interactions | Altered communication pattern within community related to lack of planning, inadequate funding, lack of coordination |
| Planning and implementing (only nursing objectives are stated) | 1. Assess contributing factors<br><br>2. Create a supportive and nonthreatening atmosphere<br><br>3. Provide client with guidance and teaching concerning communication patterns<br>4. Initiate referral if necessary | 1. Assess usual pattern of communication<br><br>2. Create conducive atmosphere for communication<br><br>3. Encourage expression of feelings about quantity and quality of interactions<br>4. Initiate referral if necessary | 1. Assess causative factors of complaints from residents<br>2. Facilitate understanding in community leaders of how residents feel<br>3. Assess community residents with appraisal of situations<br>4. Arrange consultations with appropriate agencies |
| Evaluating | Compare present response to established criteria | | |

*Step 9: State Implications for Nursing.* You could also identify implications for nursing. For example, the process concept definition has great use because it describes common patterns that nurses encounter in client situations. You may know of particular instances in which the formulated definition can be useful in interpreting client responses, identifying problems, predicting potential ones, and explaining their dynamics. These situations would be appropriate for noting in this step.

## Application of the Concept

To illustrate how process concept definitions can increase your understanding and lead to more effective interventions, let us consider the concept of loneliness. A common nursing intervention for a lonely client is to have the nurse spend 15 minutes every 2 hours speaking with the client. If you developed a process concept definition you would have additional information on which to base your nursing interventions. (Table 3–2 gives the first two steps of process concept definition).

In developing this process concept definition, you would understand that there are two different types of loneliness—each type calling for entirely different kinds of supportive nursing interventions.

Process concept definitions are useful in assessing individual clients, families, and communities (Table 3–3). They help you to determine the subjective and objective behaviors that form the pattern for nursing diagnosis. (Note that only nursing objectives are stated during the planning step.)

Even though nursing has borrowed concepts such as loneliness from other disciplines, it is no longer dependent on others for its body of knowledge. Now, nursing has established a conceptual system to provide us with clear guidelines for theory building. In the past, there was little nursing knowledge, but we face a future characterized by an acceleration of theoretical knowledge.

Now that we have identified and discussed the steps involved in defining a process concept, we are prepared to examine the relationship of theory to other processes within nursing.

## APPLICATION OF THEORIES TO NURSING PRACTICE

The importance of a theory-based practice is gaining acceptance among nurses. Theories are useful in analyzing and putting into practice the nurse's role. Nursing theories can serve as the basis for providing direct client-care activities, or they can be combined with other theories to implement a particular program. For example, Orem's theory can be implemented at the unit level by also using change theory. To practice from a theoretical base, nurses must be committed to learning more about how theories can be applied to nursing practice.

### Relationship to Nursing Process
Orem and Roy's theories will be used to illustrate how theory relates to nursing practice and the nursing process.

***Application of Orem's Theoretical Framework.*** Orem's theory has already been introduced. We will focus only on the way in which her theory applies to the nursing process. During the assessment phase, the following data are obtained: personal factors about the client, universal self-care (basic and secondary needs of man), health deviations, the medical problems and plan, and self-care deficits (the result of universal self-care disabilities and the medical problems). Nursing diagnoses are based on self-care deficits. In the planning phase, the nurse establishes goals that are compatible with the formulated nursing diagnoses and attends to the therapeutic self-care demands. Therapeutic self-care demands consist of classifying the nursing situation, selecting the method one will use to assist the client, and designing the most appropriate nursing system (i.e., wholly compensatory, partly compensatory, and supportive–educative). In

Orem's model, implementation is referred to as therapeutic self-care. The last step of the nursing process, as viewed by Orem, is evaluation (Table 3–4).

**Application of Roy's Theoretical Framework.** Roy's theory can also be used in conjunction with the nursing process. Roy divides assessment into two levels—first level and second level. During the first level, the nurse observes for signs of autonomic activity. The second level identifies the focal, contextual, and residual stimuli. The second-level assessment leads the nurse to identify adaptation problems (nursing diagnosis). Intervention is the prime nursing activity. The nursing process ends with evaluation of the effectiveness of nursing interventions (Table 3–5).

In examining both Orem's and Roy's theories, we see that both illustrate the compatibility and utility of nursing theory with use of the nursing process. In Figure 3–5,

**TABLE 3–4. APPLICATION OF OREM'S THEORY TO NURSING PROCESS**

| Assessing | | | | | |
|---|---|---|---|---|---|
| *Personal Factors* | *Universal Self-care* | *Developmental Self-care* | *Health Deviations* | *Medical Problem and Plan* | *Self-care Deficits* |
| 1. Age<br>2. Sex<br>3. Height<br>4. Weight<br>5. Culture<br>6. Marital status<br>7. Religion<br>8. Occupation | 1. Air<br>2. Food<br>3. Water<br>4. Excrements<br>5. Activity<br>6. Rest<br>7. Solitude<br>8. Social interaction<br>9. Hazards to life and well-being<br>10. Being normal | 1. Maintenance of normal growth, development, and maturation | Obvious changes in:<br>1. Human structure<br>2. Physical functioning<br>3. Behavior and habits of daily living in relation to others | The medical problem list and orders | Results of universal self-care disabilities along with medical problem |

| Diagnosing | Planning | Implementing | Evaluating |
|---|---|---|---|
| Based on self-care deficits | Nursing goals: congruent with nursing diagnosis<br>Nursing goals: therapeutic self-care demands:<br>1. Nursing situation classification<br>2. Selection of assisting method(s)<br>3. Design of nursing system<br>   a. Wholly compensatory<br>   b. Partly compensatory<br>   c. Supportive educative | Nursing action<br>Therapeutic self-care | |

**TABLE 3–5. APPLICATION OF ROY'S THEORY TO THE NURSING PROCESS**

| | | | | | |
|---|---|---|---|---|---|
| **Assessing** | | | | | |
| *First Level Assessment* | | | *Second Level Assessment* | | |
| | *Data* | | *Influencing Factors* | | |
| *Adaptive Modes* | *Subjective* | *Objective* | *Focal Stimuli* | *Contextual Stimuli* | *Residual Stimuli* |
| 1. Physiologic<br>  a. Exercise and rest<br>  b. Nutrition<br>  c. Elimination<br>  d. Fluid and electrolytes<br>  e. Oxygen<br>  f. Circulation<br>  g. Regulation<br>2. Self-concept<br>  a. Physical self<br>  b. Moral-ethical self<br>  c. Self-consistency<br>  d. Self-ideal and expectancy<br>  e. Self-esteem<br>3. Role function<br>4. Interdependence | | | | | |

| **Diagnosing** | **Planning** | **Implementing** | **Evaluating** |
|---|---|---|---|
| Problem identification | Goals, objectives | Approach to promote adaptation by manipulating stimuli | Judgment of effectiveness of interventions<br><br>Revisions on basis of evaluation |

we see that the unifying links in the relationship between the theories and nursing process are the concepts of person, environment, and nursing. The goal of all interactions is a state of health and well-being.

In addition to relating to the nursing process, there is also a link between theories and other processes important to nursing—research, teaching, decision making, and change.

## Relationship to Other Processes within Nursing

We will mention briefly other processes that will be discussed later in this book.

***Theory and Research.*** Theory and research have a reciprocal and mutually beneficial relationship. In building a theory inductively from observations, the research process becomes the source for the observations. Research methods are used to validate the con-

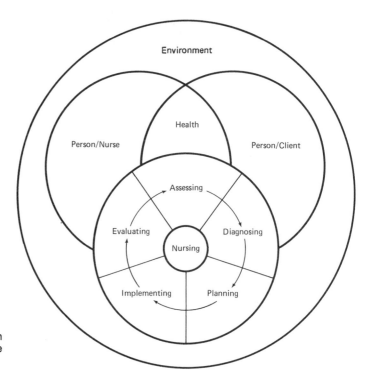

**Figure 3–5.** Relationship between the major nursing concepts and the nursing process.

cepts and the interrelationship among concepts. When validated, these concepts and relations become the foundation for theory development. Once a theory has been developed, it must be tested by subjecting hypotheses (deductions from the theory) to further research. We see that research serves a role in both theory building and testing.

There are many changes occurring within nursing every day. To ensure the success of effective and planned changes, nurses are using research to justify the need for change and to evaluate the results of the change once it has been implemented. At the onset of a change—especially one that requires additional financial support—research may be used to gather data about the existing circumstances or to establish the merit of a practice other than the one in existence. Although research may be carried out at any point in the change process, it most certainly plays an important role in evaluating the results of the change. Through evaluative research, the nurse–change agent can determine if the desired results were or were not achieved, why the desired results were not achieved, and also what changes can be made to alter the new change to obtain the desired results. Even the consequences of the change can be determined on the basis of research.

***Theory and Teaching.*** Teaching is part of nursing care activities, and as such it requires a theoretical basis. This theoretical basis provides the rationale for teaching interventions and provides a way of testing the effectiveness of these interventions.

For teaching to have impact on the quality of care, effective teaching programs must be implemented. To aid in the implementation of the teaching program, nurses use theories from other disciplines. For example, theories from psychology are used to explain behavior. Nurses also use theories from educational psychology which explain learning. The teaching strategies that are used to teach clients are based on learning theories. Although limited research is being done to test the effectiveness of particular teaching methods, research is possible since the strategies flow from psychologic, educational, and other theories.

***Theory and Decision Making.*** Decision making, an important process used by nurses, is based on theories borrowed from other disciplines. They may be used alone or concurrently with the nursing process. Decision-making theories guide nurses in making choices based on an existing body of knowledge. In nursing management, nurses use quantitative decision-making models to guide their practice. Theoretical models that either describe or explain how decisions are made in a particular setting enable testing of the models to determine effectiveness.

***Theory and Change.*** There are numerous change theories that were formulated by psychology and other disciplines outside nursing. These theories, which link together important concepts, describe and explain how nurses can cause change to come about. Theories have the power to help you predict the success, barriers, and consequences of the change before you ever implement it.

## SUMMARY

Theory development in nursing was instrumental in promoting scholarliness within the profession. The specific concepts that explain the discipline of nursing are person, environment, health, and nursing. The isolation of these central nursing concepts enables numerous nursing theorists to describe and explain the realities of nursing. Nursing also uses theories from other disciplines to guide its practice. The interdisciplinary and nursing theories can be used concurrently with the nursing process. They are particularly helpful as a framework for assessing individual, family, and community clients. There is an interrelationship between theory development and other processes used by nurses. Problem solving may be used to alter theory. Research may clarify, reformulate, initiate, verify, or even nullify theory. Existing knowledge related to teaching, decision making, and change is pulled together and summarized by theory.

## STUDY GUIDE

1. Describe your personal idea (concept) of person, environment, health, and nursing.
2. Compare your description of the central concepts of nursing with those of the nursing theorists discussed in this chapter. What are the similarities? What are the dissimilarities?
3. Develop a process concept definition for one of the following concepts using the steps discussed in this chapter: fear, anxiety, depression, or immobility.
4. Read one research article that uses a conceptual or theoretical framework. Explain how this framework guides the research discussed in the article.
5. Explain how theory relates to the nursing process.

# REFERENCES

1. Abdellah, F. G., Beland, I. L., Martin, A., & Matheney, R. V. *Patient-centered approaches to nursing.* New York: Macmillan, 1960.
2. Baker, V. Retrospective explorations in role development. In G. V. Padilla (Ed.), *The clinical nurse: specialist and improvement of nursing practice.* Wakefield, Mass.: Nursing Resources, 1979.
3. Burd, S. F. Chapter 42. In S. F. Burd, M. S. Marshall: *Some clinical approaches to psychiatric nursing.* London: Macmillan, 1963.
4. Dickoff, J., & James, P. A theory of theories: A position paper. *Nursing Research,* May–June 1968, *17,* 197–203.
5. Ellis, R. Characteristics of significant theories. *Nursing Research,* May–June 1968, *17,* 217–222.
6. Fawcett, J. A framework for analysis and evaluation of conceptual models of nursing. *Nurse Educator,* 1980, *5*(6), 10.
7. Fawcett, J. *Theory development: What, why, how?* New York: National League for Nursing, 1968, p. 26.
8. Flaskerud, J. H., & Halloran, E. J. Areas of agreement in nursing theory development. *Advances in Nursing Science,* 1980, *3*(1), 2.
9. Henderson, V. *The nature of nursing.* New York: Macmilllan, 1966.
10. Johnson, D. E. The nature of a science of nursing. *Nursing Outlook,* May 1959, *7,* 291–294.
11. King, I. M. *Toward a theory of nursing.* New York: Wiley, 1971.
12. Kramer, M. *Reality shock: Why nurses leave nursing.* St. Louis: C.V. Mosby, 1974.
13. Levine, M. E. *Introduction to clinical nursing* (2nd ed.). Philadelphia: F. A. Davis, 1973.
14. Levine, M. E. The four conservation principles of nursing. *Nursing Forum,* 1967, 45–59.
15. Nursing Theories Conference Group. *Nursing theories: The base for professional nursing practice.* Englewood Cliffs, N.J.: Prentice-Hall, 1980.
16. Oda, D. Specialized role development: A three-phase process. *Nursing Outlook,* 1977, *25,* 374–377.
17. Orem, D. E. *Nursing: Concepts of practice.* New York: McGraw-Hill, 1971.
18. Orlando, I. J. *The dynamic nurse–patient relationship.* New York: Putnam's, 1961, p. 54.
19. Paterson, J. G. The tortuous way toward nursing theory. *Theory development: What, why, how?* New York: National League for Nursing, (Pub. No. 15-1708), 1978, 49–65.
20. Reynolds, P. D. *A primer in theory construction.* Indianapolis: Bobbs-Merrill, 1977.
21. Riehl, J. P., & Roy, C. *Conceptual models for nursing practice.* New York: Appleton-Century-Crofts, 1974.
22. Rogers, M. E. *An introduction to the theoretical basis for nursing.* Philadelphia: F. A. Davis, 1970.
23. Roy, C. The Roy adaptation model. In J. P. Riehl and C. Roy (Eds.), *Conceptual models for nursing practice.* New York: Appleton-Century-Crofts, 1974, pp. 135–144.
24. Roy, C. *Introduction to nursing: An adaptation model.* Englewood Cliffs, N.J.: Prentice-Hall, 1976, p. 18.
25. Stevens, B. *Nursing theory: Analysis, application, evaluation* (2nd ed.) Boston: Little, Brown, 1984, p. 1.
26. von Bertalanffy, L. *General systems theory.* New York: Braziller, 1968.
27. Walker, L. O. Toward a clearer understanding of the concept of nursing theory. *Nursing Research,* 1971, *20,* 429.
28. Weidenbach, E. *Clinical nursing: A helping art.* New York: Springer-Verlag, 1964.
29. Yura, H., & Torres, G. Today's conceptual frameworks within baccalaureate nursing programs. In *Faculty curriculum development part III: Conceptual framework—its meaning and function.* New York: National League for Nursing, 1975, pp. 17–25.

# BIBLIOGRAPHY

Abdellah, F. G. The nature of nursing science. *Nursing Research,* 1969, *18*(5), 390–393.

Auger, J. *Behavioral systems and nursing.* Englewood Cliffs, N.J.: Prentice-Hall, 1976.

Blalock, M. H., Jr. *Theory construction.* Englewood Cliffs, N.J.: Prentice-Hall, 1969.

Bower, F. *The process of planning nursing care: A theoretical model.* St. Louis: C.V. Mosby, 1972.

Brodt, D. A synergistic theory of nursing. *American Journal of Nursing,* August 1969, 1674–1676.

Chater, S. A conceptual framework for curriculum development. *Nursing Outlook,* July 1975, 428–433.

Chinn, P. (Ed.) *Advances in nursing theory development.* Rockville, Md.: Aspen Publication, 1983.

Daubenmire, M. J., & King, I. M. Nursing process models: A systems approach. *Nursing Outlook,* August 1973, 512–517.

Dickoff, J., James, P., & Wiedenbach, E. Theory in a practice discipline: Part I, practice oriented theory. *Nursing Research,* September–October, November–December 1968, *17,* 415–435.

Dubin, R. *Theory building.* New York: Free Press, 1969.

Duffy, M., & Mullenkamp, A. F. A framework for theory analysis. *Nursing Outlook,* September 1974, *22,* 570–574.

Fielo, S. B. *A Summary of integrated nursing theory.* New York: McGraw-Hill, 1975.

Fredette, S. The art of applying theory to practice. *American Journal of Nursing,* May 1974, 856–859.

Glaser, B. G., & Strauss, A. *The discovery of grounded theory.* Chicago: Aldine Publishing Co., 1967.

Grubbs, J. An interpretation of the Johnson behavioral system model for nursing practice. In J. P. Riehl and C. Roy (Eds.), *Conceptual models for nursing practice.* New York: Appleton-Century-Crofts, 1974, pp. 160–167.

Hardy, M. E. *Theoretical foundations for nursing.* New York: MSS Corporation, 1973.

Hardy, M. E. Theories: Components, development, evaluation. *Nursing Research,* March–April, 1974, *23,* 100–107.

Hodgeman, E. C. A conceptual framework to guide nursing curriculum. *Nursing Forum,* 1973, *12*(2), 110–131.

Jacox, A. Theory construction in nursing: An overview. *Nursing Research,* January–February 1974, *23,* 4–13.

Johnson, D. E. A philosophy of nursing. *Nursing Outlook,* April 1959, 7, 198–200.

King, I. M. Nursing theory—problems and prospect. *Nursing Science,* 1964, *2*(5), 394–403.

King, I. M. Conceptual frame of reference for nursing. *Nursing Research,* 1968, *17*(1), 27–31.

King, I. M. A process for developing concepts for nursing through research. In P. Verhonick (Ed.), *Nursing research I.* Boston: Little, Brown, 1975.

King, I. M. The decision maker's perspective: Patient care aspects. In L. Schuman, R. Dixon Speas, & J. Young (Eds.). *Operations research in health care: A critical analysis.* Baltimore: Johns Hopkins University Press, 1975.

King, I. M. Health care systems: Nursing intervention subsystems. In H. Werley, A. Zuzich, M. Zajkowski, & A. Zagornik (Eds.). *Health research: The systems approach.* New York: Springer-Verlag, 1976.

King, I. M. The why of theory development. In *NLN, Theory development: What, why, and how?* New York: National League for Nursing, 1978.

King, I. M. How does the conceptual framework provide structure for the curriculum? In *NLN, Curriculum process for developing a baccalaureate nursing program.* New York: National League for Nursing, 1978.

Levine, M. E. Adaption and assessment: A rationale for nursing intervention. *American Journal of Nursing,* November 1966, *66,* 2450–2453.

Levine, M. E. Holistic nursing. *Nursing Clinics of North America,* June 1971, *6,* 253–264.

Levine, M. E. The intransigent patient. *American Journal of Nursing,* October 1970, *70,* 2106–2111.

Murphy, J. *Theoretical issues in professional nursing.* New York: Appleton-Century-Crofts, 1971.

Neumann, B. M., & Young, R. J. A model for teaching total person approach to patient problems. *Nursing Research,* May–June 1972, 264–269.

Newman, M. Nursing's theoretical evolution. *Nursing Outlook,* July 1972, *20,* 449–453.

Nightingale, F. *Notes on nursing.* New York: Dover Publications, 1969.

Norris, C. M. (Ed.). *Proceedings of the First, Second and Third Nursing Theory Conferences,* Kansas City, Kansas, University of Kansas Medical Center, Department of Nursing Education, 1969–1970.

Nursing Development Conference Group. *Concept formalization in nursing.* Boston: Little, Brown, 1973.

Parsons, T., & Shils, E. A. *Toward a general theory of action.* Cambridge, Mass.: Harvard University Press, 1959.

Paterson, J. G., & Zderad, L. T. *Humanistic nursing.* New York: Wiley, 1976.

Peplau, H. *Interpersonal relations in nursing.* New York: Putnam's, 1952.

Peterson, C. J., Hass, R. C., & Killalea, M. A. Theoretical framework for an associate degree curriculum. *Nursing Outlook,* May 1974, 321–324.

Phillips, J. R. Nursing systems and nursing models. *Image,* February 1977, *9*(1), 4–37.

Quint, J. C. The case for theories generated from empirical data. *Nursing Research,* Spring 1967, *16,* 109–114.

Quiring, J. A model for curriculum development in nursing. *Nursing Outlook,* November 1973, 714–716.

Reilly, D. E. Why a conceptual framework? *Nursing Outlook,* September 1975, 566–569.

Roy, C., & Roberts, S. *Theory construction in nursing.* Englewood Cliffs, N.J.: Prentice-Hall, 1981.

Torres, G. Florence Nightingale. In *Nursing theories: The base for professional nursing practice.* Englewood Cliffs, N. J.: Prentice-Hall, 1980, pp. 27–37.

Vaillot, M. C. *Commitment to nursing.* Philadelphia: Lippincott, 1962.

Verhonich, P. J. Clinical studies in nursing: Models, methods and madness. *Nursing Research,* November-December 1972, *21,* 490–493.

Wiedenbach, E. *Meeting the realities in clinical teaching.* New York: Springer-Verlag, 1969.

Weidenbach, E. Nurses' wisdom in nursing theory. *American Journal of Nursing,* May 1970, 1057–1062.

Zderad, L. T. From here and now to theory: Reflections on how. *Theory development: What, why, how?* New York: National League for Nursing, (Pub. No. 15-1708), 1978, 35–48.

# Nursing Process:
# Step I. Assessing

4

Assessment is, of necessity, the first step of the problem-solving method, the nursing process. This step is so closely interrelated with the other steps of the nursing process that in practice it is impossible to separate them. In order to study them in depth, each step will be discussed separately.

In this chapter, specific methods of assessing the individual client will be discussed—assessment interview, nursing health history, wellness assessment, and physical assessment. In addition, tools or guidelines for collecting information on the family or community client will be presented. Discussion of techniques and principles involved in the implementation of these methods, guidelines, and tools will be included.

Study of this chapter will help you to:

1. Define assessing as it relates to the nursing process.
2. Identify the components of the data base.
3. Discuss primary and secondary sources of data.
4. Describe guidelines to be used in the assessment interview.
5. Discuss barriers to effective communication.
6. Conduct an assessment interview on an individual.
7. Differentiate a nursing health history from a medical health history.
8. Collect a nursing health history from an individual using either a structured or semistructured format.
9. Describe the wellness assessment as it relates to the data base.
10. Describe the physical assessment as it relates to the data base.
11. Collect a family assessment.
12. Collect community data that are relevant to the care of the individual or family client.

## OVERVIEW OF ASSESSMENT PROCESS

In order to determine the health needs of the client, it is essential that information and data about the client be collected. The act of gathering, verifying, and communicating data in a comprehensive and systematic manner is **assessment**. Assessment includes the evaluation and appraisal of the whole individual, family, or community to determine the health status of each for the purpose of planning nursing care. Assessing does not end after the initial contact with the client but continues for as long as the client has need of nursing interventions.

Nursing authors, for example, Geitgey, Komorita, and McCain, describe assessment as early as the 1960s.[15,24,26] Both McCain and Geitgey developed assessment tools or guides that promoted systematic assessment. McCain's tool was directed at assessing functional abilities of individuals, and Geitgey designed a guide to assist in the identification of needs of individuals. Although neither of these assessment guides was designed to identify health problems, the emphasis on assessment of problems did evolve in the early 1970s. The concern with problem identification remained strong until the late 1970s when interest developed in the assessment of the client's level of wellness.

Today, the client is assessed to determine the existing level of wellness and the level of health care needed. A wellness assessment provides the basis for identifying potential and actual health risks and for exploring with the client the habits, behaviors, beliefs, attitudes, and values that influence levels of wellness. Aspects of wellness that should be assessed include degree of fitness, risk level for health problems, level of life-stress, life-style and health habits, level of nutrition, personal habits, and environmental sensitivity.[1,35,45,47] Potential and actual health concerns are considered when assessing the level of health care needed. Health care can be provided on three different levels: primary, secondary, and tertiary. Assessment within the **primary level** includes consideration of the client's management of developmental events and needs for health promotion; special attention is given to screening clients in high-risk groups and providing necessary health education. The obese individual, the family unit experiencing prolonged periods of stress, and the community with high levels of air pollution are in high-risk groups. Assessment within the **secondary level** includes early identification and need for treatment of an illness or injury in order to reduce its length and severity. Assessment within the **tertiary level** includes determining the client's needs for rehabilitation in order to attain the fullest physical, mental, social, and economic usefulness for the client.

Now that we have considered some of the general points on assessment, let's look at the process more closely and consider the assessment of the individual, family, and community.

## ASSESSMENT OF THE INDIVIDUAL

We will focus our initial discussion on assessment of the individual client. Much of the information presented in this section will also be applicable when you assess the family or community.

### Sources of Data

Data are information that has been gathered and organized for analysis and for use as the basis for decisions. When all of the data on one subject are compiled, it forms a body or store of knowledge known as the **data base**. In nursing, the data base is composed of all of the assessed information on the client which will be used to determine the client's health status and health care needs. Because data are the basis for decisions, they must be as complete and accurate as possible; incomplete or inaccurate data can lead to incorrect conclusions concerning the client's health status and possibly incorrect nursing interventions.

The **primary source** of data is the individual client. It is important that the total individual be assessed. Information concerning the client's physical health, mental outlook, developmental status, spiritual and cultural beliefs, communication skills, socioeconomic status, family and community life, activities of daily living, reactions to health status, and health care goals and expectations should be gathered (Fig. 4–1).

The client provides initial data during the assessment interview, nursing health history, wellness assessment, and physical assessment. (These components of the data base will be discussed in detail later in this chapter.) The assessment interview and nursing health history mainly contain subjective data; subjective and objective data are collected during the wellness assessment and physical assessment.

The term *subjective* describes that which exists only within the experiencer's mind and is apparent to or perceived by that individual only. **Subjective data** can only be provided by the client and cannot be described or verified by another person. Dizziness, nausea, thoughts, feelings, and the description of pain are examples of subjective data. When collecting subjective data, it is important to evaluate the client's ability to give accurate information. The client's age, mental and physical condition, cultural and spiritual beliefs, language and communication skills, emotional state, and former experi-

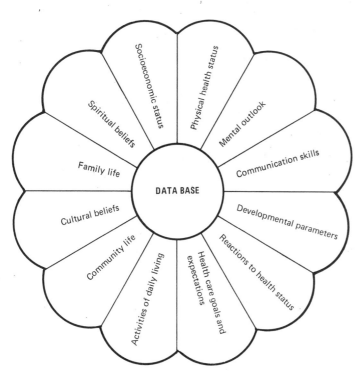

**Figure 4–1.** Components of the data base.

ence with health care providers will influence the quantity and quality of the information given.

The term *objective* is defined as something having actual existence or reality. **Objective data** can be determined by the nurse through observing, listening, feeling, smelling, or measuring. These data, such as the circumference of a forearm, skin temperature, pulse rate, skin color, or diagnostic findings, can be verified by other health team members. In the literature, when discussing the client's health status, subjective findings are often referred to as symptoms and objective findings as signs.

The following paragraph illustrates examples of both subjective and objective data.

> Mrs. P. cried occasionally during the interview; she stated that she had been having "crying spells" for the last two weeks. She never smiled during the conversation; her facial expression remained unchanged. She stated that she was "stuck" back in a corner and forgotten.

Examples of objective data include: cried during the interview, never smiled during the conversation, and unchanged facial expressions. All of the facts are observable and could be verified by another observer. The statements about "crying spells" and being "stuck" in a corner are examples of subjective data—feelings that are being experienced by the client and cannot be described by another person.

**Secondary sources** of data such as family members, significant others, other health care providers, written records, and literature can provide new information as well as serve to validate data given by the client.

Family members and significant others can provide you with their perception of the client's health status and health needs. With clients who are unable to communicate effectively, such as children or adults with physical impairment, family members and significant others may be your main source of data for the nursing health history. In some instances, family members may differ from the client in their perception of the client's response to illness and stress. In addition, they may be able to identify specific patterns of behavior and coping of which the client is unaware.

The physician, dietitian, physical therapist, social worker, respiratory therapist, and other health care providers can supply helpful information. Each of these individuals can provide information about the client from the perspective of their own disciplines.

Written records from present or prior hospitalizations, clinic visits, or home visits can provide additional information. These records may provide you with information that you will need to clarify further. They may also provide information that you were unable to attain from the client during your assessment.

Literature provides you with a textbook picture of the client's general condition, such as normal growth and developmental patterns. This information can be compared with the findings about the client. In addition, reviewing nursing literature will expand your knowledge and provide you with a theoretical basis for future assessment.

The nurse is another major source of data. You bring to the assessment situation knowledge and experience that are valuable resources for obtaining information relative to the client's needs. The quality of the assessed information depends on your expertise and skills. In order to gather complete, meaningful information, you must be *selective* in the type of data sought and yet *receptive* to all of the information offered by the client. You must not assign meaning or inferences to the information until the data base is complete and validated. Finally, you must remain objective and avoid letting your own feelings interfere with the process of data collection.

**Selectivity** is an important aspect of nursing assessment. You should seek only the information there is reason to believe will be useful in planning a particular client's nursing care. Information already available through another source should not be sought unless clarification or validation is needed. Repetitious questions are annoying to the client and might actually decrease the client's trust in health care professionals. In addition, seeking unnecessary information or duplicating information is a waste of time and energy for you and the client. Remember to use the information that is already available in the written records. Although selectivity in the type of data sought is necessary, selectivity in listening to the information given must be avoided. Four forms of selective behavior used in interpersonal relationships have been identified: selective exposure, selective attention, selective perception, and selective retention.[6,19,27,30]

*Selective exposure* implies that a person chooses messages which expose them to ideas and attitudes that reaffirm those already held. By avoiding information that conflicts with existing ideas and attitudes, the person protects and supports his or her own self-image but reduces the amount of cognitive discord that is experienced. The person also becomes less effective as a listener. For example, if the client is providing an obstetrical history and mentions a previous medical abortion, the information might be ignored if it conflicts with the nurse's attitudes on this subject.

*Selective attention* implies that a person can pay attention to only a limited number of stimuli at one time. The nurse must block out some stimuli in order to receive others. Imagine the nurse in a hospital situation who is attempting to do an admission assessment when two other clients have just returned from surgery and a third client is experiencing respiratory difficulties. The nurse's ability to receive additional input is stretched to the maximum. Some messages sent by the newly admitted client might not be received in preference to other stimuli.

*Selective perception* implies that interpretation of data usually coincides with preconceptions held about the data or idea represented. Selective perception refers to the individual's ability to perceive only selected aspects of a situation; to see only what is already known; and to see more detail in familiar than in unfamiliar situations. What effect does selective perception have on the nurse? Because of the familiarity of a situation, you might be lulled into a behavior pattern where assessment occurs in a routine manner, without thought. This will greatly reduce the amount of data collected. The client may not be viewed as an individual but perhaps as the "fifth fractured hip" admitted that week. In addition, if the client is admitted with a specific medical diagnosis, your perceptual field might be narrowed to include observation of only those symptoms known to be specific to that condition, excluding other pertinent observations.

*Selective retention* describes the process where the individuals remember only those things they want to remember. Information that reinforces one's own ideas and beliefs is usually retained with more accuracy.

These four forms of selective behavior have an impact on your ability to conduct an effective assessment. By being aware of these behaviors and by recognizing how they affect your assessment skills, you will be able to adjust the techniques that you use in data collection.

**Validity of the data** must be determined before you analyze the information and form inferences or conclusions. Failure to validate or confirm your findings will affect the quality and value of the total assessment. For example, experience can actually work against you. The nurse with advanced knowledge and experience may make earlier conclusions than the novice who feels uncertain and is more cautious.

There are several ways to validate data. One way is to clarify the information with the client. Ask specific, pointed questions or relate information back to the client for verification. For example, you observe the client not sleeping the night prior to scheduled surgery. You may infer that the client is nervous or anxious about the upcoming surgery. If you say to the client, "I see you are having difficulty sleeping tonight," the client may well indicate a concern unrelated to the surgery. You may also verify the information with family members or significant others. Determining if all cues are consistent and if other health team members have made the same observation are other methods of validation.

**Objectivity and freedom from bias** are important attributes when gathering data. Your physical and emotional state, mood, beliefs, cultural background, needs, and motivation are capable of influencing data collection. Stereotyping or distorting what is seen or heard because of preconceived ideas or past experiences must be avoided. For example, hearing difficulty is frequently ascribed to *all* elderly individuals. When health care providers talk to the aged individual in a loud voice before assessing whether a hearing loss exists, they are basing their approach on preconceived ideas or past experiences, not on documented information. You should also avoid labeling clients. Terms such as "demanding," "cranky," "depressed," "helpless," and "nervous" label the client based on situational characteristics which may not be permanent patterns of behavior.

At this point,we have discussed subjective and objective data and identified primary and secondary sources of data that are available to the nurse assessing the client. Figure 4–2 illustrates these sources and shows their relationship to subjective and objective data.

Four major tools are available for collecting subjective and objective data about the client—the assessment interview, nursing health history, wellness assessment, and physical assessment. We will discuss the assessment interview first.

## Assessment Interview
An **interview** is an exchange of verbal and nonverbal communciation by two people for the purpose of sharing information pertinent to a particular subject. Either the interviewee or or interviewer may select the subject to be discussed. The interview process may be formal and structured or informal and nonstructured. Within these two formats—formal and informal—several types of interviews exist. The various types of interviews differ as to their focus and desired outcome.

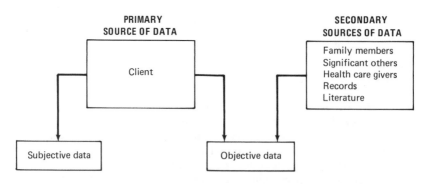

**Figure 4–2.** Sources of data.

*Types of Interviews.* Among the different types of interviews are: information-giving, problem-solving, problem-seeking, counseling, and information-gathering. The information-giving interview is used in many situations, such as panel interviews, press conferences, in-service education programs, and education classes for clients. In the problem-solving interview, the focus is on finding the solution to problems or concerns that have been identified. In addition, more information about the existing problems or concerns is sought. For example, when a client is transferred from a hospital to an extended care facility, the problem list and plan of care that accompany the client provide the basis for a problem-solving interview. In the problem-seeking interview, focus is on gathering data so that concerns might be identified. A common misinterpretation of this type of interview is that only data leading to problem identification are sought and that other data are not meaningful. All relevant data should be gathered for future analysis to ensure accuracy and comprehensiveness. A counseling interview attempts to help the client gain insight into problems. Self-understanding, discovery of solutions, exploration of feelings, and decision making are encouraged.[7,17,37,40]

The **assessment interview** is an example of an information-gathering interview. Although you may have to postpone information gathering momentarily to provide support or to give information to a client who expresses concern or who is seeking information, the main purpose of data collection must not be overlooked. During the assessment interview, therapeutic communication skills are used and the nurse is receptive to the information offered by the client. Attempts to counsel the client are postponed until the data are analyzed. Although the assessment interview primarily collects subjective data, you should note nonverbal cues, objective data, given by the client during the interview. The assessment interview can be formal or informal.

The **informal assessment interview** is shorter than the formal one and is not structured. It is usually integrated into other ongoing nursing activities and can be used to yield information that would be helpful in planning immediate nursing actions. For instance, the informal interview technique is used to assess the client's health status in emergencies: "Are you nauseated—sick to your stomach?" "Have you vomited?" "When did you eat last?" You might also use the informal interview technique to assess a client's condition during routine rounds in the hospital: "Did you sleep well last night?" "What prevented you from sleeping?" "Is there anything that we can do to make you rest better?"

The **formal assessment interview** is structured as to purpose and data to be collected; a printed form, checklist, or outline is usually followed. (Appendix B provides an example of a form that requires a formal interview setting.) Because the formal interview is longer and more complex than the informal interview, it is usually not combined with other activities. The majority of formal interviews are conducted to obtain a nursing health history. This type of interview will be more effective when the following guidelines are followed:[4,7,17,32,37,40,44]

1. Preparing and Planning for the Interview
   a. Part of your interview preparation includes analysis of your own behavior, attitudes, and responses and how they affect the nurse–client relationship. The **nurse–client relationship** is a helpful, purposeful interaction between the caregiver and the recipient of the care. In this relationship, the focus is on the client's needs and not your own. You must be cautious to maintain a professional rather than a personal relationship with the client. Your attitudes and actions should reflect your interest in and desire to help the individual. More information on the nurse–client relationship as a helping relationship is presented in Chapter 7.

    b. Other preparation and plans need to be considered prior to the interview. You should decide which type of questions will elicit the information desired. If you wish to obtain straight factual information, the *directive approach* in interviewing is used. In the directive approach, you ask a series of prepared questions. Closed-ended questions are typically used. These questions require a single word or a short phrase as a response. For example, you might ask the client, "Have you been hospitalized before?" Exploration of thoughts, feelings, and questions arising from the interview is at a minimum. The client plays a passive role while you, the interviewer, play an active, authoritative role. In this form of assessment interview, the constant barrage of questions may supply sufficient data but fail to allow the client time to reveal what the concern is. Verbal or written questionnaires are examples of this type of interview format.

    c. If you wish to allow time for exploration of thoughts and feelings, the *nondirective approach* in interviewing should be used. In the nondirective approach, you ask questions that require the client to take an active part in the interview. The interview opens with a general discussion and gradually moves to the focus point. Open-ended questions are used. The questions encourage the client to pursue his or her reactions. For example, you might state, "Tell me how you feel about your previous hospitalization." You, as the interviewer, then lead the discussion and clarify the client's statements. Most effective assessment interviews are a combination of these two approaches.

    d. You will need to familiarize yourself with any forms or guides to be used. If you are not familiar with the content on the form, you may concentrate on the interview guide to the exclusion of the client's answers.

    e. The environment also needs to be prepared. You have the responsibility of arranging the seating, determining the distance between the client and yourself, controlling interruptions, and providing privacy. External distraction or noise should be minimized. Visitors and relatives should be asked to wait elsewhere. Reduce the physical distance between you and the client by arranging your chair near the client's bed or chair. It is important to determine if you and the client will sit face to face for eye contact or be seated so that the client can see what you write during the interview. A curtain or screen may be used to promote privacy if you are in a room with other clients.

2. Initiating the Interview

    a. You should be seated during the interview unless the client's health status requires that data be collected as care is given. (Remember when this occurs, the situation is not conducive to a formal assessment interview.) The act of sitting allows both parties to be at the same level so eye contact is easier. You must create an atmosphere of warmth and acceptance. Such an atmosphere is usually more conducive to open communication. To initiate this feeling of acceptance, call the client by name; this conveys that the client is seen as a person. Whether you use the client's first or last name will vary with the situation and the client's age and preference. Children and adolescents are usually called by their first name whereas adults are usually called by their title (Miss, Ms., Mrs., Mr., etc.) and last name. In some care facilities that have contact with the same clients for long periods of time, first names are used. Next, you introduce yourself and clarify your title, role, or position. Again, whether you use your first or last name will vary with the situation. You might say, "I'm Jane Doe. I will be one of the nurses who will be caring for you."

b. You should identify how long the interview will last. For example, you might say, "I would like to speak with you for about 20 minutes."

c. You need to tell the client that any information gathered during the interview is considered confidential. Explain to the client why the information is being sought and with whom the information will be shared. The client should feel free to ask how the data relate to the client's care and should be told that it is not a requirement to answer all of the questions asked. The following explanation might be given: "I would like for us to discuss your daily routine and health history. (pause) I will use the information to plan your nursing care. (pause) It will be necessary for me to take notes as a part of your permanent record so that all the health team will have the information when they plan your care. (pause) If there is anything that you'd rather I didn't record or share with the staff, just say so." You need to pause at various times throughout the explanation to allow time for the client to absorb what is being said and to respond. If family members or other individuals are supplying the data, they must be given the same information regarding confidentiality and use of acquired information as is the client.

3. Conducting the Interview

a. One's skills in communicating and interviewing are important to the success of the assessment interview. Without appropriate interviewing skills, you may be unable to gather sufficient data on which to plan care. More information regarding communication, communication patterns, and therapeutic communication is presented in Chapter 7.

b. Questions should be asked in a clear, precise manner. Clarifying comments should be used whenever necessary. Use a vocabulary on the level of understanding of the client and avoid the use of occupational jargon. Ask questions that are well-timed and pertinent. Questions that are given too quickly produce unreliable information. Careful timing of questions allows the client time to understand and respond. This is essential.

c. You should be an attentive listener. Direct your attention to the spoken words and nonverbal cues provided by the client. The following steps will help you learn to listen more effectively:

  (1) Be Prepared to Listen. Both mental and physical preparation is needed. Your attention span is directly related to your physical and mental condition. Your actions should demonstrate interest and alertness.

  (2) Develop a Desire to Listen. Determine your purpose in the listening situation. Enter the situation because you want to hear what the client has to say. Consciously prepare yourself to listen.

  (3) Concentrate on Listening. Adjust to or dispose of distractions. Focus your attention on the client and put other thoughts or ideas out of your mind. Make listening a consciously used tool of communication.

  (4) Look at the Content of the Message. Determine the nonverbal answers to the following: Why is the client telling me this at this time? What is the meaning of the word choices, the voice inflection, the topic chosen?

  (5) Hear the Speaker Out. Do not answer too fast or ask a question too soon. Do not become impatient or interrupt. Remember that speech rate is slower than your thoughts. Suppress your desire to talk and develop a desire to learn. Remember, if you are comfortable with yourself there is no need to defend your opinions, values, or beliefs.

  (6) Focus on Ideas. Do not focus on small details; you may miss the main ideas.

The main ideas, principles, and concepts are the important things to remember.

(7) Maintain Objectivity. Try to empathize; put yourself in the client's place so that you can see the client's point of view. Do not let your own or another's biases or personal prejudices impair your data collection.

(8) Secure Clarification. Paraphrase or restate what you believe the client said. This will help you to determine your listening abilities and may help the client's self-expression.

(9) Use an Appropriate Note-taking System. Note taking may be distracting to the client and may actually prevent you from hearing much of what is said. Develop a flexible system for recording pertinent information you might not remember.

(10) Analyze Your Listening Errors. Determine why you misunderstood the client's message. Consider alternative approaches to listening situations that might enhance your listening skills.[2,29,40,50]

d. In addition to effective listening, you must remember that verbal or nonverbal indication of approval or disapproval of comments being made may alter the validity of the interview content. Avoid asking questions in a manner that implies that the client should give socially acceptable answers, such as, "You haven't experimented with drugs have you?" You should be diplomatic when asking questions about the client's home life or personal matters. Don't hesitate to change the topic if the subject meets resistance or produces anxiety in the client.

e. Avoid asking two separate questions in the same sentence: for example, "Do you have trouble seeing or hearing?" Such questions cause confusion for the client, especially if different responses are required for each question.

f. Throughout the assessment interview, assess nonverbal communication patterns. Does the client use body language—facial expressions and hand gestures—when talking? Observe for signs of anxiety, frustration, anger, or loneliness.

4. Terminating the Interview

a. As the end of the assessment interview approaches, you should indicate that the interview is almost over. An appropriate response might be, "There are two more questions I'd like to ask . . ." This approach provides structure to the situation, allowing the interview to be concluded in a planned manner instead of rambling to an unorganized conclusion. The time frame may also encourage the client to express concerns that there has been a reluctance to share.

In order to interview effectively, you must use a great deal of energy and concentration. A few techniques for conducting purposeful, meaningful communication are presented in Table 4–1. These techniques do not ensure therapeutic communication but serve as guidelines so that you can develop an effective style. Do not overuse these techniques to the exclusion of other methods that you have found effective.

There are also nontherapeutic communication techniques. Some of these are listed in Table 4–2. You may have used these techniques successfully in everyday situations, but in the interview they may create undesired or unexpected responses.

You are in the position to carry out therapeutic communication while conducting routine procedures, interviewing, teaching, counseling, or giving support. As a nurse, you will find yourself using therapeutic communication with others and teaching others

## TABLE 4–1. THERAPEUTIC COMMUNICATION TECHNIQUES

*Use Silence.* Silence gives you and the client time to organize your thoughts. This also allows the client to set the pace. During the silence, you should focus on the client and note posture, facial expressions, and gestures.

*Restate Main Ideas.* Repeating the main ideas expressed by the client in different words brings out aspects of the material that might have been overlooked by the client or yourself. For example, if the client states, "It takes effort to get out of bed every morning," you might reply, "You find it hard to get up in the morning."

*Reflection.* Paraphrase feelings, questions, ideas or key words. This indicates to the client that the client's point of view is important. For example, if the client states, "I'm not sure if I should continue taking this medicine," you might reply, "You feel unsure about continuing to take the medication."

*Seek Clarifying Statements.* To clarify comments that are vague or that you didn't completely hear or understand, you might say, "Could you explain that again?" or "I'm not sure what you mean." Often seeking clarification for yourself helps the client gain clearer self-perception.

*Use Open Body Language.* Maintain eye contact; sit with arms unfolded and body in a slightly relaxed position. Avoid facial expressions that reflect your thoughts.

*Use Leading Questions.* This technique will encourage the client to take the initiative in introducing topics and in determining the direction of conversation. You might say, "Tell me about it," or "And what else?"

*Share Perceptions.* State observations that you perceive about the person. Statements such as, "You appear . . .", "I notice that you are . . .", and "It seems to me that you . . ." will offer you and the client the opportunity to compare observations.

*Summarize.* Summarize the important points discussed, for example, the client's assets, health concerns, or perceived weaknesses. Summarizing provides a sense of closure at the end of the interview.[7,17,32,37,40]

## TABLE 4–2. NONTHERAPEUTIC COMMUNICATION TECHNIQUES

*Give Advice.* Giving advice, stating personal experiences or opinions, or telling another what should be done emphasizes yourself, elevates your self-esteem, and implies that your opinion is important or relevant. Even when the client asks for your advice or opinion, the client is usually seeking self-validation. Instead of saying, "I think that you should . . .", respond with questions such as, "What would you like to do?" or "What do you plan to do?"

*Interpret Client's Behavior.* Confronting the client with analytical meanings of the client's behavior may cause anxiety, denial, or withdrawal. Self-understanding comes from within the person and not directly from someone else.

*Change the Subject Abruptly.* This response takes control of the conservation. The client's thoughts and spontaneity are interrupted. Such behavior demonstrates a lack of empathy or the presence of anxiety on the part of the interviewer.

*Defending.* Protecting a person, place, or thing from verbal attack from the client implies that the client does not have the right to express negative impressions, opinions, or feelings.

*Belittle or Criticize Feelings Expressed.* This behavior implies that the client's feelings are not valid or that the client's concerns are mild, temporary, unimportant, or self-limiting. This behavior reflects a lack of understanding or empathy from the interviewer.

*Offer False Reassurance.* Making glib statements or indicating that there is no cause for anxiety are inappropriate ways of evaluating the client's feelings and communciate a lack of empathy and understanding. Such statements as, "Everything is OK," or "You're coming along fine, don't worry," belittle the client who feels the concerns are legitimate.

*Use Stereotyped Responses.* Using cliches and trite expressions, such as, "It's for your own good," or "The first day is always the hardest," prevent the client from expressing feelings. These also communicate disinterest and prohibit you from maintaining objectivity.

*Express Approval.* Indicating that something the client does or feels is good implies that the opposite is bad. This limits the client's freedom to think, speak, or act in ways that may not please the interviewer. Statements such as, "I'm glad that you feel that way" imply that the client should strive to please you.[7,17,32,37,40] communication patterns that will promote health for the individual, the family, and the community.

In summary, there are two types of assessment interviews—formal and informal. The informal interview is nonstructured and integrated into other ongoing nursing activities. The formal assessment interview is structured as to purpose and data to be collected; it is usually not combined with other activities. Appropriate communication skill and interviewing techniques are essential to the success of both types of interviews.

As stated earlier, most formal assessment interviews are conducted to complete a nursing health history. The nursing health history, which is the second major contributor to the data base, will be discussed next.

## Nursing Health History

You may have heard the term *health history,* even as a lay person. When going to a health facility, you were asked to supply information for the physician's history form. With this in mind, you might ask: What is a health history? What is a nursing health history? How does the nursing health history differ from the medical health history?

A **health history** is a written record of specific subjective data from the client. Neither objective data nor inferences should be included. The history includes a description of the client's present health status, past medical and surgical history, family medical history, client profile, and review of body systems. (The review of body systems (ROS) consists of the client's response to questions concerning each system. It should not be confused with the physical examination of each system.)

A **medical health history** contains the information described in the previous paragraph and concentrates on the symptoms, contributing factors, and progression of the disease process. It seeks to identify information that will aid in the diagnosis and treatment of the disease.

A **nursing health history** deals with the client's responses, physically and psychologically, to his or her health status. It focuses on the client's own perception of health status, feelings regarding the need for health care, expectations regarding this care, and the meaning of health care to the client and the family. Clues to the client's personal needs and ability to deal with health problems are sought. The nursing health history also helps you to identify past patterns of health and illness within the individual, the presence of risk factors, and the availability of resources to the individual. The health history provides you with insight into the functional status of the individual and helps to guide future data collection.

As a professional nurse, it is your responsibility to gather the nursing health history. Your educational background prepares you to use therapeutic communication skills and interviewing techniques. These skills and techniques enable you to gather pertinent data. The aide or technician may be capable of getting the history form completed but may overlook significant cues in the process and may lack the insight of knowing when to ask relevant questions.

Ideally, the nursing health history should be attained as soon as you meet the client. This may not always be possible. The client's condition and the urgency of the situation will determine when the health history can logically be gathered. Your approach should be flexible and adaptable to the situation. Remember that the nursing health history is an important portion of the data base and must be completed as soon after the initial client contact as possible.

Although a nursing health history can be collected from the client using the informal interview approach, a systematic and well-organized formal approach usually results in a more complete data base. You should use a printed form or guideline. There are a variety of forms available. Each form is developed to meet the particular needs of the nurses who use them and to be compatible with the client's age and health status. Regardless of the type of form, the following areas should be assessed: reason for contact with health care provider, past health history, family health history, activities of daily living, psychosocial history, financial status, and client's health needs. Some forms also include detailed nutritional and developmental histories.

- Reasons for Contact with Health Care Provider. You should ask the client why he came to the health care provider or facility. Assistance with health promotion, prevention of illness, or restoration of health are the primary reasons for seeking health care. If the client came for a yearly physical examination, promotion of health status is being sought. Prevention of illness is sought by the client who brings an infant for immunization, and restoration of health is sought by the client who has signs and symptoms of a disease process.
- Past Health History. You will want to determine previous hospitalizations, surgeries, and illnesses. The physician's medical record may supply dates and responses to treatment, but you will want to ask how these problems affect the client's life-style. You will also want to identify any chronic health problems and allergies and how the client copes with them.
- Family Health History. You should determine the causes of death of close family members and the presence of chronic health problems, such as diabetes mellitus, hypertension, and mental disorders, among the family members. Again, the physician's medical record may supply some of this information, but you will want to determine the effect on the client and family.
- Activities of Daily Living. Determine the client's usual routine and ability to function. Patterns of eating, sleeping, dressing, working, playing, communicating and interacting, maintaining food, shelter, and clothing, and safety should be assessed.
- Psychosocial History. You will want to assess general affect, self-concept, body image, reactions to stress, coping mechanisms, thought processes, interests and motivation, willingness to take risks and to make changes, and feelings. You will want to determine cultural patterns and beliefs. How do these affect the client's health practices, perception of wellness, and cooperation with therapies? The client's family unit should be described as well as significant others in the client's life. Determine the client's educational level and church and social affiliations.
- Financial Status. You should assess the client's financial stability; any verbalized economic concerns should be noted. You should determine any community resources being used. The client's occupation and employment record should be assessed for job-related health problems.
- Health Needs. This area includes the review of systems. Make certain that you are aware of the information already available in this area. Try to assess the client's reaction or response to the various symptoms or concerns mentioned. For example, if the client has experienced some shortness of breath, you will want to determine when the shortness of breath occurs, how long it lasts, what precipitates it, and what does the client do when it occurs. Does the client continue normal activities? Has the client sought medical treatment? Has the client tried over-the-counter medication?

*Structured and Semistructured Formats.* The nursing health history may follow a structured or semistructured format. The **structured format** may consist of a questionnaire that the client completes on entry into the health care system; a list of specific questions asked by the interviewer; or a list of specific topics to be covered by the interviewer during face-to-face questioning of the client.

*Questionnaires* save time for the individual collecting the data but allow for little input of feelings, reactions, or thoughts from the client. Figure 4–3 shows a simple, structured questionnaire which can be used to gather health history data. Some health care facilities have developed formats that allow the client to receive and complete the questionnaire prior to an appointment at the facility. This generally involves the mailing of the questionnaire to the client. Such a format allows the client ample time to answer the questions in the privacy and comfort of the home, which hopefully increases the accuracy and completeness of the client's data. The information is reviewed with the client at the facility.

Many facilities have instituted the practice of having nonnurse personnel collect the initial health history. Usually these individuals, called medical historians, use the structured questionnaire format. Appendix A contains an example of this type of health history form. When medical historians are used, you must carefully review their data and decide if more information is needed to complete the nursing health history. If in doubt about the necessity to reassess or to clarify data, remember that your observations will help to determine the validity of the information already recorded. Most clients, if they sense genuine concern in your approach, will not resent or feel uncomfortable about discussing topics previously discussed with other individuals.

When a list of specific questions is used, the directive interviewing approach is being used. You take an active part in collecting the nursing health history, but your part consists of reading a list of prepared questions to the client.

If the format includes a list of specific topics to be discussed, you must be present to interpret the form to the client. You decide how to phrase the questions in order to collect adequate data. The questions that you use may be open or closed, and thus directive or nondirective interviewing can be used.

A structured nursing health history form has been developed by the authors. This form is organized according to Maslow's[41] list of basic needs and is based on review of numerous history forms and on ideas of the authors. An outline of the major parts of the form is included in Table 4–3. The entire form may be found in Appendix B.

With the **semistructured format,** the only guide is a list of broad categories. Again, the questions to be asked may be open or closed and are developed by the nurse during the interview. Little and Carnevali developed a guide using this format. Their guide lists three main categories with appropriate topics to be discussed under each category. The main categories identified are: client perceptions, functional abilities, and resources and support systems.[25] The semistructured format can be individualized, and it allows the client an opportunity to freely express feelings and thoughts. It may also be time consuming and difficult for the beginning practitioner to use because it supplies limited guidance.

Each health history format has advantages and disadvantages. The format should be evaluated and revised periodically. The following factors should be considered: Is the form gathering the desired information? Does the nursing staff use the form? How long does it take the nurse to complete the health history? Can the information be used as a basis for nursing therapies? Does the client respond favorably or unfavorably to the interview format?

# Health History Questionnaire

## Identification Data—Please complete the following:

Please Print

Name _____     Date _____
    (Last)    (First)    (M.I.)

Address _____     S.S.#_____-_____-_____
    (No. & St.; Apt. #; Route #; Box #)

_____     Date of
(City)    (State)    (Zip)     Birth _____

Home Telephone(___)_____     Employer _____
    Area Code

Bus. Telephone(___)_____     Job Title _____
    Area Code

Marital Status (circle)    Married    Separated    Divorced
                       Widowed    Single

Education (circle last year completed)
    1  2  3  4  5  6  7  8  9  10  11  12  13  14  15  16

## General Data

1. Please check (✔) any of the following that you have right now:

| | |
|---|---|
| _____frequent headaches | _____urination problems |
| _____eye or vision problems | _____menstrual difficulties |
| _____ear or hearing problems | _____bruise easily |
| _____nosebleeds | _____aching muscles/joints |
| _____nasal congestion | _____numbness in fingers |
| _____difficulty smelling | _____frequent crying spells |
| _____persistent cough | _____family problems |
| _____coughing spells | _____work problems |
| _____difficulty breathing | _____sexual problems |
| _____dizziness | _____fever |
| _____chest pain | _____weight gain or loss |
| _____vomiting | _____fatigue |
| _____blood in stools | _____difficulty starting flow of urine |
| _____difficulty with bowel movements | |
| _____excessive phlegm | |

2. Do you have any allergies? Yes _____   No _____
(medication, food, or other substances)

  If Yes, please list_____
_____
_____

3. List *all* medications you are currently taking:
Prescription drugs:_____
_____

  Over-the-Counter drugs (aspirin, cold medicine,
laxatives, etc.): _____
_____

  Home remedies: _____
_____

4. What was the date of your last physical examination:
Month _____   Year_____

5. Do you smoke?: Yes _____No _____
If Yes, estimate number of cigarettes smoked per day: _____

**Figure 4–3.** Structured questionnaire.

**TABLE 4–3. OUTLINE OF A NURSING HEALTH HISTORY FORM**

| | |
|---|---|
| I. Client Identification | 7. Immunization |
| II. Reason Client Sought Assistance | 8. Sexual growth |
| III. Assessment of Needs of the Individual | B. Safety/Security needs |
|   A. Physiologic needs |   1. Physical safety |
|     1. Oxygenation |   2. Emotional safety |
|     2. Fluids/Electrolytes |   3. Environmental safety |
|     3. Nutrition | C. Love/Belonging needs |
|     4. Elimination | D. Esteem/Recognition needs |
|     5. Rest/Sleep | E. Self-actualization needs |
|     6. Physical/Mental comfort | |

***Recording the Data.*** When recording the data collected by directive or nondirective interviewing, be certain to use the client's words whenever possible. Recording the data in the client's words helps to convey the client's understanding of the situation, ability to recall events, and ability to organize and communicate thoughts and knowledge to others.

The client's words may be paraphrased and preceded by statements such as, "Client states the most recent visit to the clinic was in November." If direct citation is used, the client's words should appear within quotation marks: "Client described headache pain as 'constant, stabbing pain. Sometimes I want to dig my eye out.'"

It is appropriate to use contractions, phrases, and diagnostic terms if used by the client. For example, the following would be acceptable: "I have hip pain when I walk too much. Could this be rheumatoid arthritis?" You should, when appropriate, record nonverbal responses which accompany the client's words: "I get frequent headaches" (points to area over left eye).

Data must be concise, clearly stated, easy to read, and understandable to the various health personnel who will be using them. Words which are subject to individual definition or interpretation—good, bad, little, big, large, small—should be avoided unless used by the client. Uncommon terminology, abbreviations, and symbols should not be used. Abbreviations and symbols accepted by the health care facility may be used. (Most health care facilities have a procedure manual that contains a list of approved abbreviations, symbols, and terms for that institution.)

To summarize, the nursing health history is a written record of subjective data that deal with the client's responses, physically and psychologically, to the health status. A structured or semistructured health history format may be used by the professional nurse who is responsible for collecting the data. The structured format may consist of a questionnaire, a list of specific questions asked by an interviewer, or a list of specific topics to be covered by questions from the interviewer. The structured format consists of a list of broad categories.

The wellness assessment is another means of gathering information for the data base. This assessment may be considered a section of the nursing health history or as a separate contributor to the data base. Because it can be used in situations that do not warrant a complete assessment interview and nursing health history, we will discuss it separately.

## Wellness Assessment

**Wellness** is defined as a dynamic state of health. Dunn is one of the earliest authors who wrote about wellness. He believes that wellness has various levels and is a constantly changing state. He views wellness as being on a continuum with death at one end and high-level wellness at the other. Dunn indicates that we should seek to achieve **high-level wellness**—"an integrated method of functioning which is oriented toward maximizing the potential of which the individual is capable."[11] High-level wellness focuses on all dimensions of the individual—physical, mental, social, emotional, and spiritual. Because high-level wellness encourages healthful life-styles, it is viewed as a health promotion measure.

There are several aspects of wellness that should be assessed. These aspects are all interrelated and contribute collectively to the individual's level of wellness. Factors which we will consider are: degree of fitness, level of nutrition, risk level for health problems, level of life-stress, sensitivity to the environment, personal habits, life-styles, and health habits.

***Degree of Fitness.*** Both physical and mental fitness are important. Physical fitness brought about by safe and effective exercise will have a positive effect on the client's mental health. Assessment data may be collected by observation and fitness measurements or by self-reporting by the client. The client should be asked to report pattern of exercise including the type, frequency, duration, and intensity. In addition, the client should be encouraged to verbalize feelings regarding the exercise program: Is it considered a punishment or is it enjoyed?

The general appearance of the client is assessed. Muscles should be tested for strength and endurance, and muscles and joints evaluated for flexibility. Girth measurements can be taken to determine body proportions, and the percent of body fat can be calculated.[1,35,45] All of these measurements when analyzed will help you to determine the level of fitness of the client.

***Level of Nutrition.*** The inclusion of foods from the four food groups and the overall adequacy of the diet can be determined by doing a complete nutritional assessment that includes the client's 24-hour recall of food intake, general knowledge of nutrition, use of food additives, unusual dietary practices, effect of personal, family, and social beliefs, and skills in food attainment and preparation. Once this information is available, it can be analyzed for inclusion of the Recommended Daily Allowances of essential nutrients.[45,47] Appendix C contains a sample nutritional assessment tool, a form for recording the client's 24-hour recall of food intake, and a diet analysis form.

***Sensitivity to Environment.*** Assessment in this area seeks to determine how aware the client is of the personal environment. As you identify sensory stimuli and potential hazards within the client's environment, you should discuss these with the client. This will increase the client's awareness as to their impact on levels of wellness.[1,45]

***Risk Appraisal.*** Risk appraisal is a method for determining the client's risk for disease or death. Data from the client's health history, assessment interview, and physical assessment are matched against a data bank of statistics. These statistics reflect mortality rates according to the cause of death.

The risk for any given health problem generally increases with increasing number and intensity of risk factors. The purpose of the risk appraisal is to identify the client's risk factors and to provide the client with knowledge concerning threats to personal health.[35] Pender, in her book *Health Promotion in Nursing Practice,* has developed a risk appraisal form. In addition, several commercial sources for analyzing the individual's risk factors are available.

*Level of Life-stress.* The impact of stress on mental and physical well-being has been clearly documented. During the wellness assessment, you should determine the client's sources of stress, perception of stress, period of exposure to stress, and past management of stress.

Determine what sources of stress exist for your client. Stress might stem from home, family, work, community, or social activities. Life events such as the death of a spouse, divorce, marriage, or retirement are stressful and can precipitate health problems. Note the number of life changes which have occurred for the client in the past two years—changes in financial state, change in occupation, and so forth. Determine how the client perceives stress. Does the client view stress as positive or negative? As exciting or threatening? Assess your client's period of exposure to stress—hours as opposed to days and months. Finally, assess how the client managed stress in the past. What coping patterns were used? Did the client indulge in overeating? Drug or alcohol abuse? Decreased physical activity?[8,35,45]

*Life-style and Personal Health Habits.* The client's personal habits depend largely on past experiences and role models. Areas to be considered are: hours of sleep per night, dietary habits, weight as compared to recommended optimal weight, exercise patterns, alcohol and tobacco use, dental care, safety practices, and health care practices.[1,45,47]

Pender has developed a Life-style and Health-Habits Assessment tool that is intended to help you in assessing the client's life-style in terms of its impact on health. The assessment tool (see Appendix D) is divided into ten sections: competence in self-care, nutritional practices, physical or recreational activity, sleep patterns, stress management, self-actualization, sense of purpose, relationships with others, environmental control, and use of health care system. Through review of personal habits, life-style, and health habits, you can assist the client in evaluating the effects of personal behavior on health and help the client to make decisions regarding alteration of unhealthy behavior patterns.[35]

The complete wellness assessment considers the individual's degree of fitness, level of life-stress, risk level for health problems, level of nutrition, sensitivity to the environment, personal habits, life-style, and health habits. You may choose to collect only information about these areas. However, information about the client's level of wellness is more beneficial when accompanied by the other components of the data base—assessment interview, nursing health history, and physical assessment. We will discuss the fourth major contributor to the data base next—the physical assessment.

## Physical Assessment

The physical assessment provides another major source of information for the data base. In health care facilities and within literature, the terms *physical assessment* and *physical examination* are frequently used interchangeably. Both terms imply a systematic, orderly collection of information about the client. For the purpose of this chapter, **physical assessment or examination** means an evaluation of the client's health status through the use of the examiner's special senses of sight, hearing, touch, and smell. Special instruments may be required for portions of the assessment.

The physical assessment ties in with the broader concept of **medical examination,** a diagnostic evaluation of the client's health status. The medical examination includes a social, medical, and family history, a physical assessment, radiologic and laboratory studies, and other diagnostic procedures deemed necessary.

Two types of medical examinations exist: the periodic health appraisal and the diagnostic evaluation for disease. In the **periodic health appraisal,** the person being examined is apparently well. The examination is done to rule out any health problems, detect disease in an early, more treatable stage, or supply the physician and nurse with clues regarding future health problems. The examination is the basis for preventive or anticipatory health care. Annual health examinations of industrial workers, hospital employees, and school children, routine examinations of pregnant women and newborn infants, and diabetic, cancer, hypertension, and tuberculosis screening programs are examples of periodic health appraisals.

The **diagnostic examination** seeks to identify the health problem of an apparently ill person so that appropriate treatment may be initiated. Both types of medical examinations use the physical assessment as an essential means for evaluating the client's present health status, preventing future health problems, and promoting health.

In the past, the physician was the only person responsible for the physical assessment of a client. The nurse prepared the client and physical setting, gathered equipment, and assisted the physician as needed. Now, skills used in the physical assessment are recognized as important tools for the nurse also. As you assume more responsibility as a primary health care provider, you will frequently conduct a part of or the total physical assessment. When you conduct the physical assessment, you are not responsible for determining the medical diagnosis. You are responsible for recognizing and distinguishing abnormal from normal, determining client concerns, and using these findings to determine nursing diagnoses.

Whatever the work setting, you will use information obtained through the physical assessment. Knowledge of the techniques used in physical assessment will enhance your productivity and improve the client's health care. For example, a pediatric nurse practitioner will examine well infants, give immunizations, and instruct mothers about nutritional needs and expected growth and development patterns. An occupational nurse will screen for hypertension, diabetes, tuberculosis, glaucoma, and other diseases; the nurse might also conduct routine examinations of all employees. A school nurse will conduct annual hearing and visual examinations and do basic health assessments of students. In the hospital setting, the nurse will use the physical assessment as a foundation for nursing interventions.

We will not attempt to describe in this chapter the techniques to be used when conducting a physical assessment. You will need to study the references listed and to have supervised practice and experience in order to perfect physical assessment skills.

Although specific techniques are not discussed, we will consider some of the printed tools or guidelines available to the individual conducting the physical assessment. To perform a careful and complete assessment, a systematic approach is needed. Various methods for systematically inspecting and examining the client have been developed based on specific theoretical frameworks, for example, Roy's adaptation theory; on conceptual models, for example, equilibration versus disequilibration; or on approaches that are eclectic (drawn from several sources).

One method involves inspecting the client from *head to toe* in a systematic manner.

For example, all organs and structures in the region of the head and neck are examined together: the eyes, ears, mouth, nose, lymph nodes, throat, muscles, and bones. Then advancement is made to the region of the chest to assess the breasts, lungs, and heart. This pattern continues until the entire body has been examined. The actual tool or guide can be as simple or complex as desired. Only the major body regions to be examined may be listed or each of the structures or organs in that region may be included.

Another method of assessing the client is the *body systems* approach. Using this method, you observe and record data about each of the body systems: cardiovascular, respiratory, skeletal, and so forth. This approach follows the same format as the Review of Systems that occurs in the nursing health history. In the health history, however, the data are subjective, and in the physical assessment the data are objective. For instance, if during the health history the client indicated becoming short of breath when walking too fast, this information would be considered subjective data about the respiratory system. Now, during the physical assessment, you listen to the breath sounds with a stethoscope and note that some crackling sounds are present in the lower lobe of the right lung—you have collected objective data on the same body system.

The physical assessment tool may also be developed according to the *levels of organization* within the human body: subcellular, cellular, tissue, organs, organ systems, and whole organism. (Appendix E contains an example of a physical assessment tool that is organized according to this concept.)

In 1965, Faye McCain presented a physical assessment tool based on *functional abilities* of the client. This tool was oriented to nursing and was not meant to duplicate the medical history or medical physical examination; the nurse was meant to gain most of the data through direct observation and interviewing. With the growth in the knowledge base of the nurse, more in-depth assessment skills are being used and some duplication may exist. In McCain's tool, 13 functional areas are identified: social, mental, emotional, body temperature, respiratory, circulatory, nutritional, elimination, reproductive status, state of rest and comfort, state of skin and appendages, sensory perception, and motor ability.[26]

Another method was described by Doris Geitgey in 1969. This approach uses a guide based on the acronym *SELF-PACING.* Each letter represents an area to be assessed: *S*-Socialization and Special Senses, *E*-Elimination and Exercise, *L*-Liquids, *F*-Food, *P*-Pain, Personal hygiene, Posture, *A*-Aeration, *C*-Circulation, *I*-Integument, *N*-Neuromuscular control and coordination, and *G*-General condition.[15] Both the McCain and Geitgey tools can be used to gather objective and subjective data.

In some health care facilities, a combination of these methods is used. The facility may also combine the nursing health history and physical assessment on the same form; this is frequently done to decrease the time required to gather data. It is important to remember that regardless of the brevity of the form you must be open to cues given by the client and use branching questions when appropriate. Figure 4–4 shows a combined health history and physical assessment record which was developed by the authors.

***Modification of Physical Assessment Format.*** [3,21,36,39,51] Infants, children, and the aged require some modifications in the assessment format. For the infant, you must rely totally on the parents or person accompanying the infant for the nursing health history. During the physical assessment, you should gather all information attainable through general inspection or observation before touching the infant. In well infants, you initially assess those parts of the body farthest from the head. This usually decreases the

## Client's Health History and Assessment Record

Client's Name: _____ Date: _____ Time: _____

Information Provided by: Client _____ Spouse _____ Other _____

Reason for Contact with Health Care Provider _____

    Client's concept of illness (if appropriate) _____

_____

    Onset _____ Duration _____

    Symptoms _____

    Related treatments and medications _____

Client expected outcome from health care _____

Previous hospitalizations, serious illness/injury, surgery (Note approximate dates):

Current home medication/ Frequency/ Last dose/ Prescribed by:

Disposition of Medication

Allergies: (Note type of reaction and date of last reaction)

Restrictions or Limitations:

    Food _____ Prostheses _____ Cane _____ Walker _____ Special Shoes _____ Dentures _____

    (Note if full or partial) Dental Braces _____ (Upper or Lower dentures) Glasses _____

    Contact Lens _____ Hard of Hearing _____ Hearing Aids _____

    Deaf _____ Blind _____ Other Concerns _____

Family Social History:

    Occupation _____ Marital Status _____

    Children _____ Ages _____ / _____ / _____ / _____ / _____ / _____

    Others in Household _____

    Relationship _____

    Home: One Floor _____ Multilevel _____ Location of Bath _____

    Number of steps to outside _____

    Church Affiliation _____

    Membership in Social Groups _____

Social Habits:

    Alcohol Intake _____        Type _____        Amount _____

    Tobacco Use _____        What _____        Amount _____

    Drug Use _____        What _____        Amount _____

    Other Concerns _____

Dietary History:

    Type of Diet _____ Appetite _____ Wt. _____ Ht. _____

    Eating Habits _____

    Food Intolerances _____ Restrictions _____

    Food Likes _____ Dislikes _____

Liquid Intake:

    Breakfast _____ Lunch _____ Dinner _____

Hygiene and Bath:

    Bathing Habits: Frequency _____ Tub _____ Shower _____

    Special Soaps _____ Lotions _____

**Figure 4–4.** Combined nursing health history and physical assessment record.

94

Sleep:

    Falls asleep easily _____ With difficulty _____ Naps _____

    Aids used to induce sleep _____

    Usual Times: Retire _____ Arise _____

    Average number of hours of sleep _____

    Number of pillows used _____ Blankets _____

    Sleepwalks _____

Elimination Patterns:

    Bowel _____

_____

    Bladder _____

_____

Reproductive Status:

    Female—Date of last pap smear _____

    Pattern of Menses _____

    Male—Date of last testicular examination

_____

General Appearance:

    Oral Hygiene _____ Teeth _____ Dentures _____

    Hair _____ Finger Nails _____

    Alert _____ Orientated _____

    Apprehensive _____

    Confused _____

    Posture _____ Ease of Mobility _____

    Additional Observations _____

Vital Signs: BP _____ T _____ P _____ R _____

    Description of Respirations: Quality, rate and rhythm. _____

    Description of Pulse: Quality, rate and rhythm. _____

Description of Skin Color and Temperature:

Instructions: Indicate appropriate code on the anatomical diagram according to physical assessment codes:

| | | |
|---|---|---|
| A | Abrasion | Scrape |
| BL | Blister | Fluid filled vesicle |
| BR | Bruise | Purplish nonelevated area |
| C | Contusion | Injury in which skin is not broken |
| D | Decubitus | Skin ulceration caused by pressure |
| E | Erythema | Diffuse redness over skin |
| H | Hematoma | Purplish swelling elevated from bleeding |
| L | Laceration | Wound or tear of skinflesh |
| PA | Papule | Pimple red elevated area(s) |
| PE | Petechiae | Small hemorrhagic spots |
| PU | Pustule | Elevated area filled with pus |
| R | Rash | Skin eruption with little or no elevation |
| S | Scar | Mark left after healing |
| AB/ | Absent/ | Absent limb or extremity |
| O | Other | |

**Figure 4–4.** *(Continued)*

Description of Any Existing Pain or Discomfort:

Summary of Client's Strengths:

Summary of Client's Limitations:

**Figure 4–4.** *(Continued)*

fear and makes the infant easier to examine. A crying, struggling infant provides minimal information of value. For the infant brought to the health facility with a particular health problem, you may of necessity have to start with that body structure or organ involved; for example, a traumatic lesion on the head would be examined first.

The preschooler and younger school-age child can provide some history, but much reliance still must be placed on the person accompanying the child. Fear may alter the response of this age group, and examination procedures which are considered intrusive or invasive to the body (rectal temperatures, nose and ear examinations) may produce the most negative response from the child. Older children and adolescents may still be anxious during the physical assessment but are fairly reliable historians. Theories and imaginary ills usually have not influenced their interpretation of facts as frequently occurs with the adult. Examination of the male genitalia and the female genitalia and breasts will produce embarrassment and mental discomfort for most adolescents. Complete explanations must be offered and privacy provided.

Some aging people may have difficulty recalling some of the subjective data sought during the nursing health history. At the same time, they may have difficulty assuming some of the positions required during the physical assessment, such as the knee-chest position, or performing some of the tasks, such as holding their breath while heart sounds are auscultated. The aging person may also not respond as quickly to requests as younger people. Modifications of the assessment procedure should be made when necessary, and the client should be given adequate time to respond to requests.

Regardless of the age of the individual, be careful to select words that are within the client's level of understanding. Use the knowledge gained during the health history to help you formulate appropriate questions or requests during the physical assessment. Use your knowledge of normal growth and development to help you determine what physical findings should be evident for a client in a particular age group. Finally, observe the client's behavior; facial expressions, gestures, and body movements will supply information during the physical assessment. For example, you might ask the client if pain is experienced when you move the arm. If the client answers that no pain is experienced but facial expressions suggest otherwise, you will need to gather more data.

In summary, the physical assessment is a systematic inspection and examination of the client for the purpose of determining the client's health status or health problem. Various written tools or guidelines are available to the individual conducting the assessment. Regardless of the type of tool selected, it must be adapted to the particular client and clinical situation.

The overall data base for the individual client is composed of information gathered in the assessment interview, nursing health history, wellness assessment, and physical assessment (Fig. 4–5). Some information regarding the individual's family and community is included in this data base. Because the individual's need for health care extends into and affects the family and community, more data are needed. The family and community assessment will provide you with information regarding the social support groups and environment in which the individual lives.

## ASSESSMENT OF THE FAMILY

The definition of a family is dependent on many factors; they include the client's perception of family, the personal values and background of the person doing the assessment, and the guidelines of the health care facility involved. The definition can be expanded or contracted to meet the particular needs of the situation and type of family life-style being discussed.

Traditionally, family was defined as a group of people related by heredity—the nuclear family consisting of a married couple and their children by birth or adoption. The definition may be expanded to include the biologic kin networks or the family of procreation. Sociologically, the family may be considered any group of people living together. This may include the commune family, the institutional family, or the multi-generation family. Psychologically, a family is any group with strong emotional ties such as two adults, heterosexual or homosexual, sharing a common household. Regard-

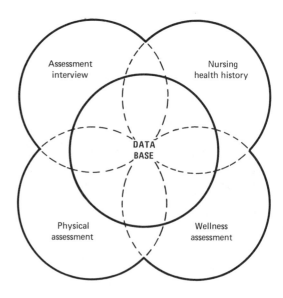

**Figure 4–5.** Composition of data base.

less of which viewpoint is used the term **family** implies a unit of interdependent individuals.

## Functions of the Family Unit

Functions describe the tasks of the family and provide the reason for its existence. Although many functions formerly performed within families are now shared with others in the community, the family's basic functions continue to meet the needs of the individual family members and the wider society.

Several theorists throughout the years have identified and described family functions. Some of the major functions are:

1. Love and Affection Function. Sharing love and affection is one of the most important functions of families. Primarily a parental role, this function deals with meeting the psychological needs of family members.[12,14,33] Love and emotional support are provided for each family member and each member can test personal emotional reactions and learn to reach and maintain emotional equilibrium.

2. Socialization Function. This function deals primarily with the socialization and social placement of children. It is aimed at making the children productive members of society. Some of this function is shared with schools, child-care facilities, and other institutions outside the family structure. Status conferring—passing on traditions, values, and privileges of the family—and transmission of the parents' cultural heritage to their children are parts of this function. Social functions of the modern family also include providing social togetherness and fostering self-esteem and a sense of social and personal identity. In addition, the family provides each member with an opportunity to observe and learn social and sexual roles. A sense of what is right and wrong is given to the growing child and essential rules, obligations, and responsibilities are instilled.[12,14,31,33,34]

3. Reproduction Function. One of the basic functions of the family is to reproduce and provide new members for society.[14,31,33]

4. Family Coping Function. This function refers to the adaptive patterns or problem-solving mechanisms used for the maintenance of stability within the inner and outer environment.[14]

5. Economic Function. This function involves the provision and allocation of sufficient resources—financial, space, and material.[14,31,33]

6. Protective Function. Families meet their members' physical needs by providing food, clothing, shelter, protection against danger, and a secure environment. In addition, health care and health care practices are relevant parts of this family function. The stability and dependability of the family unit promotes confidence, self-assurance, and a sense of security among its members.[12,14,33]

7. Security and Acceptance Function. This is an important function for the modern family. The family provides a home base and a sense of permanence, thus making its members feel secure and accepted. In a society where friends, neighbors, colleagues, and other associates do not remain constant, the family can offer a relationship that is expected to endure.[12]

As you assess a family, consider these functions. Are they evident within this particular family? Is evidence of malfunction observed? How does this affect the family?

## Characteristics of the Family Unit[13,14,16,42]

Although all families are unique, every family has certain features or characteristics that they share with other families. An understanding of these characteristics will help you to do a more complete assessment.

*Each Family Has a Separate Social System.* All members of a family are interdependent. One member's actions affect other members. For example, the mother who has abdominal surgery and must reduce her activities for 6 to 8 weeks may need help with some of her responsibilities. This will alter the family's routines as well as food preparation and eating patterns.

Families also share a complex network of communication patterns. Norms involving what is and is not shared, as well as who shares with whom, are clearly understood by all family members. Verbal, nonverbal, and behavioral interactions all occur within a family and are important aspects to be assessed. The effectiveness of communication patterns determines how well the family handles conflict and stress, provides a support system for its members, and resolves daily problems.

Families as social systems set and maintain boundaries. Boundaries mark the interface between systems. Within the boundaries, family members have the freedom to be themselves. The boundaries develop as a result of the closeness of the family relationship and will change as members come and go. These boundaries should be flexible and allow the family to function as an open system—protecting and preserving the family unity and autonomy while bringing into their system selective input from the external environment.

Families are adaptive systems. They constantly respond to internal and external stimuli which cause change within the family. As members of the family age and are exposed to new experiences and as members are added or lost from the family unit, expectations for each member change. Throughout all of the changing, the family continues to strive for an environment conducive to the development of its members.

*Each Family Has a Family Culture.* **Culture** is the term used to describe the behavior patterns, arts, beliefs, values, attitudes, and institutions that are socially transmitted from one generation to the next. Culture provides direction for daily living and a basis for decision making. A family's educational views, health care practices, dietary habits, religious practices, child-rearing practices, sex roles, and role assignments depend on their cultural beliefs and values.

Culture affects how one perceives health and illness and when and from whom health care should be sought. For example, in some cultures, a person is ill only when incapable of fulfilling a role; in other cultures, a headache may be considered a major illness. Some people do not seek health care until the dominant male or female in the family (depending on the culture) determines that a family member is in need of care.

*Each Family Unit Maintains a Structure.* The nuclear family—husband, wife, children—is usually seen as the traditional norm. There are now many variations of the nuclear model as well as other patterns of family structure. Family structures can be placed into two general categories: traditional and nontraditional.

The *traditional family structure* is the pattern with which we are most familiar. The nuclear family and the nuclear dyad (husband and wife alone either childless or after children have left home) are the most common. Single-parent family, single adult, and multigeneration families are also considered traditional families. *Nontraditional family structures* include the commune family, group marriage, unmarried couple, unmarried single parent, and unmarried couple and child family.

Each type of family structure creates different problems and therefore requires different nursing interventions. You must be careful to avoid judging by standards appropriate to your family structure or to the idealized nuclear family.

***Each Family Designates Various Roles, Responsibilities, and Tasks to its Members.*** Family roles can be classified into two categories: formal or overt roles and informal or covert roles. **Formal roles** are explicit roles which each family role structure contains. These roles represent a cluster of more or less homogeneous behaviors. Standard formal roles which exist in the family are breadwinner, cook, homemaker, house repairman, financial manager, and so forth.[14]

Along with the change in the traditional family structure has come the change in formal roles of family members. Roles have become more variable, flexible, and complex. Great variation in the roles of both sexes is possible. The female may be the breadwinner while the male in the family is the homemaker. Child-care and socialization roles are becoming the shared responsibilities of both partners in the family unit. In addition, the female's right to sexual enjoyment and fulfillment is changing the sexual roles for both males and females.

**Informal roles** are implicit and are maintained to meet the emotional needs of family members or to maintain family equilibrium. Some of the informal roles commonly seen in families are encourager, blocker, follower, dominator, recognition seeker, martyr, pal, and harmonizer.[5,38]

The status and roles of each family member change throughout that person's life cycle and the cycle of the family unit. This change in role relationships, expectations, and abilities is referred to as **role transition**.[28] Role transitions occur at definite points of family life—marriage, death, and divorce. A role change for one family member creates role changes for other family members.

***Each Family Follows a Sequential Pattern of Development.*** Families change continuously. These changes and developments occur in a predictable pattern known as the family life cycle. Duvall identifies eight stages in the family life cycle (Fig. 4–6). In order to progress through these stages, the family must perform basic functions and the developmental tasks associated with these functions. Family developmental tasks are ongoing throughout the life cycle.

Again, as you assess your client (the family), consider these characteristics. Are they evident within this particular family unit? What roles can be identified? What patterns of communication exist? Does this family have the traditional or nontraditional structure? What stage in the family life cycle exists? What developmental tasks are being met?

## Impact of Family Health Status

Family nursing should not be viewed as a function or responsibility of only the community nurse. The health of *each* member of the family will affect *all* the members and contribute to the total family's level of health. The family health will also affect the overall health of the community in which they live. With such broad ramifications, it

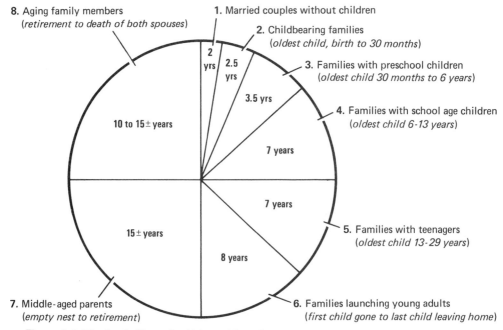

**Figure 4–6.** The family life cycle. *(Adapted from Duvall, E. M. Marriage and family development, (5th ed.). Philadelphia: Lippincott, 1977, with permission.)*

is apparent that all health care providers should be concerned with the health care needs of the whole family.

In addition, healthy families foster individual growth and resistance to disease. The family's health standards will influence each member's health practices—patterns of eating, exercise, coping with stress, rest, and sleep. Family values and decisions will determine the type of health care sought, such as immunizations, use of birth control, and preventative or maintenance dental, vision, and medical examinations.

## Sources of Data

Family data come from a variety of sources. Although the family is the client in this situation, much of the data are initially gathered through an interview with a particular family member. During the initial assessment interview and nursing health history with the family member, you determine specific information about the family unit (Appendix B, Section III. C. Love/Belonging Needs). Other sources of data include interviews with each family member, observations of the home and community, referrals, and information from health team members and agencies working with the family.

An assessment of the level of family wellness is an appropriate starting point for the family assessment.

## Wellness Assessment

Family wellness has the same elements in it that high-level wellness for the individual has. The family must be taking a forward and upward direction and must have the opportunity to develop its full potential. It is important for family wellness that the family work together as an integrated whole.

When assessing the level of family wellness, you might initially have each family member complete the individual Life-style and Health Habits Assessment (Appendix D) that was discussed earlier. You should then discuss the results with the family as a whole. During the discussion, members learn of variations in each other's perceptions—this provides greater motivation and facilitates mutual support. Discussion will also stimulate questions and feelings not previously expressed.

In addition to the individual Life-style and Health Habits Assessment, you may chose to complete a family system assessment. Kandzari has developed a tool designed to assess the family's level of wellness (see Appendix F). Unlike some wellness inventories, this tool must be completed by the nurse and not the family unit. The tool requires nurse–family interaction over a period of time—not one interview or observation. Careful observation of nonverbal behavior and evaluation of the family's reports of situations and behaviors are needed.[22] Table 4–4 shows the major areas to be assessed. Completion of this form can provide valuable information that can be shared with the family and used to determine the needs of the family unit.

## Specific Family Assessment Tools

As with the individual client, there are a variety of tools or guidelines available that will facilitate family assessment. Before selecting a tool, you must decide the purpose of the data collection. Are the data needed to determine the health concerns and needs of the entire family unit or will the data be applied toward the understanding of health needs of the individual family member? Remember that the tools are designed to serve as guides and can be altered to meet the particular situation.

A family assessment tool should be holistic—considering all things influencing the family health, including psychologic, socioeconomic, physical, and cultural factors. The format should allow for information regarding the family's level of health and assets and limitations of the family unit.

The authors have developed a tool that is organized according to Maslow's list of basic needs. The form is a compilation of numerous tools and input from the authors. An outline of the major parts of the family assessment tool is included in Table 4–5. The entire form may be found in Appendix G.

The general description of the family unit should contain the first and last names, sexes, dates and places of births and relationships to the individual client of each member of the family. Remember to include the client's interpretation of family unit. You should also record professional and volunteer persons and agencies working with the family.

**TABLE 4–4. FAMILY SYSTEM ASSESSMENT FORM**

I. Family Members Relating to One Another
  A. Individuality and autonomy
  B. Communication
  C. Bonding
II. Family Members Functioning Together
  A. Roles and role relationships
  B. Division of tasks and activities
  C. Governance and power
  D. Decision making and problem solving
  E. Leadership and initiative
III. Involvement in Outside Community

**TABLE 4–5. OUTLINE OF THE FAMILY ASSESSMENT TOOL**

| | |
|---|---|
| I. General Description of Family Unit | C. Love/Belonging needs |
| II. Assessment of Needs of the Family |    1. Marital status |
|   A. Physiologic needs |    2. Family and personal roles |
|     1. Eating habits |    3. Delegation of responsibility |
|     2. Sleeping patterns | D. Esteem/Recognition needs |
|     3. Family relationships |    1. Motivation of family unit |
|   B. Safety/Security needs |    2. Family communication patterns |
|     1. Type of health maintenance | E. Self-actualization needs |
|     2. Preventive health care practices |    1. Values and goals of family unit |
|     3. Growth and development patterns |    2. Ways in which family values are reflected |
|     4. Environmental safety |    3. Philosophical and spiritual beliefs |

*Physiologic needs* center around the client's need for food, water, rest, and sleep. You would assess the physical or emotional factors that might prevent the family from successfully meeting these needs. Information regarding any use of tobacco, alcoholic beverages, and prescribed medications by the family members should be determined. In addition, you assess the family's eating habits. If there is doubt about the family's nutritional state, use the complete Nutritional Assessment and Analysis Form (Appendix C). Sleeping patterns of individual family members are assessed; sleeping accommodations available, family members who sleep together, usual time of retiring and rising, and the room in which family members sleep are determined. Remember, each family member should be evaluated even if that member is not your primary client. Each family member should be asked their perception of family relationships that exist within the family unit, for example, how each child relates to the dominant male in the family.

*Safety and security needs* center around the need for protection. Assess the type of health maintenance facilities used by each family member. Note the location and telephone number for each facility, the particular family member using each facility, the reason for use, and the frequency with which the facility is used. You should determine the preventive health care practices that exist; dates of last eye, dental, hearing, and physical examination, immunization records, and use of over-the-counter medication are assessed for each member. Assess the type of emergency plan that the family has developed; availability of emergency telephone numbers, transportation, and support system should be noted.

Each family member should be assessed for evidence of normal developmental patterns and achievement of developmental tasks. In addition, you should determine the stage of family development (see Fig. 4–6) and the achievement of family developmental tasks. This is important since achievement of developmental expectations and tasks promotes security for the family unit.

Environmental safety is also important. Assess the employment history of each family member. Are there any potential threats to the health of family members related to their employment? Is the income adequate to meet family needs? In addition, the environment of the home and community must be assessed. Identify the type and condition of dwelling, presence of hazards, general appearance of dwelling, size of the dwelling in relation to family needs, lack of basic facilities, and size and condition of the yard. Be careful not to assess the living situation according to your personal values or preferences. Remember that the client has a right to privacy and may not want you to inspect the entire house. Characteristics of the community should be assessed to provide clues about the family's socioeconomic status, safety, available resources, and cultural and ethnic group. (Community assessment will be discussed in more depth in the next section.)

*Love and belonging needs* center around the need for love, closeness, and acceptance. The family's religion and ethnic group should be determined. Assess the marital status of each family member in the household. Assess such aspects as allocation of family and personal roles, distribution of power and authority, delegation of responsibility, and child-rearing practices. The means by which the family unit expresses kindness and consideration and the quality of interactions of the family unit should be determined.

*Esteem and recognition needs* are associated with esteem of others and self-esteem. You will need to determine the dominant language used by the family and family communication patterns. Assess the educational level of each family member and the effects these educational levels have on future health teaching. You should also determine the family's perception of its public image.

*Self-actualization needs* center around the process of making maximum use of one's abilities and potential. Determine values and goals of the family unit. Note any interfamily conflicts that arise when individual members have different values. Assess for norms of social behavior accepted by the family unit; note if these values are significant deviations from societal norms, for example, the family that supports, either implicitly or explicitly, repeated absences from school. Determine how the family's value system affects family functions and how the family's values are reflected in their wardrobe, type of reading material, residence, and health beliefs and practices.

Regardless of the guidelines being used, adequate time must be allowed in order to make an accurate, complete assessment. Time is needed to make observations, to see family interaction, and to note family communication patterns. Do not feel that all of the needed information can be gathered on the initial contact with the family.

An assessment of the family should consider functions and characteristics of the family unit plus an evaluation of the family's level of wellness and its assets and limitations. The tool or guideline that you select must be holistic and adaptable to your needs and those of the family unit being assessed.

A community assessment usually accompanies the family assessment and provides much information of value.

## ASSESSMENT OF THE COMMUNITY

*Community* is a term used in many different ways. The word may refer to a specific population living in the same locality and under the same government or a social group that has common values, interests, and needs. A community is part of a larger population group and has distinct patterns of communication and leadership which either facilitate or prevent interactions between members within the community or between the community as a whole and the larger population group.

### Functions of the Community

In order to provide for the goals and needs of the population, the community has a variety of functions. Klein identified seven major functions of the community. These are:

1. Providing and distributing living space and shelter and determining use of space for other purposes.
2. Making available the means for distribution of necessary goods and services.

3. Maintaining safety and order, and facilitating the resolution of conflicts.
4. Educating and acculturating newcomers (e.g., children and immigrants).
5. Transmitting information, ideas, and beliefs.
6. Creating and enforcing rules and standards of belief and behavior.
7. Providing opportunities for interaction between individuals and groups.[23]

Warren uses a list of community functions that is similar. This list of functions includes the following:*

1. Production, Distribution, Consumption. Goods and services are provided, distributed, and used to meet the health and welfare needs of the community's population. Service activities of industry, business, the professions, religion, education, and government are included.
2. Socialization. The process by which knowledge, values, beliefs, customs, and behavior are transmitted to the community's members.
3. Social Control. Influence of the community on the behavior of its members through norms, rules, and social sanction. This function is enforced by governmental agencies, community members, and educational, religious, and recreational systems.
4. Social Participation. Provides opportunity for members of the community to satisfy self-expression and self-fulfillment through interaction with others.
5. Mutual Support. Involves provision of support to members of the community by agencies such as health and social service departments and hospitals.[48]

These functions provide the services and activities necessary for community life. They are carried out by the subsystems of the community and must be met for the community to continue to exist. As you assess the community, consider these functions. Are they apparent within this community? Are the functions being provided in an adequate manner?

## Characteristics of the Community

Every community has certain characteristics that are common in other communities. An understanding of some of these characteristics will help you to do a more complete assessment.[9,42]

*Every Community Has Boundaries.* A community's boundaries are usually not concrete or definite; communities may overlap or intermingle, thus making boundaries difficult to identify. Boundaries are flexible, dynamic, and ever changing; they change to meet the needs of the community population. In addition, the community's boundaries may vary depending upon the nurse's focus. Boundaries, as a whole, serve to control the exchange of energies between a community and its external environment.

*Every Community Has a Structure.* The community structure is composed of several neighborhoods or population groups. Each neighborhood has its own social values, beliefs, recreational and social activities, ethnic or cultural heritage, and health concerns. Neighborhoods vary in size, leadership, cohesiveness, self-sufficiency, and relationships with the large community. Usually a neighborhood is unable to meet all the health needs of its population.

---

* Warren, R. L. The Community in America (2nd ed.). Copyright © 1972 by Houghton Mifflin Company.

*Every Community Has Service Systems.* The Service System assists the community in meeting the goals and needs of its population. These systems include: family, economy, government, religion, education, health, welfare, communication, and transportation. Each system in turn has its own role and structural patterns of behavior. The role and behavior patterns determine methods of communicating, decision making, and lines of authority within and between the systems.

Again, when assessing the community, think about these characteristics. Determine the boundaries of the community. Are they flexible? Do they change to meet the needs of the community? Assess the structure of the community. How many neighborhoods are apparent? What health needs can be met within each neighborhood? Identify the service systems and their roles. All of this information will help you determine nursing diagnoses and appropriate interventions.

## Impact of Community Health Status

The community does affect the health of people and families. Through community assessment, the health of many people may be indirectly affected without direct nursing therapies to each community member. For example, identifying and correcting inadequate sanitation measures within the community will affect everybody in the community, not just the individual or family that may have been the original client.

## Sources of Data

There are many federal, state, and local agencies and people that can supply data about the community. Federal agencies such as the National Center for Health Statistics, the National Institutes of Health, the Center for Disease Control, and the Health Resources Administration will supply health data on request. In addition, the Bureau of the Census can provide vital and demographic statistics. Biostatistics (data that delineate health or health-related events), morbidity and mortality statistics, vital statistics, and demographic statistics are also available through various state and local agencies. State health departments, the department of education, the bureau of mental health, and health service agencies are among state agencies that supply health and health-related information. Local sources include the chamber of commerce, health departments, libraries, health and welfare personnel, community leaders, and community members.[9]

You can also be a source of community data by contributing the information that you collect through interviewing and observation. Some form of community assessment is usually done in association with a family or individual assessment. In each case, you will ask questions that are directly related to the client's perception of the community. This is valuable information and should be added to the data base.

## Specific Community Assessment Tools

As with the family assessment, it is important to determine the purpose of the data collection. Is the data collection to be comprehensive in nature so that it may be used to determine health needs of the entire community population? Or are more specific data needed so that they may be applied to the health needs of a specific group within the total population?

Community assessment tools or guidelines exist. They vary according to the needs of the health facility and the data sought. A variety of conceptual models can be used as a basis for assessing the community. Several models are considered interdisciplinary models—they can be used or adapted by more than one discipline. The interdisciplinary model that we will consider is the systems model.

The **general systems theory** offers a "perspective for looking at man and nature as interacting wholes with integrated sets of properties and relationships."[16] The general systems concepts provide a language base that is understood by a variety of health professionals. Concepts such as systems, open systems, subsystems, boundaries, and feedback are applicable to the community.

The community is viewed as a *system* made up of interrelated and interdependent subsystems. The *subsystems* include economic, educational, religious, political, welfare, and recreational systems. The systems-subsystems organization reflects a *hierarchy arrangement*. Within the subsystems, there is also a hierarchy; each subsystem is organized and related to other subsystems in a specific way. The community is an *open system* that exchanges materials, services, values, and ideals with the environment outside the community. The community also has *boundaries* that separate it from other systems. *Feedback* exists as in the case of the economic system. If the output is good, it provides input and contributes to community growth.[16,43]

Assessment guidelines based on this conceptual model are organized according to the concepts just described. You should assess data about the system (the community), its environment, subsystems, and supersystems. Determine how well the community's parts are working together and if self-regulatory processes are being maintained.[18]

In addition to interdisciplinary models, a number of conceptual models have been developed by nurses. Some of these models are applicable to community assessment, for example, Roy's Adaptation Model, Orem's Self-Care Model, and Rogers' Unitary Man Model. (Refer to Chapter 3 for more discussion of these conceptual models and how they can be used to assess the community.)

An *epidemiology model* can be used to assess the community.    **Epidemiology** is the study of the occurrence, distribution, and causes of health and disease in mankind. Epidemiologic studies may analyze causes of acute or chronic health problems as well as health-related concerns such as spouse abuse and abortion. A scientific problem-solving approach is used in epidemiology.[9]

Clemen compared the nursing process directly to the epidemiologic process. In the assessment step, the investigators, nurses, physicians, statisticians, social workers, and people from other disciplines, seek data regarding factors that influence the development of the disease or health-related concern. They seek to determine characteristic signs and symptoms that occur during the progression of the problem. In addition, data concerning the people involved, the geographic distribution, and the chronological distribution of the problem are gathered. The body of knowledge gained through epidemiology serves as the basis for identifying health concerns, planning, and evaluating intervention programs aimed at primary, secondary, and tertiary health needs.[9]

If you are gathering data primarily to help identify health resources and needs for a particular individual or family, the authors suggest a tool that is organized according to Maslow's basic needs. The community assessment tool in Appendix H represents a compilation of numerous tools and input from the authors. An outline of the tool is included in Table 4–6.

Initially, you will need to identify the community being assessed, including the name of the community and its geographical boundaries. An overview of its historical development and dates of major events which affected the population's health should be noted. It is also important that you identify the sources of your information—interviews, census reports, books, and so forth.

**TABLE 4–6. OUTLINE OF COMMUNITY ASSESSMENT TOOL**

I. Identify Community to be Assessed
II. Sources of Community Data
III. History of Community Being Assessed
IV. Assessment of Needs of Community
   A. Physiologic needs
      1. Physical description of community
      2. Major concerns of community
   B. Safety/Security needs
      1. Physical safety
      2. Environmental safety
      3. Health services available
      4. Economic status of community
      5. Educational facilities available
      6. Governance
      7. Welfare agencies available

C. Love/Belonging needs
   1. Religions represented in community
   2. Religious leaders within community
   3. Community programs provided by religious groups
   4. Description of community population
D. Esteem/Recognition needs
   1. Communication patterns within community
   2. Recreational facilities available
E. Self-actualization needs
   1. Attitudes, values, and belief systems of community
   2. Goals of community
   3. Priorities of community

The *physiologic needs* of the community include data on climate, terrain, natural resources, and major concerns of the community. Answers to questions such as—what is the average temperature and precipitation? what natural resources exist? what is the crime rate? what percentage of the population is below the poverty level?—will provide important data.

*Safety and security needs* center around the need for protection. Assess the type and adequacy of the available protective services—ambulance, fire, hospital, police, social agencies. You should determine the style, type, size, and condition of the existing dwellings. Assess for environmental safety: What water sources are being used? What sewage disposal methods exist? How is solid waste handled? What forms of pollution are present? What measures are being used to eliminate the existing pollutants? The primary, secondary, and tertiary health care facilities should be noted. Discover the answers to such questions as: What are the health concerns that are prevalent in the community? Are there immunization programs available? Are there any prevalent social concerns that may affect the community's health? Assess the economic status of the community as well as the educational and transportation facilities. Determine the form of government that exists and who the key leaders are. Identify the welfare agencies that are available to the community population.

*Love and belonging needs* center around love and acceptance. The religious facilities that are available to the community's population should be noted. Identify the religious leaders of the community. Population characteristics including the number of people in the community, the age distribution, sex and race distribution, and the ethnic groups represented should be determined. You should determine: How has the population size changed during the past 10 years? Is the community urban, suburban, or rural? How mobile is the population?

*Esteem and recognition needs* can be assessed by determining the communication network of the community and the recreational facilities available to the community's population. Identifying the priorities and goals of the community and the attitudes, values, and belief systems projected by the community will help you to assess the *self-actualization needs*.

Each of these areas will provide data which will help you to obtain a total picture of the community. Remember, in order to achieve a complete community assessment, time and energy must be invested. You can collect some of the information by interviewing and observing but be sure to use the sources mentioned earlier: federal, state, and local agencies. These facilities, with the help of computers, can quickly provide you with accurate information.

## SUMMARY

This chapter has presented the first step in the nursing process—assessing. Assessing means the gathering, verifying, and communicating of data in a comprehensive and systematic manner. Communication skills are essential to this step. Through the effective use of these skills, you will be able to compile a pertinent data base.

The data base for the individual client is composed of information collected in the assessment interview, nursing health history, wellness assessment, and physical assessment. Information for the family's data base can be collected from the individual family member and the family unit by means of the well family assessment and family assessment tool. Personal observations and research, findings from the family and individual assessment, and federal, state, and local agencies all contribute to the total community assessment.

With this understanding of the first step in the nursing process, we can move on to the second step, diagnosing. In diagnosing, the data that were collected during assessing will be analyzed and conclusions concerning the health status and health needs of the client will be reached. From the conclusions, nursing diagnoses will be formulated.

## STUDY GUIDE

1. Interview a classmate using an assessment interview form of your choice. After completing the interview, analyze the interview for evidence of therapeutic and nontherapeutic communication techniques.
2. Compare two different nursing health history forms and identify their similarities and differences.
3. Select a client in a clinical setting and take a nursing health history using the form in Appendix B.
4. Obtain additional data about the client from secondary sources.
5. Select a client in a clinical setting and take a wellness assessment using the form in Appendix D. Identify potential health risks apparent in the data.

## REFERENCES

1. Ardell, D. The nature and implications of high level wellness, or why "normal health" is a rather sorry state of existence. *Health Values,* January/February 1979, *3*(1), 17–23.
2. Barker, L. L. *Listening behavior.* Englewood Cliffs, N.J.: Prentice-Hall, 1971.
3. Bates, B. *A guide to physical examination* (3rd ed.). Philadelphia: Lippincott, 1983.
4. Benjamin, A. *The helping interview* (3rd ed.). Boston: Houghton Mifflin, 1981.
5. Benne, K. D., & Sheats, P. Functional roles of group members. *Journal of Social Issues,* Spring 1948, *4,* 41.

6. Book, C. (Ed.). *Human communication: Principles, contexts, and skills.* New York: St. Martin's, 1980.
7. Carlson, R. *The nurse's guide to better communication.* Glenview, Ill.: Scott, Foresman, 1984.
8. Carnevali, D. L. *Nursing care planning: Diagnosis and management.* Philadelphia: Lippincott, 1983.
9. Clemen, S., Eigsti, D. G., & McGuire, S. *Comprehensive family and community health nursing.* New York: McGraw-Hill, 1981.
10. Dodd, M. Assessing mental status. *American Journal of Nursing,* September 1978, *78*(9), 1500–1503.
11. Dunn, H. *High level wellness.* Arlington, Va: R. W. Beatty, 1971.
12. Duvall, E. M. *Marriage and family development* (5th ed.). Philadelphia: Lippincott, 1977.
13. Eshleman, J. R. *The family: An introduction.* Boston: Allyn & Bacon, 1974.
14. Friedman, M. M. *Family nursing: Theory and assessment.* New York: Appleton-Century-Crofts, 1981.
15. Geitgey, D. SELF-PACING—A guide to nursing care. *Nursing Outlook,* August 1969, *17*(8), 48–49.
16. Hall, J., & Weaver, B. *Distributive nursing practice: A systems approach to community health.* Philadelphia: Lippincott, 1977.
17. Hays, J. S., & Larson, K. *Interacting with patients.* New York: Macmillan, 1963.
18. Helvie, C. O. *Community health nursing: Theory and process.* Philadelphia: Harper & Row, 1981.
19. Hopper, R., & Whitehead, J. *Communication concepts and skills.* New York: Harper & Row, 1971.
20. Jacox, A. Assessing pain. *American Journal of Nursing,* May 1979, *79*(5), 895–900.
21. Jones, D., Lepley, M. K., & Baker, B. *Health assessment across the life span.* New York: McGraw-Hill, 1984.
22. Kandzari, J., Howard, J., & Rock, M. *The well family: A developmental approach to assessment.* Boston: Little, Brown, 1981.
23. Klein, D. *Community dynamics and mental health.* New York: Wiley, 1968.
24. Komorita, N. Nursing diagnosis. *American Journal of Nursing,* December 1963, *63*(12), 83–86.
25. Little, D., & Carnevali, D. *Nursing care planning.* New York: Lippincott, 1976.
26. McCain, F. Nursing by assessment—not intuition. *American Journal of Nursing,* 1965, *65*(4), 82–84.
27. McCloskey, J. C., Larson, C. E., & Knapp, M. L. *An introduction to interpersonal communication.* Englewood Cliffs, N.J.: Prentice-Hall, 1971.
28. Meleis, A. Role insufficiency and role supplementation. *Nursing Research,* July/August 1975, *24*(4), 264–271.
29. Mills, E. P. *Listening: Key to communication.* New York: Petrocelli Books, 1974.
30. Mills, J., Aronson, E., & Robinson, H. Selectivity in exposure to information. *Journal of Abnormal and Social Psychology,* 1959, *59*, 250–253.
31. Murdock, G. P. *Social structure.* New York: Macmillan, 1949.
32. Murray, R. B., & Zentner, J. P. *Nursing concepts for health promotion* (3rd ed.). Englewood Cliffs, N.J.: Prentice-Hall, 1985.
33. Ogburn, W. F. The family and its function. In *Recent social trends in the United States.* New York: McGraw-Hill, 1933.
34. Parsons, T., & Bales, R. F. *Family socialization and interaction process.* New York: Free Press, 1955.
35. Pender, N. *Health promotion in nursing practice.* Norwalk, Conn.: Appleton-Century-Crofts, 1982.
36. Pilliteri, A. *Child health nursing: Care of the growing family* (2nd ed.). Boston: Little, Brown, 1981.
37. Pluckhan, M. L. *Human communication: The matrix of nursing.* New York: McGraw-Hill, 1978.

38. Satir, V. *Conjoint family therapy: A guide to theory and technique.* Palo Alto, Calif.: Science and Behavior Books, 1967.
39. Smith, M. J., Goodman, J.A., Ramsey, N. L., & Pasternack, S. B. *Child and family: Concepts of nursing practice.* New York: McGraw-Hill, 1982.
40. Smith, V., & Bass, T. *Communication for health professionals.* New York: Lippincott, 1979.
41. Sorensen, K., & Luckmann, J. *Basic nursing: A psychophysiologic approach.* Philadelphia: Saunders, 1979.
42. Spradley, B. W. *Community health nursing: Concepts and practice.* Boston: Little, Brown, 1981.
43. Stanhope, M., & Lancaster, J. *Community health nursing: Process and practice for promoting health.* St. Louis: C.V. Mosby, 1984.
44. Stano, M. E., & Reinsch, N. L. *Communication in interviews.* Englewood Cliffs, N.J.: Prentice-Hall, 1982.
45. Tulloch, J. W., & Healy, C. C. Changing lifestyles: A wellness approach. *Occupational Health Nursing,* June 1982, *30*(6), 13–21.
46. Urdang, L., & Swallow, H. H. (Eds.). *Mosby's medical and nursing dictionary.* St. Louis: C.V. Mosby, 1983.
47. Vickery, D. M. *Life plan for your health.* Reading, Mass.: Addison-Wesley, 1978.
48. Warren, R. I. *The community in America* (2nd ed.). Chicago: Rand McNally, 1972.
49. Whall, A. Nursing theory and the assessment of families. *Journal of Psychiatric Nursing and Mental Health,* January 1981, *19*(1), 30–36.
50. Weaver, C. H. *Human listening: Processes and behavior.* Indianapolis: Bobbs-Merrill, 1972.
51. Yurick, A. G., Spier, B. E., Robb, S. S., & Ebert, N. J. *The aged person and the nursing process* (2nd ed.). Norwalk, Conn.: Appleton-Century-Crofts, 1984.

## BIBLIOGRAPHY

Aiken, L., & Aiken, J. A systematic approach to the evaluation of interpersonal relationships. *American Journal of Nursing,* May 1973, *73*(5), 863–867.
Bishop, B. A guide to assessing parenting capabilities. *American Journal of Nursing,* November 1976, *76*(11), 1784–1787.
Blattner, B. *Holistic nursing.* Englewood Cliffs, N.J.: Prentice-Hall, 1981.
Burgess, W., & Ragland, E. C. *Community health nursing: Philosophy, process, practice.* Norwalk, Conn.: Appleton-Century-Crofts, 1983.
Claus, K., & Bailey, J. (Eds). *Living with stress and promoting well being: A handbook for nurses.* St. Louis: C.V. Mosby, 1980.
Ferholt, J. D. *Clinical assessment of children.* Philadelphia: Lippincott, 1980.
Flynn, P. A. R. *Holistic health: The art and science of care.* Englewood Cliffs, N.J.: Prentice-Hall, 1980.
Fromer, M. J. *Community health care and the nursing process* (2nd ed.). St. Louis: C.V. Mosby, 1983.
Getty, C., & Humphreys, W. *Understanding the family: Stress and change in American family life.* New York: Appleton-Century-Crofts, 1981.
Gordon, R. L. *Interviewing: Strategy, techniques and tactics* (3rd ed.). Homewood, Ill.: Dorsey Press, 1980.
Griffith, J., & Christensen, P. *Nursing process: Application of theories, frameworks, and models.* St. Louis: C.V. Mosby, 1982.
Holt, S., & Robinson, T. The school nurse's family assessment tool. *American Journal of Nursing,* May 1979, *79(5), 950–953.*
Jones, C. Glasgow coma scale. *American Journal of Nursing,* September 1979, *79*(9), 1551–1553.
King, C. Refining your assessment techniques. *RN,* February 1983, *46*(2), 42–47.
Mahoney, E. A., & Verdisco, L. *How to collect and record a health history* (2nd ed.). Philadelphia: Lippincott, 1982.

Marriner, A. *The nursing process: A scientific approach to nursing care* (3rd ed.). St. Louis: C.V. Mosby, 1983.

Mitchell, P. H., & Loustau, A. *Concepts basic to nursing* (3rd ed.). New York: McGraw-Hill, 1981.

Orem, D. *Nursing: Concepts of practice* (2nd ed.). New York: McGraw-Hill, 1980.

Sanders, I. T. *The community: An introduction to a social system* (2nd ed.). New York: Roland Press, 1966.

Sheahan, S. L. & Aaron, P. R. Community assessment: An essential component of practice. *Health Values: Achieving High Level Wellness,* September/October 1983, 7(5), 12–15.

Smith, C. With good assessment skills, you can construct a solid framework for patient care. *Nursing '84,* December 1984, *14*(12), 26–31.

Snyder, J. C., & Wilson, M. F. Elements of a psychological assessment. *American Journal of Nursing,* (February 1977), 77(2), 235–239.

Stoll, R. Guidelines for spiritual assessment. *American Journal of Nursing,* September 1979, 79(9), 1574–1577.

Thompson, J., & Bowers, A. *Clinical manual of health assessment.* St. Louis: C.V. Mosby, 1980.

Tinkham, C., Voorhies, E., & McCarthy, N. *Community health nursing: Evolution and process in the family and community* (3rd ed.). Norwalk, Conn.: Appleton-Century-Crofts, 1984.

Travis, J. W. *Wellness workbook for health professionals.* Mill Valley, Calif.: Wellness Associates, 1977.

# 5

# Nursing Process:
# Step II. Diagnosing

Diagnosing, the second step of the nursing process, is based on the data collected during assessing. In order to reach nursing diagnoses, you need to know and follow the diagnostic process. In this chapter we will begin with a historical review of the diagnostic process. We will then describe a diagnostic process composed of five steps: analyze data base; derive conclusion(s); assign diagnostic label(s) to conclusion(s); determine sustaining factor(s) for each conclusion; and formulate diagnostic statements. Each step will be discussed separately but as with the entire nursing process these steps cannot be considered to be independent of each other—they must be interdependent in order to make the step of diagnosing complete. The steps in the diagnostic process are appropriate whether the client is an individual, a family, or a community. Any difference that exists in the application of the step to the family or community client will be presented in Unit VII of the chapter. In addition to the discussion of the diagnostic process, a historical review of nursing diagnosis and the effect of nursing diagnoses on the nursing profession will be presented.

Study of this chapter will help you to:

1. Define diagnosing as it relates to the nursing process.
2. Describe the five steps in the diagnostic process discussed in this chapter.
3. Discuss the historical development of the nursing diagnosis.
4. Apply the diagnostic process to the individual, family, or community client.
5. Analyze data in a systematic, logical manner.
6. Describe how conclusions concerning the client's health status are derived.
7. Select an appropriate diagnostic label for each conclusion.
8. Identify sustaining factor(s) for each diagnostic label.
9. Formulate diagnostic statements composed of a diagnostic label and sustaining factor(s).
10. Discuss the effect of nursing diagnoses on the nursing profession.

A diagnosis is a statement of the conclusion(s) reached after analysis and examination of the nature of something. People in other professions and trades, such as physicians, social workers, teachers, and respiratory therapists, also diagnose. Social workers diagnose economic concerns of their clients; teachers diagnose learning difficulties in their students; physical therapists diagnose deficits in manual developmental skills; and nurses diagnose nursing needs of their clients. Differences in diagnoses arise from each practitioner's view of personal roles and responsibilities and from the knowledge necessary for the practice of each profession.

Generally speaking, in nursing a diagnosis is a clear, concise statement of the client's health status and concerns as derived from the analysis of the data from the assessment interview, nursing health history, wellness assessment, and physical assessment. For purposes of this text, a **nursing diagnosis** is a summary statement that reflects the client's healthy and unhealthy response(s) or potentially unhealthy response(s) and the sustaining factor(s) for each response. The sustaining factors are affected by interventions from the domain of nursing.

In order to help you put the current status of diagnosing into perspective, we will first discuss the historical aspect of the diagnostic process and the nursing diagnosis.

## HISTORICAL PERSPECTIVE

The aspect of diagnosing as it relates to medicine has been around for hundreds of years. Hippocrates taught physicians to observe, to keep accurate records, and to reason from facts—thus using the scientific method of solving problems and laying the foundation for the science of medicine. He described the influence of climate, soil, water, lifestyle, and nutrition on illness and emphasized the role of the environment in the spread of disease. Hippocrates believed that all of these factors were important and must be considered before an illness could be identified and treated. He followed a diagnostic process when he analyzed and examined available data before reaching a conclusion about the illness.

### Overview of Diagnostic Process

Since the days of Hippocrates, the diagnostic process has become more sophisticated. It is viewed as a dynamic process which is both systematic and flexible. The diagnostic process is composed of various steps to be followed by the investigator. These steps are designed to help the person analyze large quantities of data in the most productive manner.

As mentioned earlier, nurses are not the only people to use the diagnostic process. Other professions, as well as nursing, have proposed specific formats to be used when diagnosing. The formats vary from one discipline to another and even from one person to another within the same discipline. An overview of various diagnostic formats that are suggested in nursing literature is shown in Table 5–1. Even though these formats vary, they are all systematic and contain similar elements—data collection, organization of data, interpretation of data, and the formulation of conclusions. (It is interesting to note that the steps in the diagnostic process proposed by Chambers[6] in 1962 have slowly evolved into the steps in the nursing process.)

### Evolution of the Nursing Diagnosis

The term *diagnosis* was introduced into nursing literature years before it was acknowledged as a part of the nursing process. Initially, the literature implied that the nurse needed knowledge and skills that would ensure the diagnosis of medical problems. In-

**TABLE 5–1. VARIATION IN FORMAT FOR THE DIAGNOSTIC PROCESS**

| Chambers 1962[6] | Durand and Prince 1966[8] | Gordon 1976[15] |
|---|---|---|
| 1. Systematic collection of facts<br>2. Interpretation of facts in view of particular client<br>3. Identification of nursing problems<br>4. Determination of course of action<br>5. Evaluation of results in terms of observable client behavior | 1. Nursing investigation<br>2. Recognition of a pattern<br>3. Statement of a conclusion | 1. Collection of information<br>2. Interpretation of information<br>3. Clustering the information<br>4. Naming the cluster |

deed, nurses did diagnose for years with the emphasis on disease processes. The nurse was not academically prepared to function in this role but attempted to adapt to the expectations of society.

In 1953, Vera Fry used the term *nursing diagnosis* in an article for *American Journal of Nursing* and identified five areas of the client's needs on which the nursing diagnosis was based.[12] This was an important step in nursing. It introduced the idea that nurses were able to make a diagnosis based on the client's needs for nursing therapies, not medical therapies.

During the late 1950s and 1960s there was continuous debate and confusion over the use of the term *diagnosis* and its implied medical meaning. Because of this confusion, the terms *problems* and *needs* were used more frequently than diagnosis.[16]

In the 1950s, nursing leaders identified the need for consistency within the profession and the need to increase the quality of care through a comprehensive client-centered approach. To meet these needs, a classification of problems was proposed. In 1953, the Division of Nursing Resources of the United States Public Health Service initiated a study as the first step toward the development of such a classification. Nurses involved in this study identified "patient problems" which required nursing interventions. Because these problems required action from the nurse, the problems were soon termed "nursing problems." A second study was conducted from 1953 to 1955 in an effort to develop methods of identifying overt and covert nursing problems. From 1955 to 1958, a third study was conducted in cooperation with the National League for Nursing. The original list of nursing problems developed during 1953 was refined and compressed to 21 groups of common nursing problems. A list of nursing skills was also developed from which a classification of nursing treatments later evolved. These nursing problems and treatments were validated in 40 basic collegiate schools.[1] The list was quickly adopted by many schools of nursing as the framework for their curriculum and was soon known as "Abdellah's 21 problems" (Table 5–2).

Likewise, in 1961, Henderson described her concept of basic nursing.[18] She felt that the nurse must supply the client with what "he needs in knowledge, will, or strength to perform his daily activities." Henderson identified 14 activities or needs of the client that might require basic nursing care (Table 5–3). Neither one of these lists actually contained health problems or concerns of the client. They did serve to show nurses areas where actual or potential problems could occur.

Some progress in establishing the nursing diagnosis as a function and responsibility of the nurse was made in the 1960s. It was not until 1973 that two events occurred that helped to shape the future of diagnosing within the profession of nursing.

116

## TABLE 5–2. LIST OF 21 NURSING PROBLEMS

1. To maintain good hygiene and physical comfort.
2. To promote optimal activity; exercise, rest, and sleep.
3. To promote safety through prevention of accident, injury, or other trauma and through the prevention of the spread of infection.
4. To maintain good body mechanics and prevent and correct deformities.
5. To facilitate the maintenance of a supply of oxygen to all body cells.
6. To facilitate the maintenance of nutrition of all body cells.
7. To facilitate the maintenance of elimination.
8. To facilitate the maintenance of fluid and electrolyte balance.
9. To recognize the physiological responses of the body to disease conditions—pathological, physiological, and compensatory.
10. To facilitate the maintenance of regulatory mechanisms and functions.
11. To facilitate the maintenance of sensory function.
12. To identify and accept positive and negative expressions, feelings, and reactions.
13. To identify and accept the interrelatedness of emotions and organic illness.
14. To facilitate the maintenance of effective verbal and nonverbal communication.
15. To promote the development of productive interpersonal relationships.
16. To facilitate progress toward achievement of personal spiritual goals.
17. To create and/or maintain a therapeutic environment.
18. To facilitate awareness of self as an individual with varying physical, emotional, and developmental needs.
19. To accept the optimum possible goals in the light of limitations, physical and emotional.
20. To use community resources as an aid in resolving problems arising from illness.
21. To understand the role of social problems as influencing factors in the cause of illness.

*(Reprinted with permission from Abdellah F. G., Almeda M., Beland I. L., & Matheney R. V., Patient-centered approaches to nursing. © Copyright Macmillan Publishing Company, 1960.)*

## TABLE 5–3. LIST OF BASIC NEEDS OR ACTIVITIES

1. Breathe normally.
2. Eat and drink adequately.
3. Eliminate body wastes.
4. Move and maintain desirable posture.
5. Sleep and rest.
6. Select suitable clothes—dress and undress.
7. Maintain body temperature within normal range by adjusting clothing and modifying the environment.
8. Keep the body clean and well groomed and protect the integument.
9. Avoid dangers in the environment and avoid injuring others.
10. Communicate with others in expressing emotions, needs, and fears.
11. Worship according to one's faith.
12. Work in such a way that there is a sense of accomplishment.
13. Play, or participate in various forms of recreation.
14. Learn, discover, or satisfy the curiosity that leads to "normal" development and health and use the available health facilities.

*(Adapted with permission from the American Journal of Nursing, August, 1964, 64 (8), 62–68. Copyright © 1964, American Journal of Nursing Company.)*

First, the American Nurses' Association published the *Generic Standards of Nursing Practice* which included the nursing diagnosis as an important part of the nursing process and a function of the professional nurse. As a result of the publication, states began to include the term in their revised nurse practice acts.[5]

The second event occurring in 1973 was the first National Conference on Classification of Nursing Diagnoses. Faculty members at Saint Louis University School of Nursing and Allied Health Professions identified the need for the development and classification of diagnostic labels. Kristine Gebbie and Mary Ann Lavin were the leaders of the project. One hundred nurses from across the country participated in the First National Conference. Five additional National Conferences have been held since the fall of 1973.

One hundred nursing diagnoses were identified, but not adopted, at the first conference. In addition, a National Group for Classification of Nursing Diagnosis was established. The national group included a task force to plan succeeding conferences and to promote nursing activities in the area of diagnosing. The group also established a clearinghouse to act as a resource center for information on nursing diagnoses.[14]

The Second National Conference on Classification of Nursing Diagnoses was held in 1975. At this conference, 37 diagnoses were accepted and an additional 19 diagnoses were to be developed more completely. State and regional conference groups were formed; the major function of these groups was to generate, label, and implement nursing diagnoses.[13]

In 1978, a third national conference was held. Additional diagnoses were developed. In addition, the discussion of a conceptual framework for nursing diagnoses accelerated; the discussion had originated at the 1975 conference. At the end of the conference, a group of nurse theorists recommended that the conceptual framework of unitary man be adopted and that the term nursing diagnosis be redefined according to this framework. The recommendation was not adopted.[5]

The Fourth National Conference was held in 1980. At this conference, 42 nursing diagnoses were formally recognized. There was continued discussion on the adoption of a specific classification system and the use of unitary man as a theoretical framework for nursing diagnoses.[21]

In April 1982, the Fifth National Conference was held. K. Barnard, one of seven task force members who developed the 1980 American Nurses' Association *Social Policy Statement,* was the keynote speaker. The *Social Policy Statement* had given a major boost to the concept of diagnosing by including within its definition of nursing the function of diagnosing as an expectation of the professional nurse.

Several important issues were addressed at this conference. One main issue was the need for a classification system or taxonomy for nursing diagnoses. Standardization of nomenclature and classification of nursing diagnoses were seen as ways to facilitate communication, to allow for computer use and access of information, and to advance nursing theory, science, and education. Participants again discussed the acceptance of the unitary-man theoretical framework for the structure of the classification system. The group was still unable to reach a consensus concerning this topic and indicated that the framework needed additional theoretical development and clinical testing. A task force, which had been assigned to generate an initial taxonomy, presented a system that classified the existing National Conference list of nursing diagnoses according to four levels of abstraction. These levels of abstraction were then paralleled to nine patterns of unitary man proposed by the nurse theorists. (The unitary-man theoretical framework is discussed in Chapter 3.) The task force concluded that the taxonomy was only a beginning and many issues and questions remained unanswered.

Only eight new nursing diagnoses were approved at the Fifth National Conference. These diagnoses were accompanied by suggested etiologies and defining characteristics. Emphasis during the conference was on clarifying the existing diagnoses and determining their relationship to the unitary-man framework.

Another important event during the conference was the formation of the North American Nursing Diagnosis Association (NANDA). This organization was developed to continue the work initiated in 1973 by Gebbie and Lavin. Research, diagnosis review, and taxonomy development will be continued through the efforts of standing committees.[20]

The newly formed organization, NANDA, held the Sixth Conference on Classification of Nursing Diagnoses in April of 1984. Nearly 500 nurses, representing over 40 states and Canada, attended the conference. Unlike previous conferences, participant involvement in determining or approving new or modified nursing diagnoses did not exist. The conference participants were encouraged to develop new diagnoses or to modify existing nursing diagnoses and then share their findings with the Diagnostic Review Committee. Emphasis was given to the idea that nurses must be flexible and open in their approach to nursing diagnoses and to the development of a taxonomy for these diagnoses. Several regional nursing diagnosis organizations were represented at the conference. Although these organizations did not have formal ties with the NANDA organization, their memberships were developing and testing nursing diagnoses.

During the late 1970s and early 1980s, the influence of nursing diagnosis on education, practice, and research became more apparent. The use of nursing diagnosis as a

**TABLE 5–4. EVOLUTION OF THE DEFINITION: NURSING DIAGNOSIS**

| | |
|---|---|
| Fry (1953) | Nursing diagnosis is based on five areas of client's needs—"treatment and medication needs, personal needs, personal hygiene needs, environmental needs, guidance and teaching needs, human or self needs."[16] |
| Abdellah (1957) | "The determination of the nature and extent of nursing problems presented by the individual patients or families receiving nursing care."[1] |
| Chambers (1962) | " . . . an investigation of the facts to determine the nature of a nursing problem . . . limited to those activities legally interpreted as being within the province of the professional nurse."[6] |
| Komorita (1963) | " . . . involves discriminative judgment, based on a body of scientific knowledge, and is a process which provides nursing with a systematic way of assessing patient problems and needs."[22] |
| Durand and Prince (1966) | " . . . a statement of a conclusion resulting from a recognition of a pattern derived from a nursing investigation of the patient."[8] |
| Roy (1975) | " . . . the summary statement or judgment made by the nurse about the data she has gathered in her nursing assessment."[29] |
| Mundinger and Jauron (1975) | " . . . statement of a patient problem which is arrived at by making inferences from the collected data. The problem is one that can be alleviated by nursing intervention."[25] |
| Gordon (1976) | " . . . made by professional nurses, describe actual or potential health problems which nurses, by virtue of their education and experience, are capable and licensed to treat."[15] |
| Carlson, Craft, McQuire (1982) | " . . . statement of a potential or actual altered health status of a client(s) which is derived from nursing assessment and which requires intervention from the domain of nursing."[5] |
| Pinnell and de Meneses (1986) | "a summary statement that reflects the client's healthy/unhealthy response(s) or potentially unhealthy response(s) and the sustaining factor(s) for each response." |

part of the nursing process was included in the curriculum of schools of nursing and in continuing education programs. Inclusion of the concept of diagnosing in the education of nurses was reflected by changes that the nurses implemented in their clinical settings. Nursing care plans and chart forms were altered to include the aspect of nursing diagnosis. In addition, more articles and books on nursing diagnosis appeared in the nursing literature.

Table 5–4 shows how the definition of nursing diagnosis was expressed by various nurse–authors over a 20-year period. Many of the earlier authors actually described the diagnostic process instead of defining the term nursing diagnosis. Legal definitions of nursing diagnosis are found in nurse practice acts of most states. These definitions vary from state to state and implications associated with them change over time.

Now that we have a basic understanding of the evolution of the diagnostic process and nursing diagnosis, let us turn our attention to the five steps of the diagnostic process: analyze data base; derive conclusion(s); assign diagnostic label(s) to conclusion(s); determine sustaining factor(s) for each conclusion; formulate diagnostic statement(s) (Fig. 5–1).

It is recommended that initially you write out all of the steps in the diagnostic process. As your knowledge and skills increase, the act of diagnosing becomes easier, data analysis may become a mental exercise, and only diagnostic labels and sustaining factors need to be recorded.

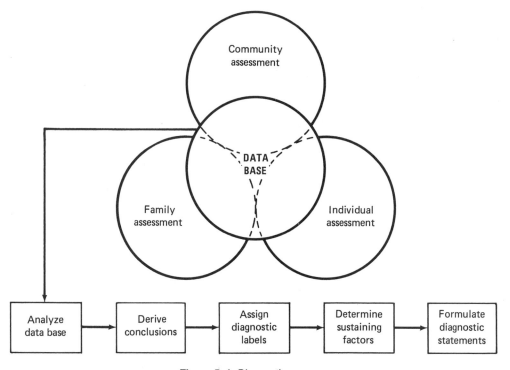

**Figure 5–1.** Diagnostic process.

## ANALYZE THE DATA BASE

The data base at this point is composed of the information from the assessment interview, nursing health history, wellness assessment, and physical assessment. This information must now be analyzed. Analysis of data allows you to organize, separate relevant from irrelevant information, identify inconsistencies and omissions, establish patterns within the data, and compare the data with norms, standards, and theories (Fig. 5–2).

The idea of analyzing data to determine health concerns of the client is not new. Komorita described a systematic approach to data analysis in 1963.[22] As the nurse's knowledge base grew with the advances in the field of nursing and medicine, the process of analyzing has become more complicated.

**Analysis** literally means to dissect, to pull apart, to examine each component of the whole separately in order to better understand the whole and to identify inconsistencies and gaps. You should examine each piece of assessed data, interpret it, and then compile the data in an organized, meaningful manner. Critical thinking, problem solving, and decision making must be used to determine what are essential data and how to use the data productively. (Refer to Chapters 2 and 11 for more discussion on the problem-solving and decision-making processes.) As with other parts of the nursing process, data analysis is influenced by your background knowledge and your nursing experiences. In addition, your values and beliefs will affect data perception. You must therefore strive for objectivity to ensure accuracy of data interpretation.

The data are analyzed for indications of the client's level of health and health needs. For the individual and family, you will be analyzing data specifically for three levels of health needs: primary, secondary, and tertiary. **Primary health needs** are related to the management of normal growth and developmental changes; to health promotion and wellness aspects; and for assistance with self-care management of minor or controlled health disruptions. **Secondary health needs** require specialized attention during an episode of illness or injury. The episode is either resolved or becomes a long-term health concern. **Tertiary health needs** are related to the concerns of a health condition of an ongoing nature.

Strengths, assets, abilities, weaknesses, and liabilities, as well as healthy and unhealthy responses, are considered. Using the approach that considers both healthy and unhealthy responses prevents you from identifying only *problems*. Instead, it allows the identification of nursing diagnoses that stress maintenance of health and that support positive, healthy responses.

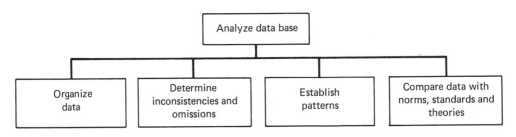

**Figure 5–2.** Analyze data base.

Now that we have discussed some of the general aspects of data analysis, we will consider the separate components of this step.

## Organize Data

As the data base is analyzed, it is organized, grouped, or sorted in a logical, systematic way. Data may be organized or categorized according to the structure of conceptual models or frameworks, basic needs, body systems or developmental stages, or tasks.

There is no one method of data organization that is the best. You will probably decide to use the conceptual model, theoretical framework, or other organizational structure that is most familiar to you. Remember that not all methods are adaptable to every clinical setting. In some instances, because of time restraints, you may elect to use the quickest and simplest method to organize data. In other situations, you may chose a more sophisticated but lengthier method.

The following two examples of data organization according to Orem's self-care theoretical framework and the basic needs approach will demonstrate this step.

*Examples of Organizing Data.* Dorothea Orem views nursing as a special type of health care service based on the values of self-help and help to others. Her concept of nursing was first published in 1959 and a more formalized development of her model was initiated in 1965. This model, which is still used in nursing service and nursing education, states that the focus of nursing is to help the individual achieve health through therapeutic self-care. (For more information on Orem's theoretical framework, refer to Chapter 3.)

Orem defines self-care as the practice of activities that individuals personally initiate and perform on their own behalf in maintaining life, health, and well-being. To engage in self-care activities, the person must have the ability and skills to initiate and sustain self-care efforts as well as the knowledge and understanding of self-care practices and their relationship to health and disease.[26,27]

The practical application of Orem's theory to the organization of data can be illustrated by the following:

G. K., a 26-year-old, married, male Caucasian, lived with his wife and three children. He was employed; his employment required him to service typewriters and laboratory equipment. He had two brothers and one sister who were living and well. Both parents died of cancer. His admitting medical diagnosis was acromegaly, posthypophysectomy of 1 year with resultant adrenal insufficiency and diabetes insipidus. At the time of the assessment interview and nursing health history, Mr. K. indicated that it was difficult for him to recall some of his pre-illness living patterns. He attributed this problem to his long periods of hospitalizations and to the fact that his illness had affected his activities for at least 1 year prior to his condition being diagnosed. He was quite informed about his surgery and his most recent health problems created by the surgery. He used complex medical terms correctly, and he accurately described his illness and surgery, recalling dates, medications, and physicians.

### Fluid and Food Intake

Prior to surgery, Mr. K. ate three meals daily. Breakfast consisted of cereal, fruit or fruit juice, eggs, toast, and two 12-ounce glasses of milk. Meat, potatoes, vegetable, dessert, iced tea, and two glasses of milk usually constituted his noon and evening meal. During the day, he did not snack; but in the evening, he usually drank two 16-ounce sodas. Since his surgery, he had experienced a decreased appetite. He had an increased preference for sweets and a decreased intake of solid foods. He had been placed on a 2 g NaC1, 60 g protein diet by the physician.

### Sleep and Rest Habits
Prior to surgery, Mr. K. required at least 8 hours of sleep every night. After his evening meal, he would frequently nap for 30 minutes. Since his surgery, he had experienced "excessive fatigue" and a need for more frequent naps. Recently, he had been awake every 1 to 2 hours during the night to void.

### Elimination
Prior to surgery, Mr. K. had a daily bowel movement and urinated aproximately four to five times daily. His urinary output had increased during the last 2 months, and he voided at least every 2 hours.

### Physical Assessment
Mr. K.'s speech was clear and distinct. He was alert and talkative throughout the assessment interview. Mr. K. weighed 92.5 kilograms and was 193 centimeters tall. He had many of the physical changes associated with acromegaly: thickened and lengthened mandible, protrusion of the lower jaw, enlarged tongue, enlarged nose, thickened lips, deepened voice, enlarged thoracic cage, enlarged hands and feet. (Mr. K. indicated that his ring size had increased three sizes in the past 3 years.) He showed signs of muscle wasting and weakness. His skin was dry, pale, and coarse; his hair and nails were dry and brittle. He had experienced visual problems with his right eye since surgery; he complained of diplopia (double vision) and light sensitivity.

### Diagnostic Findings
His serum potassium was 3.4 mEq/L; his serum chloride was 91 mEq/L. His chest film and electrocardiogram were within normal limits. His urine specific gravity was 1.000.

To initiate this step in data analysis, you would organize your data in terms of Orem's theoretical framework (Table 5–5). You would then look at these data to (1) determine if the client needs nursing assistance, (2) design a plan of assistance, and (3) initiate, conduct, and direct actions to achieve the client's goals.

If these data are organized according to basic needs, such categories as physiologic, psychological, sociocultural, spiritual, nutritional, and financial are used (Table 5–6).

Organization of the family and community data base differs from the organization of data for the individual client; these differences are discussed later in this chapter. Once the data concerning the individual, family, or community have been organized, you should review data to determine inconsistencies and patterns within the data and to compare the finding with norms, standards, and theories.

## Determine Inconsistencies Within Data
Once data have been appropriately organized or categorized, they must be reviewed for inconsistencies. The word "inconsistent" can be applied to information that is contradictory or illogical. It also refers to a lack of uniformity in content, for example, when two or more accounts of a single event differ in important details. Gordon also states that inconsistencies arise when the nurse's expectations are not what is actually assessed.[16] The nurse's expectations are formed as a result of educational background and work experiences.

To determine inconsistencies within data, you ask yourself how your present observations compare or contrast with those made previously by other health team members. Are there contradictory or illogical data? Did the client tell one health care provider one version of his health problem and another version to another health team member? Did the client identify different concerns, strengths, or weaknesses for various team members?

**TABLE 5–5. ORGANIZATION OF DATA USING OREM'S THEORETICAL FRAMEWORK[26,27]**

| Assessment and Nursing Diagnosis Guidelines Based on Orem's Theoretical Framework | Information from Client's Data Base |
|---|---|
| **A. Therapeutic self-care** | |
| 1. *Universal self-care* | |
| a. Air, water, food | Three balanced meals a day. At least 3000 cc fluids daily. Decreased appetite since surgery Increased fluid intake. Special diet ordered |
| b. Excrements | Daily bowel movement Increased urinary output Urine specific gravity 1.000 |
| c. Activity and rest | 8 hours of sleep needed. Naps after supper Increased need for rest since surgery |
| d. Solitude and social interaction | Frequent and long hospitalizations. Employed |
| e. Hazards to life and well-being | Fatigue, weakness, muscle wasting |
| 2. *Health-deviation self-care* | |
| a. Changes in human structure (disease derived) | Multiple physical changes (large hands, feet, etc.) Increased urinary output and need for rest |
| b. Changes in physical functioning (medically derived) | Data not known at present* |
| **B. Self-care agency** | |
| 1. *Knowledge* | |
| a. Knowledge about physical and social environment | Used complex medical terms; could recall past medical–surgical therapies |
| b. Knowledge about self-care goals and practices | Balanced meals, adequate rest patterns before illness |
| c. Knowledge about scientifically derived health information | Used complex medical terms |
| 2. *Skills* | |
| a. Skills in utilizing available resources | Data not known at present* |
| b. Skills in interaction with others | Communicated easily with nurse |
| c. Skills in activities of daily living | Employed; works with hands servicing equipment |
| 3. *Motivation* | |
| a. Psychologic maturity | Married |
| b. Self-concept | Data not known at present* |
| 4. *Orientation* | |
| a. Culturally derived roles and practices | Data not known at present* |
| b. Placement in family | Husband, father, sibling |
| c. Membership in social groups | Data not known at present* |
| d. Developmental maturity | Married, employed, father |
| **C. Self-care deficits** | |
| 1. *Knowledge deficits* | Difficulty recalling preillness patterns |
| 2. *Skills deficits* | Data not known at present* |
| 3. *Motivation deficits* | Data not known at present* |
| 4. *Orientation deficits* | Oriented, alert |

*Any area with incomplete data would require further assessment before accurate interpretation could be achieved.

Some slight degree of inconsistency can be expected when more than one person has contributed to the data base. There may have been actual changes in the client's health status in the interim between assessments, one nurse's assessment skills may have been more sophisticated than those of another nurse, or perhaps the client's level of recall was different during the two periods of contact. These inconsistencies should be minor; major or glaring inconsistencies are not expected and must be investigated.

**TABLE 5–6. ORGANIZATION OF DATA USING BASIC NEEDS APPROACH**

| Physiological | Social |
|---|---|
| Many physical changes | Married |
| Weak: easily fatigued | Three children |
| Required increased rest and sleep | Recent long periods in hospitals |
| Increased urinary output | Requires more sleep and rest |
| Serum potassium 3.4 mEq/L | Many physical changes |
| Serum chloride 91 mEq/L | **Spiritual** |
| Urine specific gravity 1.000 | No data |
| Alert | **Nutritional** |
| **Psychological** | Balanced meals prior to surgery |
| Some difficulty recalling preillness living | Decreased appetite |
| patterns | Increased fluid intake |
| Clear, accurate description of medical problem | 2 g NaC1, 60 g protein diet |
| Many physical changes | |
| Recent long hospitalizations | |
| **Cultural** | |
| No data | |

Inconsistencies can also arise when verbal data given by the client are misunderstood or incorrectly recorded. There may be inattentive listening or selective inattention on the part of the nurse during the assessment interview and health history. In this situation, the nurse selects what to hear during the process of data collection and discards the rest.[28] In either case, the nurse must review the technique for collecting data and validate the information more carefully with the client.

Inconsistencies can also arise if the person giving the information is not reliable. Perhaps the client's physical or mental status prevents the collection of clear, accurate information or perhaps the family's level of anxiety is so high that accuracy is not possible. When the reliability of the data source is questioned, you should seek validation through other sources.

During this step you must also analyze data for gaps, omissions, or incomplete information. Obtaining missing data is necessary before patterns can be determined. When omissions are found, further assessment is needed. Necessary data may be gathered at this point in the diagnostic process or, if this is not possible, they may be added later.

Referring back to the analysis of data utilizing Orem's theoretical framework (see Table 5–5), it is apparent that many gaps and omissions exist. How have the physical changes produced by the client's medical disease affected self-concept? Do these changes interfere with the client's ability to perform the manual skills required by employment? What social activities did the client participate in prior to illness? Have these activities changed since the illness?

## Establish Patterns within Data

The data base, both objective and subjective information, must be examined to determine if the client's behavior is an isolated incident or a regularly occurring response. Does the individual react negatively to all attempts at health teaching or just to teaching concerning the new medical diagnosis of diabetes insipidus? Does the family continue to function effectively under most stressful situations?

Data are also analyzed to determine if the response appears in more than one category—thus making the result of the response more supportive or more detrimental to the client's well-being. At this point, ask yourself questions to determine the relationships between facts. Could the client's decrease in appetite be related to psychological factors such as depression or anxiety? Is the family's role disturbance related to the recent death of a family member? Gradually, your thought processes draw these facts into a pattern.

To illustrate this point, examine the data base presented earlier and organized according to basic needs (see Table 5–6). It becomes apparent that some patterns do exist. Notations concerning the client's physical changes appear under the physiologic, psychological, social, and economic categories. The client did not actually voice concerns about his appearance or how these changes did or did not affect his social, family, or economic status. Relying on theoretical knowledge concerning self-concept and body image, you might ask if G. K.'s body image is altered. If so, does this altered body image affect his social or family life? You might also ask if his enlarged hands have decreased his manual skills, thus threatening his economic status. For these reasons, data should be listed under more than the one category, physiologic. Analyzing the data at this point, you would realize that the one aspect, physical changes, may be a major concern for the client and requires further investigation.

Do not approach this step in data analysis in an unorganized manner. Data must be examined carefully, using professional judgment and decision-making skills. Using such an approach will enable you to discover patterns of responses or patterns of concern within data.

## Compare Data with Norms, Standards, and Theories

It is during this step that comparisons are made between the collected data and norms, standards, and theories. Developmental, physiologic, and psychological norms and values applicable to nursing can be drawn from such sciences as psychology, sociology, anthropology, anatomy, physiology, pathology, and bacteriology. Formal education in these sciences serves to form your background knowledge. Regular referral to current literature will keep you informed of new findings.

Scientific knowledge is reinforced and expanded by clinical experience. In addition, feel free to consult resource people, such as other members of the health team, that is, other nurses, dietitians, social workers, and physical therapists. These people may provide additional comparative data.

The findings of the physical assessment, assessment interview, wellness assessment, nursing health history, family assessment, and community assessment serve as bases for the comparison. Organized data are compared to standards such as normal ranges of vital signs, laboratory values, nutritional requirements, and height and weight charts. For many of these standards and norms, you must make certain that data are compared with the appropriate norms for the client's age, sex, height, or other measurements. For example, a 26-year-old male who is of medium frame and 193 centimeters tall should weigh between 78 and 86 kilograms; a 26-year-old male who is of large frame and 193 centimeters tall should weigh between 84 and 93 kilograms. Developmental status, role function, family patterns, family characteristics, community structure, community function, communication patterns, and reaction to stress are examples of other assessed data that can be compared to norms and theories found in literature. (Refer to Chapter 4 and the earlier portion of this chapter for discussion of family and community structure, role, and function. Also, refer to the Bibliography at the end of this chapter for readings concerning the various theories.)

While comparing data with norms, standards, and theories, be careful not to misinterpret the findings. It is important to remember that although literature can provide you with what is considered normal or expected, you must not overlook the individuality or uniqueness of the individual, family, or community. One way to prevent the client from becoming lost in the maze of quoted norms and standards is to clarify the client's self-perception of normal. Compare the assessed data with the client's standards for optimal physical, mental, and emotional functioning. How does the client define health? What is the client's self-regard? What was the client's self-regard 6 months ago? What is the client's self-regard now? How does the family unit feel about itself? Does the family unit perceive itself as "different" from other families? How does the community see itself?

To illustrate the aspect of comparing data, again refer to the analysis of data utilizing Orem's theoretical framework (see Table 5–5). It is apparent that not all of the data are "normal." The client's physical changes are not within the norms. His need for increased rest and sleep is not compatible with the developmental expectations of this age group; his urine specific gravity is decreased, and he has low serum potassium and chloride levels. His weight is within the normal range for his height and body frame. He is meeting some of his developmental tasks in that he is married, a father, and employed. He has also demonstrated the ability to use manual, intellectual, and communication skills. Even in this brief comparison, you have considered several norms—laboratory values, height and weight norms, growth and development expectations.

This step, analyze data base, allows you to organize data, to separate relevant from irrelevant information, to identify inconsistencies and omissions, to establish patterns within data, and to compare data with norms, standards, and theories. Initially, to help clarify and reinforce this step, you will need to write down all or portions of the process. With this step completed, you are ready to derive conclusions concerning the individual's or family's health status and the concerns of the community.

## DERIVE CONCLUSIONS

Deriving conclusions, a part of data analysis, requires a high level of cognitive functioning. The cognitive processes discussed in Chapter 2, synthesis, inductive reasoning, and deductive reasoning, are especially important to the success or failure of this step.

Up to this point, the data base has been analyzed—each fact examined separately. It is now time to synthesize the information—to pull it together and integrate it so that conclusions or inferences can be reached. Synthesizing will also help you to establish the patterns that were suggested in the first step in the diagnostic process.

After data have been synthesized, inferences or conclusions concerning the client's health status are reached through inductive and deductive reasoning processes. You will recall that **inductive reasoning** or **thinking** proceeds from particular facts to a general conclusion while **deductive reasoning** or **thinking** proceeds from general to specific.

The diagnostic process represents inductive reasoning. For instance, you are caring for Mr. J., a 71-year-old who is on bed rest and cannot turn himself without help; you conclude that the client will be prone to skin breakdown. You used inductive reasoning to reach your conclusion. When you apply general principles in a theoretical framework to a specific client, you are using deductive reasoning.

## Formulate Conclusion(s) Concerning Health Status

Because you are concerned with *all* of the responses of the individual, family, and community, conclusions containing healthy as well as unhealthy responses will be made. Conclusions, which are generalizations or summary statements, should reflect the client's health status and the locus of decision making in the nurse–client interaction. By locus of decision making, we mean that decisions regarding health management rest with the client, the client and nurse, or the nurse. When the client is demonstrating healthy responses that require minimal supportive action from the nurse, the client makes the decisions regarding health management. When the client is demonstrating responses, healthy or unhealthy, that require some degree of supportive action from the nurse, the decision-making process regarding health management is shared by the client and nurse. If the client is demonstrating only unhealthy responses that require supportive action from the nurse, the nurse makes the decisions regarding health management.

## Conclusions Involving the Individual

The following are examples of conclusions that may be reached concerning the individual's health status:

1. Only healthy responses are evident; minimal supportive actions are needed from the nurse.
2. Only healthy responses are evident; supportive action from the nurse is needed to assist the individual to sustain these responses.
3. Healthy and potentially unhealthy responses are evident; present coping mechanisms are effective and no supportive action is needed from the nurse.
4. Healthy and potentially unhealthy responses are evident; present coping mechanisms are not effective and supportive action is needed from the nurse.
5. Healthy and unhealthy responses are evident; present coping mechanisms are effective and no supportive action is needed from the nurse.
6. Healthy and unhealthy responses are evident; present coping mechanisms are not effective and supportive action is needed from the nurse.
7. Only unhealthy responses are evident; supportive action must be given by the nurse.

These seven conclusions are not meant to reflect all the possible conclusions that exist. Responses can occur in varying degrees and some overlap of conclusions may exist. Do not force the data to conform to a standardized set of conclusions; use the list as a guide and adapt the conclusion to the data.

Conclusions one, three, and five require no supportive action from the nurse, and, therefore, the decisions concerning health management should rest with the individual client. Conclusion two requires supportive action from the nurse to help the individual client sustain healthy responses. In this case, decisions concerning health management are shared by the individual client and nurse. Usually the nurse would make the decisions regarding health management for the remaining conclusions since the individual client's coping mechanisms are not effective or only unhealthy responses exist.

Conclusions related to the family and community will be discussed later in this chapter. Once conclusions have been reached, conclusions are assigned a diagnostic label.

## ASSIGN DIAGNOSTIC LABELS TO CONCLUSIONS

While the conclusion represents a summary statement, the diagnostic label and eventual diagnostic statement are more specific. You may decide to use standardized labels; for instance, those labels developed by the National Conference on Classification of Nursing Diagnoses, Lunney, Shortridge and Lee, or Campbell[4,20,23,30] (Table 5–7).

To help you to select the most appropriate standardized diagnostic label, the National Conference on Classification of Nursing Diagnoses has established etiologies and defining characteristics. For example, etiologies for the diagnostic label *Anxiety* include: threat to self-concept, threat to or change in role functioning, situational and maturational crises, and unmet needs. The defining characteristics include: apprehension, uncertainty, shakiness, overexcitedness, restlessness, poor eye contact, facial tension, increased perspiration, and trembling or hand tremors. If we consider a diagnostic label involving the family—*Alteration in Family Process*—the etiologies include: situation transition, and/or crisis and development transition, and/or crisis. The defining characteristics include: family system unable to meet physical needs for its members, inability to express and accept feelings of members, inability of family members to relate to each other for mutual growth and maturation, rigidity in function and roles.[20]

These etiologies and defining characteristics will help you to select appropriate diagnostic labels. Do not feel restricted by standardized diagnostic labels. Instead, use the labels as a guide to assist in the development of individualized labels that may be better suited to your particular situation. Remember that most standardized labels do not recognize healthy responses from the individual, family, or community and therefore may not be helpful when forming this type of diagnostic label. Diagnostic labels that reflect

**TABLE 5–7. STANDARDIZED DIAGNOSTIC LABELS**

| National Conference on Classification of Nursing Diagnoses*[20] | Shortridge and Lee (1980) |
| --- | --- |
| Activity intolerance | Disruption of the integument |
| | Inadequate activity |
| Activity intolerance, potential | Alterations in sleep patterns |
| | Pain |
| Anxiety | Increased susceptibility to injury |
| | Increased susceptibility to infection |
| Family process, alteration in | Respiratory insufficiency |
| | Circulatory insufficiency |
| Fluid volume, alteration in: excess | Inadequate nutrition |
| | Inadequate elimination |
| Health maintenance, alteration in | Alterations in temperature |
| | Alterations in sensory perception |
| Oral mucous membrane, alteration in | Changes in sexual function |
| | Anxiety |
| Powerlessness | Depression |
| | Anger and hostility |
| Social isolation | Alterations in thought processes |
| | Alterations in family dynamics |
| | Inadequate community health practices |
| | Grieving |

*This table contains only those diagnostic labels accepted at the Fifth National Conference. See Appendix I for a complete list of the diagnostic labels approved by the National Conference on Classification of Nursing Diagnoses.
*(From Shortridge, L. & Lee, E., Introduction to nursing practice. New York: McGraw-Hill, 1980, with permission.)*

healthy responses from the client do not negate the need for nursing interventions. You will want to support, promote, or maintain these responses.

Conclusions concerning healthy responses of clients that require little if any supportive action from the nurse should have diagnostic labels that reflect **maintenance, preservation, or protection** of the existing health status. Examples of this type of diagnostic label are: maintenance of effective coping patterns, maintenance of parent–infant bonding, and maintenance of the support system.

Some healthy responses do not lend themselves to diagnostic labels. Griffith suggests that these responses be considered strengths and assets of the individual, family, or community and that they should be listed with the conclusions.[17] These strengths would be used when planning nursing interventions and might include such aspects as adequate finances, adequate housing arrangements, low levels of environmental stress, and knowledge and acceptance of health status.

Diagnostic labels for conclusions concerning potentially unhealthy responses should reflect that potential state. **Potential** implies that the client may develop unhealthly responses unless the nurse intervenes. Identification of potential areas of concern frequently stems from the nurse's prior experiences. In addition, the term can be assigned in areas where there is evidence of previous unhealthy responses. For instance, if the health history indicated that your surgical client had developed pneumonia during the last postoperative period, you might conclude that pneumonia may develop during the current postoperative period. An appropriate diagnostic label would be: potential respiratory insufficiency. Other examples of this type of diagnostic label are: potential fluid imbalance, potential altered parenting, and potential mismanagement of care at home.

Diagnostic labels for conclusions concerning unhealthy responses that are supported by existing assessed data are classified as **actual.** If data are not complete enough for a definite conclusion, they are classified as **probable.** Probable implies that more data are needed; the conclusion should be written in the form of a conjecture and the diagnostic label must reflect this state of uncertainty. Actual and probable diagnostic labels are stated: threat to self-esteem (probable), interruption in play activity (actual), impaired skin integrity (actual), nonacceptance of developmental tasks (probable), and lack of preventive health care (actual).

To help clarify the diagnostic process up to this point, look at Table 5–8. This table illustrates the synthesizing of data, the designating of conclusions, and the assigning of diagnostic labels.

At this point in the diagnostic process, we have discussed the first three steps: analyze data base, derive conclusions, and assign diagnostic labels. We now need to determine what factors are contributing to the conclusions that we have reached.

## DETERMINE SUSTAINING FACTORS

**Sustaining factors** are those contributory elements that cause or perpetuate the response(s) designated by the diagnostic label. They are usually determined by a reanalysis of the assessed data. The same data base that supplied the needed information for conclusions concerning the client's health status should also give you clues as to the sustaining factors of those responses.

In some instances, it may be difficult to identify definite sustaining factors for each diagnostic label. In that case, you should state possible factors that have been *suggested* by the data. If, after working with the client longer, new data support other sustaining

**TABLE 5–8. DEVELOPMENT OF DIAGNOSTIC LABELS FROM DATA BASE**

| Data Base | Conclusions | Diagnostic Labels |
|---|---|---|
| Medical diagnosis: Small bowel bypass 9 months ago for obesity | | |
| 38 year old, white female<br>Married<br>Housewife<br>Four children | Healthy responses evident in the area of developmental tasks of young adult; supportive action from the nurse not needed at this point | Maintenance of developmental task of intimacy |
| Frequent visits from family<br>Cards and flowers in room<br>Mother, father, one sister are obese<br>Frequent phone calls<br>Ht 5'1" (153.75 cm) | Healthy responses evident in the area of support systems; action from the nurse may be needed to assist individual to sustain these responses | Maintenance of active support system |
| Wt 198 lbs (90 kilograms). Was 255 lbs–115.9 kilograms before surgery<br>Referred to herself as "us fat people" | Unhealthy responses evident in the area of self-concept; supportive action needed from the nurse | *Disturbance in self-concept (actual) |
| Consumes 2500 calories daily<br>Eats many small meals throughout day<br>States she eats more now than before surgery | Unhealthy responses evident in the area of nutritional needs; supportive action needed from the nurse | *Alteration in nutrition: more than body requirements (actual)<br><br>*Probable knowledge deficit concerning nutritional needs |
| Does not take medication as prescribed (potassium, calcium, magnesium)<br>Did not keep follow-up appointments | Unhealthy responses evident in the area of health maintenance; supportive action needed from the nurse. | *Health maintenance alteration (actual) |

*Diagnostic labels from National Conference on Classification of Nursing Diagnoses.[20]

factors, you restate the diagnosis to correlate with the new findings. It is possible that one sustaining factor may be related to several diagnostic labels. It is also possible that the diagnostic label may become a sustaining factor and vice versa. For example, the diagnostic label "Fear" may also be the sustaining factor for "Impaired Verbal Communication."

Analysis of the data base may not even reveal possible sustaining factors or the factors may be too complex to be stated in a brief phrase. Do not feel constrained by a diagnostic format requiring the inclusion of sustaining factors. List the diagnostic label only, alerting everyone to the conclusions previously reached concerning the client's health status.

A universally accepted format for stating the sustaining factor of the nursing diagnosis does not exist; some general guidelines, however, can be identified. These same considerations are applicable to the entire diagnostic statement and will be discussed in the next section. Table 5–9 illustrates the steps in determining sustaining factors.

**TABLE 5–9. IDENTIFICATION OF SUSTAINING FACTORS**

| Data Base | Diagnostic Labels | Sustaining Factors |
|---|---|---|
| Frequent visits from family<br>Cards and flowers in hospital room<br>Frequent phone calls | Maintenance of active support system | (Complex factors not stated) |
| Ht 153.75 cm<br>Wt 90 kilograms<br>Consumes 2500 calories daily<br>Eats many small meals per day<br>Eats more now than before surgery | Alteration in nutrition: more than body requirements (actual) | Inappropriate eating patterns<br><br>Excessive caloric intake |
| Does not take prescribed electrolyte replacements | Potential electrolyte imbalance | Failure to take prescribed medications |
| Did not keep follow-up appointments after surgery | Health maintenance alteration (actual) | Possible lack of knowledge concerning need for medical management |

After completing the first four steps of the diagnostic process, we have all of the information necessary to formulate the diagnostic statement: the nursing diagnosis.

## FORMULATE DIAGNOSTIC STATEMENT

It is appropriate at this point to restate the definition for nursing diagnosis. A **nursing diagnosis** is a summary statement that reflects the client's healthy and unhealthy response(s) or potentially unhealthy response(s) and the sustaining factor(s) for each response. A nursing diagnosis reflects responses to or effects of the health condition on the individual or family. The diagnosis can also reflect factors that affect or have the potential for affecting the attainment and maintenance of optimal wellness. Nursing diagnoses about the community might incorporate health needs that exist; health needs that are or are not being met; community dynamics which influence health action; and deficiencies in the existing health care delivery system.

A nursing diagnosis differs from a medical diagnosis. The medical diagnosis does not consider responses from the individual, family, or community but focuses on the disease, the progression of the disease, and the treatment of the pathology. For instance, the physician will diagnose and treat someone for diabetes mellitus. The nurse will diagnose and treat the individual's and family's response to the disease process: Will lifestyle changes be necessary? Is menu planning a problem? Does the client understand the reason for insulin injections?

Although nursing and medical diagnoses are different, they are both reached by use of the diagnostic process. Both you and the physician must have assessment and interview skills and a strong theoretical background. Basically, you and the physician have the same overall goal; you are both interested in improving the client's level of health and assisting the client to return to optimal wellness. For these reasons, neither health care provider should try to function independently of the other. You, as the nurse, can and do make independent nursing diagnoses that require independent nursing therapies, but many nursing therapies are dependent on the physician's diagnostic workup and written orders. All health care disciplines must function together in order to provide holistic care for the client.

## Format for Stating Nursing Diagnoses

As indicated by the definition, the nursing diagnosis is a two-part statement. The first part of the diagnosis consists of the diagnostic label. Only one diagnostic label is addressed in each nursing diagnosis. The second part of the diagnosis consists of the sustaining factor(s) that contributed to or are sustaining the responses. More than one sustaining factor may be present in the diagnostic statement.

The two parts of the diagnosis are joined or connected by "related to" or "associated with" clauses. "Due to" or "caused by" are not used; these expressions imply a direct cause and effect relationship that might be difficult to establish with certainty.[25]

To illustrate the formation of the two-part diagnostic statement, refer to the diagnostic labels and sustaining factors shown in Table 5–9. Nursing diagnoses stemming from this information would be stated:

- Alteration in nutrition: more than body requirements related to inappropriate eating patterns and excessive caloric intake.
- Potential electrolyte imbalance related to failure to take prescribed medications.
- Health maintenance alteration related to possible lack of knowledge concerning the importance of medical management.
- Maintenance of active support system.

The completed nursing diagnoses need to be evaluated and redefined periodically. One or both parts of the diagnostic statement may require change as the data base for the client changes—this change may be needed days after the original diagnosis was made or within minutes. Changes are made in the diagnoses to indicate significant responses that the client has made concerning personal health care and to give a more accurate picture of the client. When new diagnoses reflect a positive change by the client, the change can serve as a motivating factor for both the client and nurse. Do not be tempted to wait until the client's condition stablizes to write nursing diagnoses. Even though initially they may require frequent changes, the diagnoses direct the plan of care and are needed throughout the client's contact with the health care provider. You should consider nursing diagnoses as hypotheses to be tested. If proved to be ineffective or inaccurate, they are changed or discarded.

Each current list of nursing diagnoses is ranked (placed in order according to which diagnosis requires the most immediate attention) and a plan of care developed. Nursing interventions are directed at reducing and eliminating the effect of the sustaining factors. This aspect of the nursing process—ranking, stating nursing interventions, and developing a plan of care—will be discussed in the next chapter.

## Characteristics of Nursing Diagnoses

The following summarization of characteristics should help you in the development of the diagnostic statement.

1.  The nursing diagnosis is a statement reflecting the client's response to personal health condition. It is not a restatement of a medical diagnosis, diagnostic test, treatment, or piece of equipment.

Incorrect:  Potential for impaired skin integrity related to diabetes mellitus.
Correct:    Potential for impaired skin integrity related to decreased peripheral circulation secondary to diabetes mellitus.
Incorrect:  Potential for infection related to cholecystectomy.
Correct:    Potential for infection related to interruption of the body's first line of defense secondary to abdominal incision.

The preceding two incorrect examples focus your attention on complex medical diagnoses and do not identify precise sustaining factors that can be affected by interventions from the domain of nursing.

Incorrect:  Tube feedings.
Correct:    Impaired oral intake related to decreased sucking reflex.
Incorrect:  High levels of environmental lead.
Correct:    Increased risk for lead poisoning related to inadequate enforcement of housing regulations.
Incorrect:  Gall bladder x-rays.
Correct:    Anxiety related to lack of knowledge concerning scheduled gall bladder x-rays.
Incorrect:  Foley catheter.
Correct:    Disturbance in self-concept related to need for and presence of Foley catheter.

These last four incorrect examples do not identify the client's response to the situation or the affect the situation has on the client; they simply identify diagnostic tests, treatments, or existing conditions. This approach does not individualize the diagnosis and provides minimal direction for nursing interventions.

2.  The nursing diagnosis is usually a two-part statement; both parts must be amenable to nursing therapies.

Incorrect:  Alterations in nutrition related to diabetes mellitus.
Correct:    Alterations in nutrition related to possible lack of knowledge concerning 1800 calorie diabetic diet.

In the preceding example, the incorrect nursing diagnosis is stated in such a manner that the nurse must direct therapies at the complex disease process, diabetes mellitus. In the correct diagnosis, the sustaining factor—"possible lack of knowledge concerning 1800 calorie diabetic diet"—is amenable to nursing therapies, as is the diagnostic label "Alterations in nutrition." In addition, the sustaining factor is specific enough to give direction to those nursing therapies.

3.  The nursing diagnosis reflects healthy, unhealthy, or potentially unhealthy responses of the client. It should not reflect needs; the diagnostic statement is broader than a need.

Incorrect:  Need for activity.
Correct:    Impaired skin integrity related to lack of body movement.

4.  The nursing diagnosis may consist of only the diagnostic label when the sustaining factors cannot be determined or are too complex to be stated in a brief phrase.

    Correct:    Lack of self-esteem.
                Family communication deficit.
                Maintenance of effective coping patterns.

5.  The nursing diagnosis contains only one diagnostic label; it may have one or more sustaining factors.

    Incorrect:  Potential for injury and impaired physical mobility related to decreased coordination, unsteady gait, and loss of movement of the right leg.
    Correct:    Potential for injury related to decreased coordination, unsteady gait, and loss of movement of the right leg.
                Impaired physical mobility related to loss of movement of the right leg.

When more than one diagnostic label is included in a nursing diagnosis, the identification of goals, objectives, and interventions is hampered and the plan of care becomes more difficult to develop and follow.

6.  The nursing diagnosis reflects a pattern—not a single sign or symptom.

    Incorrect:  Shortness of breath related to an increase in respiratory secretions.
    Correct:    Ineffective breathing patterns related to an increase in respiratory secretions.
    Incorrect:  Crying related to loss of loved one.
    Correct:    Grieving related to loss of husband.

7.  The nursing diagnosis is a clear, concise statement. It should be in terminology that is generally understood by all health care providers. Jargon and abbreviations should be avoided. Remember that nursing diagnoses provide a basis for communication within the profession and therefore must be meaningful to all members of the profession.

    Incorrect:  Parental anxiety related to neonatal "dying spells."
    Correct:    Parental anxiety related to instability of their newborn's condition.

In this case, "dying spells" applies to periods where the neonate's heart rate decreases and apnea and cyanosis occur. This is a term used in some neonatal care units but is not universally understood by all health care providers.

8.  The nursing diagnosis is individualized for a specific client. The statement must be specific enough to direct the planning, implementing, and evaluating aspects of the nursing process.

    Incorrect:   Self-care deficits related to decreased mobility.
    Correct:     Self-care deficits in the area of bathing and dressing related to immobility of the left arm.
    Incorrect:   Environmental hazards.
    Correct:     Increased risk for respiratory impairment related to inadequate enforcement of air control regulations.
    Incorrect:   Impaired parent–infant bonding related to hospitalization.
    Correct:     Impaired parent–infant bonding related to hospitalization of new mother.

9. The nursing diagnosis is client centered—not nurse centered. For instance, the fact that an individual is in isolation is a concern to the nurse and to the client. Isolation requires specific nursing therapies, but these should not be reflected in the diagnostic statement unless the client's response is reflected.

    Incorrect:   Gown-and-mask technique related to need for isolation.
    Correct:     Alteration in family dynamics related to decreased contact with family members.
                Sleep pattern disturbance related to decreased meaningful sensory input.
                Inability to adjust to the need for gown-and-mask isolation related to ineffective coping patterns.

10. The nursing diagnosis should be worded so that it does not reflect negative aspects of client care. Such statements have legal implications.

    Incorrect:   Potential impairment of skin integrity related to incorrect positioning.
    Correct:     Potential impairment of skin integrity related to inability to turn self.

11. The diagnostic label and sustaining factors should not reflect the same idea.

    Incorrect:   Decreased appetite related to anorexia.
    Correct:     Alteration in nutrition: less than body requirements related to decreased appetite.

## DIAGNOSING FAMILY AND COMMUNITY NEEDS

Organization of the family and community data base and the resulting conclusions regarding their health needs will be discussed at this time.

***Analyze Family Data Base and Organization of Data.*** Data concerning the family can also be analyzed and organized according to conceptual frameworks. The most frequently used frameworks for family study are: structural–functional, interactional, institutional, developmental, balance theory, game theory, social exchange theory, and general systems theory. A brief overview of some of these frameworks will help you to select the one that meets your needs. (Since it is beyond the scope of this book to give an in-depth coverage of each framework, you should refer to appropriate references for more information on the particular framework you want to use.)

The **structural–functional** framework was developed by the disciplines of sociology and social anthropology. This approach views the family as a social system that interacts with other social systems, such as school, work, or health care systems. Emphasis is placed on examining the functions that society performs for the family as well as the functions that the family performs for society. The family and its members are seen as reactive and passive instead of active elements capable of producing change. Ultimately, family structure is evaluated by determining how well the family fulfills its family functions.[9,10,19]

The **interactional** approach comes from the disciplines of sociology and social psychology. This approach views the family unit as a relatively closed system composed of interacting personalities. Family members are viewed as interacting with their environment through symbolic communication. Emphasis is placed on how family members relate to one another and the overall relationship between the individual family member and the family group. The family is perceived as an internal organizational structure instead of a social institution.[9,10] This approach provides a narrower basis for analyzing data about the family.

The third framework for analyzing the family is the **institutional** approach. This approach views the family as an institution and analyzes how it relates to other institutions such as religion, education, and government. Emphasis is on the functions that the family performs for society and how these merge with the functions provided by other institutions for the family. Within this framework, the family is also analyzed as to how its functions have changed over time.[10]

The **developmental** approach to family study was based on theories from a variety of disciplines such as sociology, child psychology, and human development. This approach views the family as a unit that progresses and changes as it moves through a life cycle. Developmental tasks and role expectations for children, parents, and the family, as well as how these aspects change throughout family life, are examined.[9]

The **social exchange theory** was developed by sociologists and behavioral psychologists. This approach studies human behavior from a social exchange relationship viewpoint. The theory believes that human beings follow the principle of reciprocity—in order to receive, they are willing to give. For a relationship to last, a person must believe that the rewards (the receiving aspect) are equal to or greater than the costs (the giving aspect). The exchange theory has been used to determine why certain behavioral patterns have developed between individual family members.[3,9]

In the **general systems theory,** the family is viewed as an open social system with boundaries, self-regulatory mechanisms, interacting systems, and subcomponents. This approach operates on the premise that all systems have inputs or resources which, once processed, assist the system to achieve its goals or output. Feedback from within the system or the environment provides data which help the system determine if goals are being met. This approach analyzes the family as a whole instead of by means of a cause and effect relationship.[7,10] Because of this, the general systems theory is being used more frequently as the basis of study of the family. It is one conceptual framework that is consistent with the holistic approach used in health care; it offers a logical way to integrate all the factors that affect family functioning.

These theoretical frameworks (structural–functional, interactional, general systems, etc.) will help you to analyze family structure and processes. They promote analysis of data so that the information is presented in a logical, organized manner that makes the identification of family strengths and needs easier. Without such frameworks, it is difficult to organize or group data and to identify the relationships that exist between variables and the family as a whole or between individual family members. In some situations, nurses use a combination of several frameworks. This combined approach is effective because the needs of different family units are varied.

***Analyze Community Data Base and Organization of Data.*** Community data can also be organized according to a variety of approaches. The information can be grouped or organized into specific categories such as existing social groups, environmental factors, systems of health care delivery, or existing communication patterns. The structure of the specific assessment tool (interactional, general systems, etc.) used to gather data or an epidemiologic approach can also be used as a basis for organizing data.

As with the analysis of data concerning the individual or family, analysis of community data in an organized, logical manner will increase the value of the data collected. As you follow a systematic analysis, it enables you to see the assessment data as a whole rather than as loosely related pieces of information. From the assessed data, you must determine (1) overall community strengths, (2) major community concerns, (3) major health concerns within the community, and (4) community action being taken, or planned, to resolve the concerns.[7,11]

For a nurse, it is rare that a community assessment would be done without considering the families of the community. Information learned from the community analysis, therefore, will help you to plan more effectively for the individuals or families under your care. You will know the resources and concerns of the community and this will assist in the identification and ranking of nursing needs of families of the community.

As with the individual client, once the data base has been analyzed, you must reach conclusions concerning the health status and health needs of the family and community client.

## Conclusions Involving the Family

Tapia and Meister contributed to a tool that can be used to derive conclusions about the family's health status and need for nursing interventions. Tapia developed a model for family nursing based on a continuum of five levels of family function: Level I—Infancy; Level II—Childhood; Level III—Adolescence; Level IV—Adulthood; Level V—Maturity (Fig. 5–3). A Level-I family is disorganized and fails to provide for support and growth of its individual members. The family demonstrates depression and a feeling of failure. A somewhat lesser degree of disorganization is displayed by the Level-II family. Members of this family remain alienated from the community but are slightly more capable of meeting their own security and physical survival needs. This type of family is still unable to support and promote growth of its members. Parents are immature, and role distortion and confusion exist. A Level-III family has more than the usual amount of conflicts and problems but is capable of meeting the physical survival and security needs of its members. Children from this type of family have less difficulty adjusting to changes but may have more emotional conflicts. Confusion for the children is created because one parent is usually more mature than the other. A family at Level IV may be described as stable and healthy. It is capable of providing physical security and psychosocial functions of the family. Parents are mature and confident; role confusion is not present. In Level V, all tasks are met by the family unit. There exists a balance of individual and group goals, activities, participation, and concerns.[31]

**Figure 5–3.** The nursing process in family (*From Nursing Outlook, 20(4):268. Copyright © 1972, American Journal of Nursing Company, with permission.*)

| Nursing Activities / Continuum of Nursing Skills | Trust | Counseling | Complex of Skills | Prevention | None |
|---|---|---|---|---|---|
| Continuum of Family Functioning | Nurse and Family—Partners<br>Acceptance and trust, maturity and patience, clarification of role, limit setting, constant evaluation of relationship and progress. | Partnership<br>Based on trust relationship, uses counseling and interpersonal skills to help family begin to understand itself and define its problems. Nurse uses honesty and genuineness, and self-evaluation. | Partnership Stressing Family's Ability<br>Information, coordination, teamwork, teaching; uses special skills; helps family in making decisions and finding solutions. | Nurse—Expert and Partner<br>Anticipated problem areas studied, teaching of available resources, assistance in family-group understanding, maturity and foresight. | Family Independent<br>Nurse not Needed |
| | Nurse—"Good Mother" to Family<br>Chaotic family, barely surviving, inadequate provision of physical and emotional supports. Alienation from community, deviant behavior, distortion and confusion of roles, immaturity, child neglect, depression-failure. | Nurse and Family—Siblings<br>Intermediate family, slightly above survival level, variation in economic provisions, alienation but with more ability to trust. Child neglect not as great, defensive but slightly more willingness to accept help. | Nurse—Adult Helper to Family<br>Normal family but with many conflicts and problems, variation in economic levels, greater trust and ability to seek and use help. Parents more mature, but still have emotional conflicts. Do have successes and achievements, and are more willing to seek solutions to problems, future oriented. | Nurse—Expert and Partner with Family<br>Family has solutions, are stable, healthy with fewer conflicts or problems, very capable providers of physical and emotional supports. Parents mature and confident, fewer difficulties in training of children, able to seek help, future oriented, enjoy present. | Ideal family, homeostatic, balance between individual and group goals and activities. Family meets its tasks and roles well, and are able to seek appropriate help when needed. |
| Family Levels | I. Infancy | II. Childhood | III. Adolescence | IV. Adulthood | V. Maturity |

Meister developed behavioral characteristics for each of these five family levels. They are as follows:

Level I—Infancy
 1. Demonstrates family organization in some areas
 2. Meets essential security and survival needs
 3. Shows orientation to community involvement
 4. Trusts those within the family
 5. Exhibits no socially deviant behavior (family defined)
 6. Displays adequate parent role models
 7. Parents interpret their roles appropriately
 8. Members feel adequate within the family
Level II—Childhood
 9. Trust extends to the community
 10. Meets all physical needs
 11. Exhibits no socially deviant behavior (family and community defined)
 12. Members display acceptance of self and family members
 13. Shows awareness of community resources
Level III—Adolescence
 14. Meets physical needs (community defined)
 15. Utilizes some community resources
 16. Becomes future oriented
 17. Functions socially
 18. Experiences normal amount of problems
 19. Possesses one mature parent
Level IV—Adulthood
 20. Has fewer problems than usual
 21. Is secure in emotional and social functions
 22. Possesses two mature parents
 23. Demonstrates normal concern over problems
 24. Shows flexibility in family organization
 25. Plans for future
Level V—Maturity
 26. Meets needs of members
 27. Needs nursing only during severe crises[24]

Assessed data are compared to these behavioral characteristics to determine which ones are being met by the family. The characteristics of any level must be considered as a group. As you evaluate the family's ability to perform each behavior, you will eventually determine the level at which the family is functioning. For example, you would begin with the first behavioral characteristic, *Demonstrates family organization in some areas*. From the organized data, you would determine if the family being assessed was accomplishing this behavior. If you felt that the family did demonstrate family organization in some areas, you would move on to the second behavioral characteristic. You would continue this process until you arrived at a behavior not existing in this family. For purposes of the example, we will indicate that the family was not meeting number 11—*Exhibits no socially deviant behavior (family and community defined)*. This means that your data base contained information indicating deviant social behavior in the family. Even though the family has achieved most of the behaviors for the childhood family, the family will be classified as functioning at Level II until all of the behaviors are achieved (Fig. 5–4).

Determination of the family level will assist you in deriving conclusions concerning the health needs of the family. General conclusions that might be made are:

1. The family is functioning at Level I and experiencing disorganization in all areas of family life. The family would need the nurse to assume decision-making functions regarding health management.
2. The family is functioning at Level II, and although slightly more organized, they would still require the nurse to make the decisions regarding health care.
3. The family is functioning at Level III and requires a variety of nursing skills. The family is capable of sharing with the nurse decision-making functions regarding health care.
4. The family is functioning at Level IV and primarily requires preventive health teaching. The family is capable of sharing with the nurse decision-making functions regarding health care.
5. The family is functioning at Level V and requires no nursing therapies unless a crisis arises. The family is capable of making their own decisions regarding health management.

As with the conclusions concerning the health status of the individual, these conclusions are not meant to reflect all the possible conclusions that exist.

## Conclusions Involving the Community

Conclusions concerning the community fall within the four areas previously identified: overall community strengths; major community concerns; major health concerns within the community; and community action being taken, or planned, to resolve the concerns. General conclusions that might be made are:

1. Health care services are comprehensive; care is available and accessible to all people in the community.
2. Health care is continuous and coordinated; primary, secondary, and tertiary settings are available and used.
3. Health care facilities, personnel, and finances are used.
4. Major health concerns are identifiable; methods for resolving the concerns are established.
5. Health care facilities, personnel, and finances are inadequate.
6. Health care is not continuous or coordinated; care is focused at the secondary level to the exclusion or neglect of prevention and rehabilitation.
7. Health care services are not comprehensive; care is not available or accessible to portions of the community population.

Most decisions made regarding community health care should be shared between the population of the community and appropriate resource personnel. When decisions about health care management are made independently by the community, health care services are frequently inadequate or inappropriate. This situation arises because the community as a whole is not adequately educated in all aspects of comprehensive health care. On the other hand, when decisions about health care management are made inde-

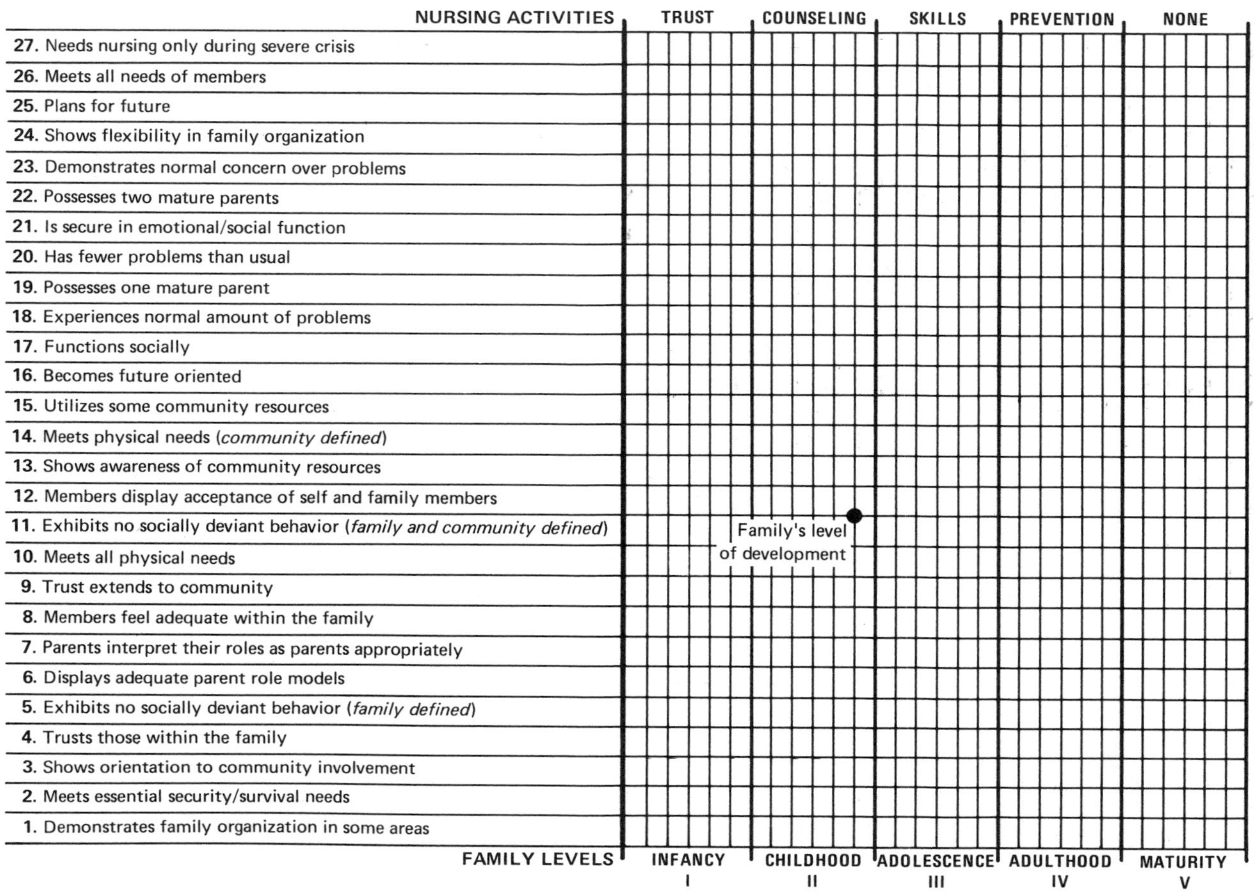

NURSING ACTIVITIES

TRUST   COUNSELING   SKILLS   PREVENTION   NONE

27. Needs nursing only during severe crisis
26. Meets all needs of members
25. Plans for future
24. Shows flexibility in family organization
23. Demonstrates normal concern over problems
22. Possesses two mature parents
21. Is secure in emotional/social function
20. Has fewer problems than usual
19. Possesses one mature parent
18. Experiences normal amount of problems
17. Functions socially
16. Becomes future oriented
15. Utilizes some community resources
14. Meets physical needs (community defined)
13. Shows awareness of community resources
12. Members display acceptance of self and family members
11. Exhibits no socially deviant behavior (family and community defined)
10. Meets all physical needs
9. Trust extends to community
8. Members feel adequate within the family
7. Parents interpret their roles as parents appropriately
6. Displays adequate parent role models
5. Exhibits no socially deviant behavior (family defined)
4. Trusts those within the family
3. Shows orientation to community involvement
2. Meets essential security/survival needs
1. Demonstrates family organization in some areas

Family's level of development

FAMILY LEVELS   INFANCY I   CHILDHOOD II   ADOLESCENCE III   ADULTHOOD IV   MATURITY V

**Figure 5–4.** Family assessment and nursing intervention identifier. (Adapted from Meister, 1977, with permission[23])

pendently by health care providers, the needs, as seen by the community, may be overlooked.

We have looked at the diagnostic process and how nursing diagnoses can be made for the individual, the family, and the community client. How has the concept of nursing diagnoses affected the profession of nursing? We will consider this aspect next.

## IMPACT ON NURSING

The acceptance of diagnosing as a separate step in the nursing process has had a definite impact on the nursing profession. Although there are still issues to be resolved, nursing diagnoses have, overall, been beneficial to the profession.

### Effects on Practice

Perhaps the most apparent benefit from the use of nursing diagnoses is the impact on the nursing process itself. Diagnosing makes the transition from assessing to planning easier. The diagnostic process helps you, the nurse, to analyze large quantities of data and to draw conclusions regarding the client's health status. This provides you with a sound foundation for the development of the nursing care plan.

This approach also provides for less fragmentation of care. Because you have looked at each piece of the data closely, a better understanding of the client exists. Nursing interventions become goal oriented instead of task oriented. The end result is more comprehensive and individualized health care.

Nursing diagnoses are also a means of communication within the profession. They allow nurses in education, practice, and research to speak the same language; this facilitates teaching, consultation, and the transfer of information. When one nurse relates information to another, reference to the nursing diagnoses of the client should produce mental images of the client's health status just as medical diagnoses do. Nursing diagnoses also help communication among nurses and other care providers as well as the general public.

Another area of practice that has been affected by the use of nursing diagnoses is the area of accountability. Nursing diagnoses have helped to delineate independent nursing functions. Diagnoses must be within the domain of the nurse; both the diagnostic label and the sustaining factors must be conducive to independent nursing therapies. As the nurse functions within this framework, independent nursing functions become clearer and more universally accepted. You cannot, however, seek an independent function without accepting the responsibility for your actions. Acceptance of responsibility implies being accountable for your actions.

### Effects on Education and Research

Nursing diagnoses have provided a basis for theory development. Nurse researchers are conducting research studies to determine the appropriateness of specific diagnostic labels and to determine the etiology and identifying characteristics of these labels. All of this information helps to establish an independent body of knowledge for the nursing profession.

The effect on nursing education can be seen in many areas. Curriculum changes have been made in some schools of nursing to make certain that the diagnostic process and nursing diagnosis are being taught. In addition, some of the processes necessary for diagnosing are being included: critical thinking, problem solving, and analytic thinking. Some educational programs use nursing diagnoses as the format for curriculum development. This helps to move nursing education away from the medical model that was taught for many years. In addition, nursing textbooks are being written using the nursing diagnoses format instead of the medical model. All of these activities expand the body of nursing knowledge and widen the framework for nursing education.

## SUMMARY AND STUDY GUIDE

This portion of the chapter will serve two purposes. First, it will be used as a summary or review of the major points discussed in this chapter. Secondly, the section will serve as a study guide to facilitate your understanding of the diagnostic process. In order for the section to be of benefit as a study guide, you will be asked at various points to perform certain activities before you read any further information provided by the authors. Your activities will be marked by an arrowhead (▶).

We will apply each of the steps in the diagnostic process to the following data base.

### Data Base

Mrs. P. H., a 46-year-old, white, Catholic female, was admitted to the hospital with the symptom of rectal bleeding. The assessment interview and health history revealed that Mrs. H. had been married for 22 years and was the mother of three boys and one girl, ages 10 to 20.

Mrs. H. lived with her husband and three of her children in a six-room apartment in a portion of the city heavily populated with Italians. Her husband's family was born in Italy, but she and her husband were American born. Mrs. H. and her husband were unable to work, and her husband was on compensation. Mrs. H. had had numerous hospital admissions, approximately 21, and was being followed by various clinics at a local hospital. She had been treated for hypertension and cardiac problems in the past and was still being treated for diabetes mellitus.

Mrs. H. reported that at home she was having difficulty sleeping. She took Dalmane 30 milligrams nightly for sleep and Valium 5 to 10 milligrams for nervousness. She also took insulin at home.

Mrs. H. was alert and responded quickly to questions. Her answers were related to time and place; she easily recalled her past health care experiences. Her speech was distinct, and she used simple, noncomplex words. She smiled frequently and stated that she enjoyed talking with people. She had frequent visits from her husband and children.

The physical assessment revealed that Mrs. H. was 161 centimeters tall and weighed 114.5 kilograms. She stated that she did not follow her 1800 calorie diabetic diet at home. She found it hard to prepare the special foods since her family enjoyed Italian food. She did not tolerate gas-forming, rich, or spicy foods. Mrs. H. complained of general tiredness and weakness. Her respiratory rate ranged between 18 and 32, and she had slight orthopnea. She complained of diarrhea, abdominal pain and cramping, nausea, and back and leg pain. Her blood pressure was 150/100 mm of mercury. Severe scars covered her neck, arms, and chest; the scars were the result of burns sustained when she was four years of age.

Her chest x-ray revealed cardiomegaly, and the liver and spleen scan showed hepatosplenomegaly. The serum LDH (lactic dehydrogenase) was 310 mU/ml; the SGOT (serum glutamic oxaloacetic transaminase) was 110 mU/ml; and the serum alkaline phosphatase was 43.2 mU/ml.

The first step in the diagnostic process is data base analysis. You must organize the data in a logical, systematic manner so that irrelevant information, inconsistencies, omissions, and patterns of responses can be identified. After this has been accomplished, the data are compared to norms, standards, and theories.

▶Organize the data base according to basic needs. After you have completed this portion of the step, identify areas of concern (data that conflict with accepted norms, standards, or theories) with an asterisk.

Using basic needs as the organizing framework, the data base could be sorted and organized in the following manner. (The asterisks indicate areas of concern.)

**Physiologic**
Alert
Difficulty sleeping*
Wt 114.5 kg*
Ht 161 cm
Diarrhea*
Tired and weak*
Orthopnea*
Abdominal pains and cramping*
Nausea*
Back and leg pains*
Blood pressure 150/100*
LDH 310 mU/ml*
SGOT 110 mU/ml*
Alkaline phosphatase 43.2 mU/ml*

**Psychological**
Recalled past medical experience
Husband on compensation*
Many physical complaints*
Difficulty sleeping*
No difficulty recalling living patterns
Scars on neck, arms, and chest*
Lives in Italian community

**Cultural**
Italian background
(More data needed)

**Spiritual**
Catholic
(More data needed)

**Social**
Married
Four children
Housewife
Multiple hospital admissions*
Frequent visits from family
Scars on neck, arms, and
   chest*
Lives in Italian community

**Nutritional**
Takes NPH insulin*
Not following 1800 calorie dia-
   betic diet at home*
Avoids gas-forming, rich, or
   spicy foods
Prepares Italian food for family

**Economic**
Husband on compensation*
Multiple hospital admissions*
Rents apartment

The second step in the diagnostic process involves deriving conclusions based on the analyzed data. Remember that conclusions are summary statements or generalizations concerning the health status of a client.

▶Develop conclusions regarding the health status of Mrs. H. Supply data that support your conclusion(s).

The following are examples of conclusions that could be reached based on the information supplied.

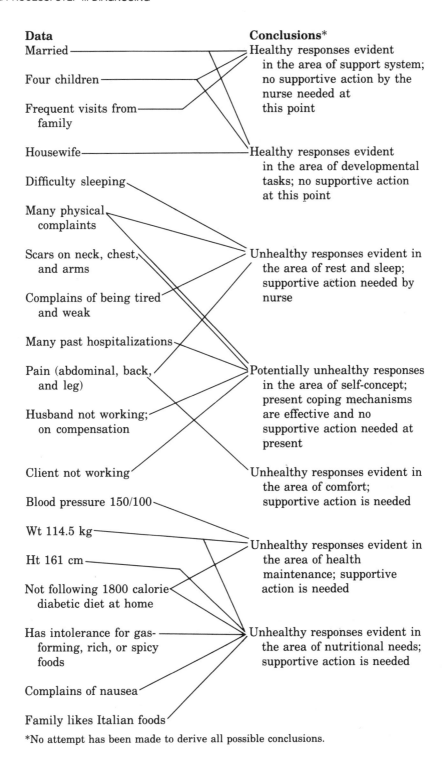

**Data**

Married

Four children

Frequent visits from family

Housewife

Difficulty sleeping

Many physical complaints

Scars on neck, chest, and arms

Complains of being tired and weak

Many past hospitalizations

Pain (abdominal, back, and leg)

Husband not working; on compensation

Client not working

Blood pressure 150/100

Wt 114.5 kg

Ht 161 cm

Not following 1800 calorie diabetic diet at home

Has intolerance for gas-forming, rich, or spicy foods

Complains of nausea

Family likes Italian foods

**Conclusions***

Healthy responses evident in the area of support system; no supportive action by the nurse needed at this point

Healthy responses evident in the area of developmental tasks; no supportive action at this point

Unhealthy responses evident in the area of rest and sleep; supportive action needed by nurse

Potentially unhealthy responses in the area of self-concept; present coping mechanisms are effective and no supportive action needed at present

Unhealthy responses evident in the area of comfort; supportive action is needed

Unhealthy responses evident in the area of health maintenance; supportive action is needed

Unhealthy responses evident in the area of nutritional needs; supportive action is needed

*No attempt has been made to derive all possible conclusions.

Assigning a diagnostic label to the conclusion is the third step in the diagnostic process. Standardized labels are available and should be used when possible to promote consistency within the profession. Do not be restricted by the labels or force your conclusions to conform to them. Individualize the diagnostic labels as much as possible.

►Assign diagnostic labels to the conclusions that you reached.

The following are examples of diagnostic labels that could be assigned to the conclusions derived from the data base.

| Conclusions | Diagnostic Labels |
| --- | --- |
| Healthy responses evident in the area of support system | Maintenance of active support system |
| Healthy responses evident in the area of developmental tasks | Maintenance of developmental status |
| Unhealthy responses evident in the area of rest and sleep | Sleep pattern disturbance (actual) |
| Potentially unhealthy responses in the area of self-concept | Potential self-care deficit  Potential disturbance in self-concept |
| Unhealthy responses evident in the area of comfort | Alteration in comfort level |
| Unhealthy responses evident in the area of health maintenance | Health maintenance alteration (actual) |
| Unhealthy responses evident in the area of nutritional needs | Alteration in nutrition: more than body requirements (actual)  Probable knowledge deficit concerning nutritional needs* |

*No attempt has been made to identify all possible diagnostic labels.

The fourth step in the diagnostic process is the identification of sustaining factors. The data base is reexamined for possible or actual causes of the client's responses. These sustaining factors are then combined with the diagnostic label to form the diagnostic statement—nursing diagnosis. This is the fifth step in the process. Sustaining factors and diagnostic labels are connected by "related to" or "associated with" clauses.

►Develop diagnostic statements for your diagnostic labels. Underline the sustaining factors to help you separate the two components of the statement.

The following are nursing diagnoses that have been formed by combining diagnostic labels and sustaining factors.

- Maintenance of active support system. Sustaining factors too complex to state.
- Maintenance of developmental status. Sustaining factors too complex to state.
- Sleep pattern disturbance related to difficulty breathing while in lying position, pain, and nausea.
- Potential self-care deficit related to weakness, fatigue, and pain.
- Potential disturbance in self-concept related to ineffective coping with physical scars and inability to work.
- Alteration in comfort level related to pain and nausea.
- Health maintenance alteration related to lack of resources, incomplete knowledge base, and decreased motivation to follow nursing and medical therapies.
- Alteration in nutrition: more than body requirements related to possible lack of information regarding 1800 calorie diabetic diet and desires to meet cultural preferences of family.
- Probable knowledge deficit concerning nutritional needs. Sustaining factors not known.

Now that we have discussed the diagnostic process and the formulation of the diagnostic statement, we must develop a plan of care that will provide appropriate nursing interventions. The fourth step in the nursing process, planning, will be discussed in the next chapter.

# REFERENCES

1. Abdellah, F. Methods of identifying covert aspects of nursing problems. *Nursing Research,* June 1957, *6*(1), 4–23.
2. Abdellah, F., Beland, I., Martin, A., & Matheney, R. *Patient-centered approaches to nursing.* New York: Macmillan, 1961.
3. Broderick, C. B. Beyond the five conceptual frameworks: A decade of development in family theory. *The Journal of Marriage and the Family,* February 1971, *33* (1), 139–159.
4. Campbell, C. *Nursing diagnosis and interventions in nursing practice* (2nd ed.). New York: Wiley, 1984.
5. Carlson, J. H., Craft, C. & McGuire, A. *Nursing diagnosis.* Philadelphia: Saunders, 1982.
6. Chambers, W. Nursing diagnosis. *American Journal of Nursing,* November 1962, *62* (11), 102–104.
7. Clemen, S. A., Eigsti, D. G., & McGuire, S. *Comprehensive family and community health nursing.* New York: McGraw-Hill, 1981.
8. Durand, M. & Prince, R. Nursing diagnosis: Process and decision. *Nursing Forum,* 1966, *5* (4), 50–59.
9. Eshleman, J. R. *The family.* Boston: Allyn and Bacon, 1978.
10. Friedmen, M. *Family nursing: Theory and assessment.* New York: Appleton-Century-Crofts, 1981.
11. Fromer, M. J. *Community health care and the nursing process* (2nd ed.). St. Louis: C.V. Mosby, 1983.
12. Fry, V. The creative approach to nursing. *American Journal of Nursing,* March 1953, *53* (3), 301–302.
13. Gebbie, K. (Ed.). *Summary of the second national conference: Classification of nursing diagnoses.* St. Louis: Clearinghouse-National Group for Classification of Nursing Diagnoses, 1976.
14. Gebbie, K., & Lavin, M. A. *Classification of nursing diagnoses: Proceedings of the first national conference.* St. Louis: C.V. Mosby, 1975.
15. Gordon, M. Nursing diagnosis and the diagnostic process. *American Journal of Nursing,* August 1976, *76* (8), 1298–1300.

16. Gordon, M. *Nursing diagnosis: Process and application.* New York: McGraw-Hill, 1982.
17. Griffith, J., & Christensen, P. *Nursing process: Application of theories, frameworks and models.* St. Louis: C.V. Mosby, 1982.
18. Henderson, V. The nature of nursing. *American Journal of Nursing,* August 1964, *64* (8), 62–68.
19. Hill, R., & Hansen, D. The identification of conceptual frameworks utilized in family study. *Marriage and Family Living,* November 1960, *22,* 299–311.
20. Kim, M. J., McFarland, G., & McLane, A. *Classification of nursing diagnoses: Proceedings of the fifth national conference.* New York: McGraw-Hill, 1984.
21. Kim, M. J., & Moritz, D. E. (Eds.). *Classification of nursing diagnoses: Proceedings of the third and fourth national conferences.* New York: McGraw-Hill, 1982.
22. Komorita, N. Nursing diagnosis. *American Journal of Nursing,* December 1963, *63* (12), 83–86.
23. Lunney, M. Nursing diagnosis: Refining the system. *American Journal of Nursing,* March 1982, *82* (3), 456–459.
24. Meister, S. B. Charting a family's developmental status—for intervention and for the record. *Journal of Maternal–Child Nursing,* January/February 1977, *2* (1), 43–48.
25. Mundinger, M. O. & Jauron, G. D. Developing a nursing diagnosis. *Nursing Outlook,* 1975, *23* (2), 94–98.
26. Orem, D. E. *Nursing: Concepts of practice* (2nd ed.). New York: McGraw-Hill, 1980.
27. Orem, D. E. (Ed.). *Concept formalization in nursing: Process and product* (2nd ed.). Boston: Little, Brown, 1979.
28. Peplau, H. *Interpersonal relations in nursing.* New York: G. P. Putnam's Sons, 1952.
29. Roy, C. A diagnostic classification system for nursing. *Nursing Outlook,* February 1975, *23* (2), 90–94.
30. Shortridge, L., & Lee, E. J. *Introduction to nursing practice.* New York: McGraw-Hill, 1980.
31. Tapia, J. The nursing process in family health. *Nursing Outlook,* April 1972, *20* (4), 267–270.

## BIBLIOGRAPHY

Aspinall, M. J. Nursing diagnosis—the weak link. *Nursing Outlook,* July 1976, *24* (7), 433–436.
Baer, C. L. Nursing diagnosis: A futuristic process for nursing practice. *Topics in Clinical Nursing,* January 1984, *5* (4), 89–96.
Bower, F. L. *The process of planning nursing care: A model for practice* (3rd ed.). St. Louis: C.V. Mosby, 1982.
Brill, E. L., & Kilts, D. *Foundations for nursing.* New York: Appleton-Century-Crofts, 1980.
Burgess, W. & Ragland, E.C. *Community health nursing: Philosophy, process, practice.* Norwalk, Conn: Appleton-Century-Crofts, 1983.
Carnevali, D. Nursing diagnosis: An evolutionary view. *Topics in Clinical Nursing,* January 1984, *5*(4), 10–20.
Eshleman, J. R., & Clarke, J. N. *Intimacy, commitments, and marriage: Development of relationships.* Boston: Allyn and Bacon, 1978.
Gaines, B. C., & McFarland, M. B. Nursing diagnosis: Its relationship to and use in nursing education. *Topics in Clinical Nursing,* January 1984, *5* (4), 39–49.
Gebbie, K. Nursing diagnosis: What is it and why does it exist? *Topics in Clinical Nursing,* January 1984, *5* (4), 1–9.
Gebbie, K., & Lavin, M. A. Classifying nursing diagnoses. *American Journal of Nursing,* February 1974, *74* (2), 250–253.
Gordon, M., Sweeney, M.A., & McKeehan, K. Nursing diagnosis: Looking at its use in the clinical area. *American Journal of Nursing,* April 1980, *80* (4), 672–675.
Herrington, J. & Houston, S. Using Orem's theory: A plan for all seasons. *Nursing and Health Care,* January 1984, *5* (1), 45–47.
Marriner, *The nursing process: A scientific approach to nursing care* (3rd ed.). St. Louis: C.V. Mosby, 1983.

McManus, R. L. Assumption of functions in nursing. In *Regional Planning for Nurses and Nursing Education*. New York: Teacher's College Columbia University, 1951.

Narrow, B., & Buschle, K.B. *Fundamentals of nursing practice*. New York: Wiley, 1982.

Oelbaum, C. H. Hallmarks of adult wellness. *American Journal of Nursing,* September 1974, *74* (9), 1623–1625.

Popkess, S.A. Diagnosing your patient's strengths. *Nursing '81,* July 1981, *11* (7), 34–37.

Price, M. R. Nursing diagnosis: Making a concept come alive. *American Journal of Nursing,* April 1980, *80* (4), 668–671.

Putzier, D.J., & Padrick, K.P. Nursing diagnosis: A component of nursing process and decision making. *Topics on Clinical Nursing,* January 1984, 21–29.

Shamansky, S., & Yanni, C. In opposition to nursing diagnosis: A minority opinion. *Image: The Journal of Nursing Scholarship,* Spring 1983, *15* (2), 47–50.

Sorensen, K., & Luckmann, J. *Basic nursing: A psychophysiologic approach*. Philadelphia: Saunders, 1979.

Tinkham, C., Voorhies, E., & McCarthy, N. *Community health nursing: Evolution and process in the family and community* (3rd ed.). New York: Appleton-Century-Crofts, 1984.

# 6

# Nursing Process:
# Step III. Planning

Planning is the third step in the nursing process. This step involves the development of a plan which directs the client's care. In order to develop an appropriate plan of care, priorities must be established, prognoses determined, goals, objectives, and outcome criteria established, and nursing interventions identified. Each of these aspects will be discussed in this chapter.

Study of this chapter will help you to:

1. Define planning as it relates to the nursing process.
2. Describe the purposes of nursing prognoses.
3. Identify factors affecting nursing prognoses.
4. Define goals and objectives.
5. Discuss the purposes of goals and objectives.
6. Describe the characteristics of goals and objectives.
7. Write goals and behavioral objectives in client-behavioral terms.
8. Write outcome criteria that will evaluate the effectiveness of the plan of care.
9. Describe independent, interdependent, and dependent nursing interventions.
10. Write specific, individualized nursing orders.
11. Develop an individualized plan of care that includes goals, behavioral objectives, and nursing orders.

A plan is a specific aim or purpose; it is a detailed scheme or method developed for the accomplishment or attainment of a desired end. **Planning** describes the nursing strategy or scheme designed to assure goal-directed care for the client. Planning begins as a mental process, but ultimately the plan must be recorded to ensure continuity of care. The first step toward this written plan is the establishment of priorities.

## ESTABLISH PRIORITIES

"To establish priorities" or "to rank" means to place in order of importance or urgency, according to or based on criteria. The term implies that preferential attention will be given one thing over competing alternatives. You set priorities at several stages in the nursing process. Priority must be determined for nursing diagnoses, objectives, and interventions. In addition, when caring for a group of clients, you set priorities when you decide which client requires your attention first.

At present, you are concerned with ranking the nursing diagnoses that have been identified for a particular client. All diagnoses are considered. By means of a triaging or sorting process, the nursing diagnoses are ranked to determine which diagnoses receive immediate, delayed, or no attention from the health care professional. The diagnoses are ranked so those with the greatest urgency, greatest threat, or gravest consequence are considered first.

Priorities are constantly changing. As the client's condition changes, the ranking of needs will change. Since these needs are reflected in the nursing diagnoses, the actual list of diagnoses as well as the ranking of these diagnoses will change. During the acute phase of an illness or in a crisis, high priority needs are the primary concern. At other times, your plan may contain interventions that will meet both low and high priority needs at the same time. Priorities will also change as diagnoses of high priority are met and diagnoses of low priority shift upward. Classifying a diagnosis as a high-priority diagnosis does not guarantee goal achievement and resolution of the client's concerns. High-priority diagnoses may have low likelihood of goal achievement because of the client's overall condition or other factors affecting the situation.

### Factors Affecting Priority Setting

Some of the factors affecting the setting of priorities include: conflicting goals, external factors such as time, personnel, and money, agency policy, and value systems of the people involved.[3,12,25]

*Conflicting Goals.* Conflicting goals may affect priority setting when consensus among client, family, and health care providers is not gained. An understanding of the client's goals can be achieved by reviewing the data base. Even though the client's goals and perception of priorities may differ from yours, the client should still be involved in setting priorities whenever possible. Generally, what is important to the client is considered high priority. If this does not seem to be in the client's best interest, assess the client's decision-making ability, talk to the client, and provide information regarding the possible consequences of each alternative goal. Decisions made by a well-informed client should direct your future course of action.

In some instances, the client is not capable of making decisions regarding priorities; the client may be too young or incapacitated. At other times, the client may elect to leave the decision in the hands of the care provider. Your priority setting will be based upon your theoretical knowledge, background experience, and information gathered from the family or significant others. Do not hesitate to consult with colleagues concerning their interpretation of appropriate actions.

You must also consider the goals of each discipline involved in the care of the client. The physician, physical therapist, occupational therapist, and so forth, will each set different priorities. These priorities will be based on their understanding and interpretation of the client's health needs and their goals for the client's care. In addition, the health agency or facility involved will also have goals that will affect priority setting. For instance, if the physician's goal of therapy is directed at rehabilitation, this must be considered when you and the client discuss priorities. If the health facility's goals focus on custodial care instead of curative or rehabilitative care, priority setting and your interventions will be affected.

*Value Systems.* Value systems will affect priority setting. Values have either implicit or explicit effects on one's life and are important determinants of priorities. The type of health care accepted—promotive, preventive, palliative, curative, or rehabilitative— may depend on the value placed on age, physical health, mental status, and dependency.

You have some knowledge of the client's value system based on the data collected in the nursing health history and assessment. Remember that the values of the health care provider and client may differ. Do not impose values on the client. If the client's value system is preventing appropriate health care, encourage the client to reexamine personal values after exposure to various views on the issue.

*External Factors.* External factors such as time, money, facilities, and knowledge will affect priority setting. As a nurse, you function within a time frame. Your contact with the client may be as brief as a few minutes in an emergency room or as long as an 8-, 10-, or 12-hour shift in a hospital. In a community care facility your contact with the client may last for days, weeks, months, or years. Regardless of the setting or the length of contact with the client, your therapies will be restricted by time. The possibility of achieving objectives during the length of time to be spent with each client will affect the rank order given to that client's nursing diagnoses.

Personnel, resources, and the financial status of the client may also determine the rank order given to nursing diagnoses. What is the size of the health care staff? How many clients are involved? What is the ratio of health care providers to clients? A health care provider assigned to four clients will perceive priorities differently than one assigned to 12 clients. The availability of equipment, specialized consultants, and specific resources will affect priority setting. Does the facility have a physical therapist or occupational therapist? Is a social worker available at all times or just on certain days of the week? Can certain therapies be conducted if the needed equipment is not available?

Obviously, the client's financial status does not affect the overall quality of care to be given or the priority of that care when crises arise. When conferring with the client, family, or significant others concerning priority setting, however, financial concerns may become important. Review the assessed data and determine the type of health care affordable to the client. Note the client's health insurance coverage, financial responsibilities, and stability of employment. Can the client afford the nursing therapies involved with a particular nursing diagnosis? If not, are there other alternatives open to the client? With the assessed data available, you will be able to discuss this aspect of priority setting more effectively with the client.

The knowledge base of each person involved in the decision-making process regarding priorities will have an effect. For this reason, it is important to provide the client with information that will facilitate the setting of priorities. In addition, you, as the nurse, must be well informed concerning the alternatives available to the client.

***Agency Policies.*** In some health care facilities or agencies, policies set certain priorities. Some agencies set high priorities on specific types of health problems; this may even dictate their acceptance of people as clients. The general philosophy of care in a facility (acute versus chronic, palliative versus rehabilitative) must be considered before determining priorities. In addition, the health care facility can determine what independent actions can be taken by the health care provider. What nursing interventions can be initiated by the nurse independently of physician's orders and agency policies? Can the physical therapist or the dietitian see the client without specific orders from the physician?

## Criteria for Setting Priorities

Criteria are needed to assist in the setting of priorities. Criteria for setting priorities for the individual or family client include preservation of life, basic human needs, and developmental tasks.[3,12,25]

***Preservation of Life.*** Those needs necessary for preservation of life assume priority over comfort measures. Most physical discomforts must be met before the individual can handle other needs. One method of ranking nursing diagnoses according to this criterion is to assign a rating of high, medium, or low priority to each diagnosis.

A **high-priority need** is life threatening. For the individual client, respiratory obstruction or severe loss of blood would be considered high priority. For the family, a high-priority need represents a threat to family life, for example, an alcoholic mother or father.

**Medium-priority needs** do not directly threaten the life of the client although they may produce unhealthy or destructive physical or emotional changes. A breakdown in communication within the family structure or imposed immobility of the individual represent medium-priority needs. Changes which arise from normal growth and development or needs which require minimal supportive actions from the health care provider are considered **low priority.** The family that can not function as a unit or the individual who is experiencing body image changes related to recent surgery may represent this level of priority.

With this criterion, the rank order of each nursing diagnosis is established in relation to other diagnoses. The rank order goes from the most important to the least important and is reflected in the examples in Table 6–1.

***Basic Human Needs.*** Abraham Maslow is credited with the initial research in the area of basic needs. He asserted that human beings are dominated by basic needs that direct their behavior. This direction of behavior continues until each need is satisfied.[16]

The basic needs are interrelated but hierarchical—arranged or organized according to rank. Usually the lower-level needs must be met before the higher-level needs are considered. It is possible for higher-level needs to not emerge until lower-level needs are at least minimally met or satisfied. The higher the need the less necessary it is for survival, the longer fulfillment can be delayed, and the easier it is for the need to disappear.[15] Maslow ranks the needs as physical needs, safety needs, love needs, needs for self-respect, and self-actualization needs; the hierarchy begins with physiologic needs and progresses upward to self-actualization.[16]

Physical needs include the need for oxygen, food, water, sleep, shelter, activity, and sex. Nursing diagnoses which reflect these needs would usually be considered high priority. Safety needs include a desire for a safe, secure, orderly, predictable world. As

**TABLE 6-1. RANKING NURSING DIAGNOSES ACCORDING TO PRESERVATION OF LIFE CRITERION**

| Diagnoses | Ranking | Rationale |
|---|---|---|
| Impaired breathing patterns related to increased secretions in the respiratory tract. | 1 | Represents a life-threatening need with potential air-way obstruction: a high-priority diagnosis. |
| Interruption in play activity related to decreased mobility and pain on movement. | 2 | Play activity is needed for growth and development; the sustaining factors support the fact that interventions are needed to prevent unhealthy or destructive physical or emotional changes: a medium-priority diagnosis. |
| Altered body image related to difficulty accepting the sudden adolescent growth spurt. | 3 | A normal growth and development event that probably requires minimal supportive actions from the nurse: a low-priority diagnosis. |

physical and safety needs are met, love needs emerge. The person or family has a need to give and receive love and to experience a sense of belonging. The need for self-respect is reflected in the client's need for self-esteem and the client's esteem of others. Desire for recognition, attention, prestige, importance, and independence are experienced. Self-actualization emerges when other needs have been satisfied and centers around the desire to fully realize one's potential.[16]

The following nursing diagnoses exemplify the use of Maslow's Hierarchy of Needs as the criterion for establishing priorities.

Physical Needs:       Loss of appetite related to fatigue and lack of interest in eating alone.

Safety Needs:         Potential for injury related to decreased vision and dizziness.

Love Needs:           Loneliness related to decreased support system (death of husband and sister).

Self-Esteem Needs:   Threat to self-esteem related to role losses.

Self-Actualization    Decreased motivation related to lack of family support
   Needs:             of perceived goals.

There may be exceptions to this method of setting priorities. The hierarchy is not absolute, and each client must be viewed separately. For example, the medical diagnosis, failure to thrive, refers to the abnormal retardation of growth and development in infants resulting from conditions that interfere with normal metabolism, appetite, and activity.[23] Since the most prominent visual indication of this condition is failure to gain weight, you might be tempted to consider the physical need for food as this client's high-priority need. The infant does need food, but research has shown that infants with failure to thrive are frequently lacking love. The infant may be suffering from maternal deprivation.[24] In this instance, the love needs must be met before the infant will take adequate quantities of nourishment.

When considering this set of criteria, remember that most people who have barely met low-level needs for years may lack the drive for higher-level needs. Therefore, do not establish your priorities without conferring with the client. In addition, because most people do manage to satisfy many or most of their lower-level needs with minimal outside assistance, they may not be receptive to your identifying these areas as high-priority needs. During illness or time of increased stress, more needs may be unmet, and the client becomes more receptive to your interventions.

***Developmental Tasks.*** Erik Erikson's stages of man and Robert Havighurst's developmental tasks for each stage provide[8,9] another way of determining priorities for the individual client.[8,9] **Developmental tasks** are physical or cognitive skills that an individual must accomplish during a particular age period in order to continue developing.[23] Successful achievement of these tasks prepares the person for later tasks in a later stage. Although not all nursing diagnoses will relate directly to these tasks, using developmental tasks as criteria for setting priorities may assist you to understand the client's perception of health and health care priorities. In addition, skills that have not been achieved would be given priority over those accomplished.

The following is an example of how developmental tasks affect priorities. One of the developmental tasks of the preschooler is to master physical skills of large and small muscle coordination and movement.[9] If the child was immobilized for some reason (confined to bed after a fractured femur), his ability to achieve this task would be hampered. Based on this knowledge, the nursing diagnosis, *Inability to achieve developmental task of mastering physical skills of large and small muscle coordination and movement related to immobility,* could be considered a high-priority diagnosis.

Duvall identified family developmental tasks. "A **family developmental task** is a growth responsibility that arises at a certain stage in the life of a family. . . ."[7] Family developmental tasks must be achieved successfully in a sequential pattern or the family will have difficulty with later developmental tasks. As with the individual client, these tasks can be used as criteria to determine priority needs for the family unit.

Criteria for setting priorities for the community have also been identified. Stanhope and Lancaster have identified six criteria to assist you when ranking problems and needs of the community. These criteria include: (1) community awareness of the problem; (2) motivation of the community to resolve or manage the problem more effectively; (3) your ability as a nurse to influence the problem's solution; (4) availability of expertise relevant to the problem; (5) consequences and severity of consequences if the problem is not solved; and (6) speed with which the solution can be accomplished.[19] These criteria can be weighted—assigned numbers from 1 to 10. Each nursing diagnosis is rated according to the criteria. (Remember nursing diagnoses reflect the responses of the client and will therefore reflect any problems or needs.) The number(s) assigned to each diagnosis is computed; the scores of the various diagnoses are compared, and priorities are determined. The most significant nursing diagnosis will have the highest rating and thus the highest priority.[19]

For this example, let us assume that each criterion is assigned a point value ranging from 1 to 6. To simplify the example, assign the points in the same order as the

| | 1 | 2 | 3 | 4 | 5 | 6 | TOTAL |
|---|---|---|---|---|---|---|---|
| DIAGNOSIS #1 | X | | | X | X | | 10 |
| DIAGNOSIS #2 | | X | X | X | X | X | 20 |

**Figure 6–1.** Ranking community diagnoses.

criterion is numbered—criterion number 1 will be assigned one point and so forth. Two nursing diagnoses will be used: (1) Potential for an increase in respiratory disease in the community related to high levels of air pollution from a local industry, and (2) increased risk for lead poisoning related to inadequate enforcement of housing regulations. You would then review your assessment data. Based on these data, you would examine each diagnosis to determine its relation to the criterion—do your assessment data show that the community is aware of the risk of lead poisoning and respiratory disease, is the community motivated to resolve the problem, and so forth. Your analysis may be placed on a grid as shown in Figure 6–1. Once you have totaled the numbers assigned each diagnosis, you would rank the diagnoses. In this example, the diagnosis concerned with lead poisoning would be ranked as a high-priority diagnosis based on its total number of points.

Another method of ranking nursing diagnoses associated with the community is to determine those that are of high, medium, or low priority. Health needs or problems that affect the life of members of the community usually take first priority. An influenza outbreak in the community would be of high priority. Health problems that threaten to destructively change the lives of the community population, for example, high pollution levels within the community, are considered medium priority. Nursing interventions are required but the urgency of the situation is less than seen with high-priority concerns. Problems or needs associated with the normal developmental growth of the community are viewed as low priority. For instance, a lack of innovative programs or inadequate recreational facilities would be classified as low priority.

As with the individual client, the family and community should collaborate when possible in setting priorities. The attitude, preference, and knowledge base of the people involved will determine their degree of participation.

Once priorities for the client's nursing diagnoses have been established, you are ready to determine nursing prognoses.

## DETERMINE NURSING PROGNOSES

The **nursing prognosis** is a prediction or forecast of the probable course of events or outcome associated with a particular nursing diagnosis. It contains a prediction of what changes you expect to occur and the rate at which these changes might occur. The prognosis should not be allowed to shape the outcome of the situation. Do not set yourself or the client up for failure based on an unfavorable prognosis. The prognosis is a statement of probability—a prediction; it is not made with certainty and is not a statement of expectation.

Although the nursing prognosis is usually not written, it should be shared with the client and health team. A prognosis is made for each individual nursing diagnosis and for the overall client situation. These prognoses are the bases for planning goals, objectives, and nursing interventions. In addition, prognoses may help to establish rationale for assigning client care to particular health care providers or for using the services of other disciplines.

## Factors Affecting Prognoses

Prognoses are affected by several factors including the client's overall health status; the client's resources, abilities, and strengths; and the health care provider's knowledge and experience.

*Overall Status.* The client's overall health status will affect nursing prognoses. Review the wellness assessment and identify what health promotion measures are used by the client. Consider the client's abilities, strengths, weaknesses, and limitations that were identified in the health history and physical assessment. If no actual disease state exists, consider the incidence of disease, genetic and developmental disabilities, environmental or traumatic health problems associated with the client's age or ethnic group. What are the client's health risks? Is the client a candidate for genetic diseases such as sickle cell anemia or Tay-Sachs disease? What health problems are most frequently seen in the middle-aged person? What health needs are associated with the family in the childbearing stage of the family life cycle? What are the health needs of a community that has experienced an economic decline?

If a disease state exists, consider the structural or functional changes produced by the pathology. Is the disease considered acute or chronic? Are there curative, palliative, or rehabilitative therapies involved? Are there structural changes that occur as a result of the pathology—loss of a limb, decreased muscle mass, residual scars? Will the disease interfere with the client's ability to function as before? Will there be decreased vision, hearing, strength, endurance, or emotional stamina? All of this information about the client's overall health status will assist you in making nursing prognoses.

*Resources, Abilities, and Strengths.* The client's resources, abilities, and strengths will affect nursing prognoses. You should again consider the assessed data and look for information that reflects the resources available to the client—financial status, support system, coping abilities. Look for data that would indicate if the client is willing and able to follow a treatment regimen, to participate in self-care, or to understand health teaching.

*Knowledge and Experience.* In addition, the health care provider's knowledge and experience will affect nursing prognoses. Your knowledge concerning the usual course of the pathology or the possible threats to the client's health status will help to determine the type of prognosis you assign to each nursing diagnosis. Your experience with similar health needs and problems and the resources available to you will also have an influence.

## Relationship to Other Disciplines

Other disciplines involved in the client's care also will establish prognoses. The medical prognosis is a predictive statement concerning the probable outcome of the disease or pathology. The nursing and medical prognoses influence one another but are not completely dependent upon one another. Both types of prognostic statements must be considered independently and interdependently. The nursing and medical prognoses may both be positive or negative—or one may be positive and the other negative.

To illustrate the relationship between nursing and medical prognoses, consider the following examples.

Mrs. V. S., a 40-year-old executive vice-president of an advertising company, was seen in the clinic after an acute attack of epigastric pain. She had been a widow for the past 5 years and was the sole support of two teenage children, ages 15 and 17 years. Her health history showed that she had been experiencing gnawing-type epigastric pain and heartburn after eating for the past 10 days. The symptoms were usually relieved by milk or a commercial antacid. Mrs. V. S. frequently skipped meals or ate quick meals on the run. Recently she had been under increased pressure at home and work. She refused to discuss the events producing the recent stress and stated they had nothing to do with her health problems. The medical diagnosis of acute gastritis was made after gastrointestinal x-rays failed to reveal any pathology. Mrs. V. S. was placed on Librax and a bland diet. She was receptive to the diet instructions given her.

After reviewing the assessed data, the physician's medical prognosis was favorable. There was nothing to indicate that the client's life was threatened by the episode of gastritis or that she should not recover completely. Since Mrs. V. S. was receptive to diet teaching, the nursing diagnosis, *Impaired nutritional state related to lack of knowledge about bland diets and proper eating patterns,* also had a positive or favorable prognosis. However, the nursing diagnosis, *Increased stress levels related to ineffective or inappropriate coping patterns,* had a negative or unfavorable prognosis. Since the client was unwilling to discuss the stress-producing events in her life and felt that they had no effects on her health problem, it might be difficult to gain adequate client cooperation so that this nursing diagnosis might be resolved.

After the nursing diagnoses have been ranked and prognoses determined, it is time to assemble the various elements in the plan of care: nursing diagnoses, goals, objectives, and nursing interventions (Fig. 6–2).

## ESTABLISH GOALS

A **goal** is a broad statement of what is to be accomplished. It indicates what is desired—the outcome, end state, or point to be achieved.

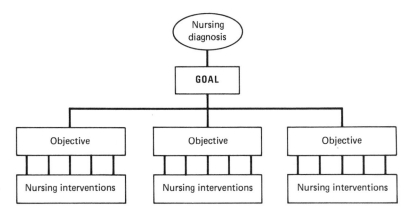

**Figure 6–2.** Elements of the plan of care.

In nursing, goals arise from the nursing diagnoses. Each nursing diagnosis has a goal. These goals serve several purposes. They give direction to nursing interventions and communicate the intent of the plan of care. In addition, goals pace activities with each client and provide a sense of achievement for the client when the goal is reached.

## Factors Affecting Goal Setting

Information within the data base is important and will affect goal setting. You should review the data base and evaluate the client's resources, abilities and disabilities, assets and limitations, and medical and nursing prognoses. The data base should also provide information on the client's health goals and expectations.

As with priority setting, the client should be involved in setting goals. You and the client have different value systems, backgrounds, and experiences. From these differences arise a variety of concerns and ideas. It is important that the plan of care includes goals that primarily reflect the client's concerns. If input from the client is not sought or is ignored, the nurse–client relationship will be threatened, and the client's willingness to participate in the plan of care may decrease.

The client may feel anger, hostility, loss of control, anxiety, altered self-esteem, depression, or dependency when conflicting goals exist or the client disapproves of the goals. Observation of the client's behavior might be the only means to determine these feelings. The client might refuse or forget to perform activities identified within the care plan; an unenthusiastic response to ideas, activities, or the health care provider might be exhibited; angry, resentful, or aggressive responses to suggestions might be made, or nonverbal body and facial cues might be evident.[13]

Your behavior may also transmit disapproval, irritation, or frustration when there is disagreement with the client's goal selection or goal-directed behavior. You must not, through overt or covert measures, try to force the client to comply with goals identified by the health team. When conflict or disagreement concerning goal selection exists, every person involved in the situation must make an effort to resolve the differences.

The client's family or significant others should be involved in goal setting. These people may need to take an active part in implementing the client's plan of care. They may be more willing to participate in and continue with the plan of care if they agree with the goals of the plan. In addition, they may be able to give you insight into how the client handled goal setting in the past.

The physician and other members of the health team will affect goal setting. Members of each discipline that participates in the plan of care for the client will have their own goals. Your goals as a nurse identify what you want to achieve with a particular client or in a particular situation. Every client situation should be approached with goals in mind. What do I want to accomplish today? What activities must I complete during my time with the client? Although the goals of the various disciplines are important, they should not take priority over the client's goals. Whenever possible, these disciplines need to coordinate their goals and plans with and for the client.

Finally, the educational and work background of the nurse will affect goal setting. If you are a new graduate or have had limited experience, you may have difficulty identifying realistic goals with the client or may have insufficient knowledge of what is available to the client. In addition, your philosophy of nursing will influence goal setting. If you believe that the individuals with whom you are working are in a "patient role" (one who is a *recipient* of a health-care service), you may feel that you are obligated to set the health care goals and control the locus of decision making. If viewed as *consumers* of health care, however, the individuals will be considered clients—the ones who employ the services of the health care provider. As such, the clients have the right to know and understand the options available and to assist in the goal setting.[13]

## Components of Goal Statements

A well-constructed statement of a goal should contain a verb, a description of the content area involved, and the expected time when the goal will be achieved or accomplished. Modifiers to describe the action more specifically may be used.

Goals contain verbs that reflect responses to be observed in the client, not activities to be performed by the nurse. Goals are client-centered, not nurse-centered. This does not, however, negate the need for you to assist the client in accomplishing goals.

Since goals are broad statements, the verbs are broad and do not describe the exact process necessary to reach the goal. Verbs such as improve, develop, maintain, promote, increase, decrease, and restore are appropriate for use in goals.

Initially, you may feel more comfortable starting the goal statement with "Client will." Since this is the client's goal, these words are not actually necessary, but this approach will decrease the chance of your including verbs that do not denote client responses.

Goals contain a description of the content area involved. Depending on the goal, this portion of the statement will indicate what the client is to improve, develop, maintain, and so forth. The content area should be precise and exact so that the client and health care providers know what to expect.

Within goal statements, time elements are identified. This portion indicates the time frame for the achievement of the goal and provides motivation and direction for the client and nurse. Goals are either long-, intermediate-, or short-range. The time element is determined by considering the client's health status, resources, and the complexity of the health need. Although the time element is important, if not met it should not become a stumbling block or deterrent for the client. The entire plan of care, including the goal and the client's progress toward its achievement, will be evaluated and changes made where necessary.

The following examples illustrate how these components formulate goal statements.

Client [will increase] [adherence to drug therapy] within [1 month].
    *Action Verb*    *Content Area*    *Time Frame*

Client [will have improved] [body image] by [2 weeks].
    *Action Verb*    *Content Area*    *Time Frame*

Client (family) [will restore] [interfamily communication] within [3 months].
    *Action Verb*    *Content Area*    *Time Frame*

Client (community) [will develop] [plans to reduce pollution level] within [6 months].
    *Action Verb*    *Content Area*    *Time Frame*

## Guidelines for Writing Goals

Now that we know the components of a goal, it is possible to write client-centered goals for each of the client's nursing diagnosis. The following summary of characteristics and examples of goals will help to clarify this portion of the plan of care.

Goals should be directed toward the first part of the nursing diagnosis. The conclusions drawn from the data base are summarized and assigned a diagnostic label; this label is the first part of the diagnostic statement. Since the diagnostic label represents the client's response or need that is to be changed or supported, the goal must reflect it.

Nursing Diagnosis:   Inability to perform activities of daily living related to stiffness, fatigue, and joint pain in knees and hands.

Incorrect Goal:   Client will increase endurance level within 1 month.

Correct Goal:   Client will improve ability to perform activities of daily living within 1 month.

Goals should be written according to what is expected of the client, not what you will do. Remember that these are client-centered goals and include client response.

Nursing Diagnosis:   Anxiety related to fear of or lack of knowledge about the medical diagnosis.

Incorrect Goal:   I will help to reduce the client's anxiety level.

Correct Goal:   Client will have decreased anxiety levels within 6 days.

Goals should be written in positive terms. Negative terms focus on weaknesses instead of strengths. A goal written in positive terms promotes direction for more effective, positive therapies or interventions.

Nursing Diagnosis:   Depression related to self-imposed social isolation.

Incorrect Goal:   Client will not be depressed.

Correct Goal:   Client will have decreased level of depression within 2 weeks.

Goals must be realistic. Remember to take into account the nursing prognosis and the medical diagnosis and prognosis. Write goals that are attainable and practical. Include expectations that incorporate the client's and health care provider's resources and capabilities.

Nursing Diagnosis:   Lack of family preventive health care related to insufficient money to cover cost.

Incorrect Goal:   Client (family) will establish preventive health program for each family member within 1 week.

Correct Goal:   Client (family) will increase participation in preventive health program within 2 months.

Although goals are broad statements, they should be stated in specific, concise terms. They should be as clear and simple as possible. Avoid unnecessary or redundant words; lengthy, wordy goals lose their meaning and effectiveness.

Now that priorities, prognoses, and goals have been established, let us focus our attention on behavioral objectives.

## ESTABLISH BEHAVIORAL OBJECTIVES

Although client-centered goal statements contain time frames and modifiers, they are not quantitative because they are too broad and general. Behavioral objectives which are more specific are needed to accurately measure the client's progress.

A **behavioral objective** is a statement containing observable behaviors. These behaviors describe the change that should be evident in the client. To be effective, behavioral objectives must be stated in specific, measurable terms.

Each nursing diagnosis will have at least one goal. Each goal will have several objectives that reflect the steps leading to the accomplishment of the goal. Evaluation outcome criteria or performance criteria which are developed from objectives are the basis for analyzing the effectiveness of the plan of care and for determining if goals and objectives were accomplished.

Like goals, behavioral objectives give direction to and pace nursing interventions. They motivate both the client and the nurse, and once accomplished, provide the client with a sense of achievement. Behavioral objectives are also affected by the data base, the client's and significant others' input, the attitudes and knowledge of other health team members, and the educational and work background of the nurse. Objectives should be understood and accepted by the client, the client's family or significant others, and the nurse; they should be developed cooperatively between the client and nurse whenever possible.

### Components of Behavioral Objectives

Various formats for behavioral objectives have been proposed. Usually the choice of format is determined by how the objective is to be used—instructional objective, informational objective, planning objective, performance objective, and so forth.

Behavioral objectives may contain the following components:

1. A description of the learner—the person who is to perform the desired behavior.
2. A statement of the actual behavior to be employed—the desired behavior the person will exhibit.
3. A description of the result of the behavior that will be evaluated to determine if the objective was achieved.
4. A description of conditions under which the desired behavior will be demonstrated.
5. A statement of standards or criteria of acceptable performance.[5,10,14,18,22]

An example of an objective that contains all of these components is:

*4*           *1*         *2*

[Given a list of food], the [client] will [plan]

3                                        5

[meals for one day] that [reflect his dietary restrictions in terms of serving size and preparation].

Some of these components are merged to produce a format that can be used in the planning step of the nursing process. To ensure that the behavioral objectives used in the plan of care are specific and measurable, they should contain four elements.

1. Description of the client.
2. Statement of the behavior to be accomplished.
3. Statement of the content to which the behavior relates.
4. Statement of time frame for the achievement of the objective.
   Example:   G.P. will verbalize feelings of self-worth within 2 weeks.

The first element in the objective is a **description of the client.** You may state "Client will," or use the initials or name of the individual client. As with the goal, this portion of the statement is not actually necessary since it is the client's objective. Inclusion of the client's name or initials will make it easier to write client-centered objectives and to make the objectives more individualized.

The second part of the objective is a **statement of the behavior** that the client is to accomplish. Behavioral objectives contain verbs that describe an action by the client that can be seen, felt, heard, or assessed by another person.

Action verbs that denote learning behavior can be used. Bloom, Krathwohl, and others have divided learning behavior into three domains—cognitive, affective, and psychomotor. (Refer to Chapter 10 for further discussion of learning behavior.) Within each domain, levels of thinking, ranging from simple to complex, have been identified.[2,10,11]

Objectives written to include behavioral terms from the **cognitive domain** will reflect changes in knowledge or intellectual abilities. These objectives will include behavior ranging from simple recall to the complex processes of synthesis and validation. Six levels of cognitive behavior have been identified: knowledge, comprehension, application, analysis, synthesis, and evaluation. Although behavioral terms that reflect cognitive function at all six levels may be used, verbs from the first three levels—knowledge, comprehension, and application—are the ones most frequently used.

**Knowledge** is defined as the ability to recall previously learned material. Action verbs that reflect this level of cognitive function include: define, name, list, recall, underline, record, and tell. **Comprehension** is defined as the ability to translate from one form to another—to grasp the meaning of material. Action verbs that represent this level of cognitive function are: discuss, describe, translate, recognize, explain, identify, locate, restate, and report. **Application** refers to the ability to use what is learned in a new situation. Verbs that might be used in stating cognitive outcomes in this level are: interpret, demonstrate, practice, illustrate, apply, use, employ, schedule, and prepare.

**Examples**
Cognitive Domain
   Knowledge:       C. J. will list at least six foods high in sodium by to-morrow.

   Comprehension:    Sara will explain how to adjust her daughter's home feeding schedule by the time of discharge.

Application:          The family will use at least two preventive health mea-
                      sures within the next month.

Objectives written to include behavioral terms from the **affective domain** will reflect such concepts as attitudes, beliefs, and values. Action verbs that might be used in
stating affective function are: listen, touch, express, share, provide, support, relate,
judge, act, and regard.

**Example**
Affective Domain:    The community will express an awareness of the need to
                     increase recreational facilities within 1 month.

Objectives written to include behavioral terms from the **psychomotor domain** will
reflect the client's ability to perform a manual or motor skill. It must be kept in mind
that performing a psychomotor skill includes cognitive and affective behaviors as well
as psychomotor. Action verbs that might be used are: use, administer, take, demonstrate, measure, practice, inject, and assist.

**Example**
Psychomotor Domain:    P. T. will administer her own insulin within 3 days.

Other action verbs that do not necessarily fit into the framework of cognitive, affective, and psychomotor domains are also used. These verbs denote observable and therefore measurable behavior—walk, eat, drink, sleep, laugh, cough, turn, read, speak. In
some instances, modifiers describing how the client will perform the action might be
used. Modifiers make the objective more graphic and descriptive. They help to identify
what is to be observed. For example, walk slowly, eat without help, and speak clearly
are more explicit than the verbs walk, eat, and speak.

**Example**   T. P. will eat foods from each of the four food groups daily start-
              ing tomorrow.

When caring for children or an individual who is disabled or incapacitated, the
verbs may describe the expected behavior of a family member or of a significant other.
The verbs may also reflect the desired physiologic response of the individual's body. For
example, the objective may be, Client's breath sounds will be clear to auscultation
within 1 week. Such objectives are frequently used with people who are confused, unconscious, or unable to demonstrate independent physical or verbal action.

The third part of the objective is a **statement of the content** to which the behavior
relates. This portion of the objective will depend on the nursing diagnosis. The content
area of the objective can be directed at either part of the nursing diagnosis but usually
reflects the second part, the sustaining factors.

Nursing Diagnosis:   Inability to perform activities of daily living related to
                     stiffness, fatigue, and joint pain in knees and hands.

Goal:                K. P. will improve ability to perform activities of daily
                     living within 1 month.

Objective:         K. P. will discuss two measures to decrease joint pain in
                   knees and hands within 4 days.

By directing the objectives at the sustaining factors, nursing interventions can be developed that eliminate, maintain, or reduce the effects of the elements that are sustaining the client's response. (This aspect of the nursing process will be discussed later in this chapter.)

**Time elements** are the fourth part of the behavioral objective. This portion indicates the time frame for the achievement of the objective and provides motivation and direction for the client and nurse by setting an end point. The time element must be exact. It may be stated in terms of hours, days, weeks, or months. When establishing the time frame, it is important that you and the client consider the feasibility of accomplishing the objective in that period of time. As with the goals, the objectives and the client's progress toward their achievement will be evaluated and altered as necessary.

Nursing Diagnosis:   Self-care deficits in the area of bathing and dressing related to decreased movement of left arm.

Goal:                J. N. will improve ability to perform self-care within one month.

Objectives:          J. N. will wash own face, hands, and arms by 5/21.
                     J. N. will button own robe by 5/23.

## Guidelines for Writing Objectives
The following summary of characteristics and examples of behavioral objectives will help to clarify this step in the plan of care.

Behavioral objectives express the intended outcome, not outcomes. Each objective contains only one behavior. This practice will prevent confusion and facilitate identification of desired behaviors.

Incorrect Objective:   Client will define and list the symptoms of diabetes mellitus in own words by 5/30.

Correct Objective:     M. P. will define diabetes mellitus in own words by 5/28.
                       M. P. will describe in own words the symptoms of diabetes mellitus by 5/30.

The first example includes two cognitive behaviors: define and list. A client may define diabetes mellitus but may not be able to list the symptoms associated with the disease. It is therefore difficult to evaluate the outcome.

An inclusion of a **methodology** statement within the behavioral objective is not necessary. Methodology states how the objective is to be accomplished. This practice limits the client and the nurse because it states that there is only one way that a particular behavior can be accomplished.

Incorrect Objective:   Client will demonstrate communication patterns
                       [through use of effective interpersonal interactions]
                       within 1 week.

The information that appears in the brackets in the above example represents the use of methodology within an objective. The methodology in this behavioral objective suggests that only one aspect reflects communication patterns: effective interpersonal interactions. It ignores many other actions that could be used to accomplish the behavior.

Incorrect Objective:   Client will develop [through group discussion] an awareness of his health risks within 3 days.

This objective suggests that the client's learning can only be attained in terms of one procedure: group discussion. It eliminates other sources of learning. You should avoid words such as *through* or *by* when writing behavioral objectives. These words usually precede a statement of methodology.

Write the behavioral objective according to what is expected of the client, not what you will do. Remember that the goals and objectives are client centered and include client behavior.

Incorrect Objective:   I will have the client list four examples of foods high in Vitamin C by 5/30.

Correct Objective:   M. S. will list four examples of foods high in Vitamin C by 5/30.

Make the behavior or verb in your objective clear and measurable. Words such as know, understand, believe, recognize, appreciate, grasp significance of, and learn are open to many interpretations and cannot be measured.[10,14]

Incorrect Objective:   Client will *know* four examples of foods high in Vitamin D by 5/30.

Correct Objective:   L. M. will *list* four examples of foods high in Vitamin D by 5/30.

In this example, list is more specific and measurable than *know* and is open to fewer interpretations.

A behavioral objective should be stated in specific, concise terms.

Incorrect Objective:   Client will demonstrate methods to increase pulmonary ventilation within 3 days.

Correct Objective:   T. H. will demonstrate pursed-lip breathing within 3 days (6/23).

The correct example specifies the method the client is expected to learn.

The behavioral objective should be written in positive terms. It must be realistic and reflect the capabilities and limitations of the client and health care providers.

## Outcome Criteria

A **criterion** is a statement of a standard, rule, or model used in judging. **Outcome criteria** are standards used to determine the responses to or results of nursing interventions. The client's objectives are the foundation for the outcome criteria. As stated earlier, in some formats the criteria may be written as a part of the behavioral objective instead of a separate statement. Although outcome criteria are used in the evaluating step of the nursing process, they should be established in the planning step. (Refer to Chapter 8 for a discussion of the evaluating process.)

Outcome criteria may contain:

1. A description of the change, specific behavior, or response that must be evident as a result of the nursing action.

   Example:   Mrs. O. fed herself.

   This portion of the criterion may be written in behavioral or performance terms. Behavior implies physiologic, social, psychological, and intellectual activities. In addition, the criterion may be written in terms of the change expected in the environment or community or the response as reflected by x-rays and laboratory tests.
2. A statement of the conditions under which the behavior, change, or response occurs. This would include any restrictions, situations, or requirements. Inclusion of these factors decreases the chance for misunderstanding, error, or ambiguity. Perhaps the most commonly used limitation is time. The limitation should indicate when the outcome should occur.

   Examples:   Mrs. O. fed herself with her affected hand. (The condition in this statement is a restriction.)
   Mrs. O. fed herself, unassisted, before going home. (The conditions in this statement represent both a restriction and a time limitation.)
   Mr. T stated the correct schedule for his medications by 6 PM today. (The condition in this is a time limitation.)

3. A statement defining the limits of acceptable performance or behavior. Time limits, minimum number of correct responses, and accuracy are measures of acceptable performance. At times it may be difficult to decide if a statement is a restriction or a description of an acceptable performance. As long as the outcome is clearly stated, this differentiation will not create any difficulties.

Each of the three items discussed will make the outcome more specific; it is not necessary to include all items in each evaluative criterion. Your aim is to write criteria that communicate the expected outcome of the nursing intervention so that it is possible to determine if the care has accomplished what it was designed to do.[3,14,26]

Several characteristics of criteria have been identified.[14,26] These include:

1. Each outcome criterion relates to an established client objective.
2. The criterion must identify the act (outcome) that will be accepted as evidence that the client has achieved the objective.
3. The outcome stated in the criterion must be achievable. It must also be important or critical. For example, a 14-kilogram weight loss within 6 weeks would be a critical criterion for a moderately obese client.
4. Each criterion should contain a single behavior or outcome. If a criterion includes more than one outcome, it is difficult to determine if the criterion is met.

The statement "loss of 14 kilograms and 5 centimeters at the waist within 6 weeks" should be written as two separate criteria.

5. Each criterion should be as specific as possible.
6. A criterion must be measurable; the outcome can be observed, heard, felt, assessed, or measured by another person. A statement such as "The client's appetite improved" is not mesurable. To make the statement measurable you should change the criterion to read "J. N. ate 1200 calories in a 24-hour period." Outcomes may frequently be measured by means of rating scales or instruments. For example, you can use scales to determine the client's weight loss or gain or a thermometer to determine the client's temperature. You can also ask the client how he or she feels emotionally, rated on a scale from 1 to 10.
7. A criterion is stated in positive rather than negative terms. Positive criteria describe outcomes or responses that should occur. By stating the criterion in positive terms, you are describing a condition that can be observed. The statement "No signs of dehydration" is more appropriately stated "M. N.'s skin is moist and supple in 2 days."

When the nursing diagnosis, goal, objectives, and outcome criteria are viewed together, the evaluation process becomes clearer.

Nursing Diagnosis:    Fluid imbalance (dehydration) related to decreased fluid intake and nausea.

Goal:    M. R. will have improved hydration within 1 week.

Objective:    M. R. will drink 200 ml of water every 3 hours.

Outcome Criteria:    M. R.'s oral mucous membranes are moist and pink within 1 week.
M. R.'s oral intake was at least 1600 ml/24 hours.

To clarify this portion of the planning step, we will develop goals, objectives, and outcome criteria for some of the nursing diagnoses developed in Chapter 5 (Table 6–2).

At this point, nursing interventions must be identified that will assist the client to achieve the established goals and objectives.

## IDENTIFY NURSING INTERVENTIONS

The term **intervention** is applied to any action that prevents harm from occurring to a client or that maintains or improves the mental, physical, or psychological function of a client. The term is frequently used interchangeably with nursing actions, therapies, and strategies. Although interventions are identified at this point, the actual performance of the interventions occurs during the fourth step in the nursing process—implementing.

### Types of Nursing Interventions

There are three types of interventions: dependent, independent, and interdependent. Dependent interventions stem from the physician's orders. The physician's orders are directed at the medical diagnosis or problem, not the nursing diagnosis. These **depen-**

TABLE 6–2. EXAMPLES OF GOALS, OBJECTIVES, OUTCOME CRITERIA

| Nursing Diagnoses | Goal | Objectives | Outcome Criteria |
|---|---|---|---|
| Maintenance of active support system. | Client will continue to maintain active support network with family throughout period of hospitalization. | Client will utilize measures to maintain contact with family daily. | Contact with family member at least once per day occurred. |
| Sleep pattern disturbance related to difficulty breathing in a lying position and back and leg pain. | Client will have an improved sleep pattern within two weeks. | Client will discuss today measures used at home to promote sleep. (Since this was not a part of the data base, it should be considered at this point.) | Discussed without hesitation her usual bedtime routine by 2/18. |
| | | Client will identify within the next 4 days measures to reduce back and leg pain. | Stated two measures that effectively reduced her discomfort by 2/22. |
| | | Client will sleep uninterrupted, 5 hours a night by 1 week. | Statements of feeling more rested by 1 week were made. |
| Health maintenance alteration related to lack of resources, incomplete knowledge base, and decreased motivation to follow nursing and medical therapies. (Diagnosis based on failure to follow diabetic diet, excessive body weight, and elevated blood pressure.) | Client will have improved health maintenance program within 3 months. | Client will identify basic health practices that she should follow by 1 week. | Stated two basic health practices that she should follow by 2/25. |
| | | Client will discuss effects of excess weight and elevated blood pressure on overall health status by 1 week. | Described how excess weight increases fluid retention by 2/25. |
| | | Client will plan menus for 1 day within the next week. | Prepared menu that reflected her dietary restrictions for an 1800 calorie diabetic diet by 2/25. |

Note: These are only examples of objectives and outcome criteria that would be appropriate for this client. More objectives and criteria would be needed to ensure achievement of the goal.

**dent interventions** include actions needed to implement the physician's or medical order. Diagnostic procedures, medications, activity regulation, dietary restrictions, therapeutic procedures such as hot and cold applications, enemas, urinary catheterizations, and restraints are some of the therapies usually controlled by physician's orders.

Even though the physician's orders are directed at the medical problem, in some instances they help the client to achieve the goals and objectives associated with nursing diagnoses. For example, the client with the nursing diagnosis of *Depression related to prolonged bed rest* will be helped psychologically by the medical order to "dangle the client three times daily." The physician's determination that activities should be increased was probably based on the client's signs and symptoms and evidence of physical improvement. Regardless of the goal of the medical order, it may help the client to achieve the personal goal: client will have decreased level of depression within 1 week.

Usually dependent interventions cannot be initiated by the nurse without a written order from the physician. Most institutions have established policies governing verbal orders received directly from the physician or by telephone. In addition, in some institutions **standing orders** are used. These orders are based on specific criteria and are supported by policies within the institution. Nurses in emergency rooms, delivery rooms, intensive care units, nursing homes, or areas with decreased access to physicians frequently use standing orders. Examples of standing orders might include:

| Situation | Criteria | Standing Orders |
|---|---|---|
| Coronary intensive care unit | Premature ventricular contractions (PVC's) of more than 6/minute or runs or bursts of 3 or more. | Lidocaine 1% 50 mg intravenous push and lidocaine drip of 2 Gr. added to 500 ml 5% D/W; infuse at 15 to 60 microdrops/minute. |
| Emergency Room | Anaphylaxis (allergic reaction) with history of exposure to allergen, urticaria, respiratory distress, and hypertension. | Administer epinephrine 0.3 to 0.5 ml of 1:1000 SQ or IM; Oxygen 6 to 10 liters/minute by mask. |
| Community health nurse—family nurse practitioner | Otitis externa as diagnosed by pain in ear, partial occlusion of external canal by edema or discharge, no swelling over mastoid, tympanic membrane normal, injected, or covered with flecks of exudate.[19] | Gentle and thorough removal of debris from canal; acetominophen or aspirin as appropriate for age; cortisporin otic drops 4 in affected ear four times daily.[19] |
| Nursing Home—elderly client with foley catheter | Encrustations are felt within the lumen of the catheter; leakage of urine around the catheter has developed; the catheter is no longer soft and pliable. | Change foley catheter as needed based on any one of the criteria. |

Medical orders initiate dependent interventions, but critical thinking and sound judgment are still needed by the nurse. No order should be implemented blindly. You must use your own theoretical knowledge to assist you in determining if these are the correct actions in this particular situation. No one is infallible. An incorrect drug dose or treatment might inadvertently be prescribed for a client. Through careful examination and interpretation of orders prior to implementation, the chances of errors occurring can be reduced.

**Interdependent interventions** include those actions which the nurse performs in collaboration with multidisciplinary health team members. For example, the physician may order physical therapy to perform range-of-motion exercises twice daily on the client's left arm and leg. You, as a nurse, are responsible for making certain that the physical therapy department is informed and for organizing the client's other activities so that the therapy can be given. In addition, you should collaborate with the physical therapist so that you can determine the client's response to the exercises.

**Independent nursing interventions** include the actions described in nursing orders or the actions needed to implement the order. (Nursing orders will be discussed later in this chapter.) These interventions are based on your knowledge base, and they do not require a physician's order. Independent interventions provide the methodology for achieving goals and objectives—the how, where, when, and by whom it will be done.

## Levels of Interventions

In previous chapters, we indicated that you must be mindful of the three levels of health needs—primary, secondary, and tertiary—when assessing and analyzing the assessed data. Independent, dependent, and interdependent interventions will arise from the client's needs at each of these levels. Interventions on the primary level might include measures to promote health—arranging an immunization schedule—or to assist the client to manage developmental changes—talking with the client about peer pressure. Secondary level interventions might include measures directed at any episode of illness or injury—talking with a mother about the care of her child's chicken pox lesions or administering prescribed medications to the client with pneumonia. Interventions on the tertiary level might include measures that would promote rehabilitation—teaching range of motion to the client's spouse so that care can be continued at home. As you identify interventions for your client, you should keep these three levels of care in mind so that more of the client's health needs are met.

## Determine Appropriate Independent Interventions

The first intervention that comes to mind may not be the best. It is therefore important to generate as many alternative interventions as possible. Generating a list of possible interventions for a particular situation has several advantages. First, it will help you to develop the best possible plan for a particular client. If one intervention fails to meet the needs of the client, other alternatives are available for immediate incorporation into the plan. This will prevent lapses in care. In addition, generating various alternative interventions will help you to develop a creative approach to client care rather than relying on a few basic interventions.

Several sources of alternative solutions or interventions have been identified. These sources include: (1) past experience and knowledge; (2) experiences and opinions of colleagues; (3) opinions and data from the individual, family, or community affected; and (4) advice or consultation from experts.[1] In addition, you should check references (journals and books) for ideas. (Chapter 11 on decision making will help you to understand the process of deriving alternative solutions.)

As with any aspect of the plan of care, you should confer with colleagues for advice and ideas. Their clinical experience and theoretical background will complement and support your own knowledge base and should enable you to develop a more comprehensive plan of care. Ideas can be gathered from colleagues by informal inquiry or through brainstorming. Brainstorming is a group process. In brainstorming, ideas stimulate other ideas—one person's suggestion stimulates another person to think of an idea. It is important that each person in the group feels free to express an idea; judgment or criticism of the ideas generated should not occur during the brainstorming session.

You must also discuss the plan of care with the client involved. Remember that the client's opinions were sought during establishing priorities and goal setting; the client should not be left out of this portion of the plan. If the client is not able to participate in the identification of possible interventions, the client's family or significant others should be involved.

Your next step is to analyze the various alternatives and to select the ones that seem the most appropriate. Each intervention may have positive and negative effects. Weigh the merit of each proposed alternative and consider its predicted outcome. The most appropriate alternatives will produce the greatest benefit to the client with the least amount of risk. Ask yourself the following questions about each intervention:

- Is this intervention based on scientific rationale?
- Has this intervention been used before in a similar situation? If so, what was the outcome?
- Is this intervention safe? What might be some undesirable consequences if this alternative is used?
- Is this intervention realistic in terms of the available resources?
- Does this intervention reflect the client's life-style, attitudes, religious and cultural beliefs, and ability to adapt?
- Does this intervention reflect the client's choices and opinions?
- Will this intervention help the client to meet personal goals and objectives?

If you were to ask a group of nurses to brainstorm and to list interventions that might be used to promote the healing of a decubitus ulcer, you would receive a variety of responses. Based on the experience and knowledge base of each nurse, the list might include the following responses:

- Turn the client every two hours.
- Massage the area around the decubitus.
- Use Maalox and Merthiolate on the decubitus.*
- Spray the ulcer with benzoin.*
- Apply granulated sugar to the area.*
- Use a heat lamp on the area.
- Increase protein and vitamin C in the diet.
- Use a rubber ring or donut around the area.*
- Debride the ulcer with enzyme ointments.
- Massage the adjacent area with alcohol.*
- Cover the decubitus with Op-site.
- Apply insulin to the decubitus.*
- Place an air mattress on the bed.

If you were to consider each of these alternatives in view of the previous set of questions, you would find that many of them do not have a scientific basis. (The asterisk indicates alternatives not presently supported by a scientific rationale.) Other interventions might have to be eliminated for other reasons—perhaps in your institution some of the alternatives would not be considered independent nursing interventions. Although brainstorming in this case produced a variety of alternatives, not all of the interventions were considered appropriate.

After analyzing each intervention and eliminating those not considered appropriate, you will have a concise list of interventions. Priorities should now be set for items on the list to reflect which one you and the other people involved in the plan feel will best achieve the stated objectives and goal. This intervention will be the one that you try initially. It is not easy to decide which intervention to use first. The ability to select the best of several alternatives comes gradually with acquired knowledge and experience.

It is possible that several interventions might be necessary to contribute to the success of a plan. These interventions might be so interrelated that they depend on each other for their effectiveness. In this case, all the interventions would be started at the same time. An example of this aspect can be seen in the list of possible interventions for the decubitus ulcer. Used alone, a diet high in protein and vitamin C will probably not heal a decubitus ulcer. The decubitus ulcer may heal, however, when the diet is combined with some of the other appropriate interventions.

The interventions that are to be used on the plan of care should be written as nursing orders.

## Write the Interventions as Nursing Orders

Nursing orders contain descriptions of the actions needed to *implement* independent behavior of the nurse, medical orders (dependent behavior), or collaboration with other health team members (interdependent behavior). Nursing orders provide nurses with specific directives for the behaviors they are to perform. These behaviors are based on a scientific rationale whenever possible and directed toward the second part of the nursing diagnosis, the sustaining factors.

Nursing orders are not repetitious of medical orders and are directed at the nursing diagnosis, not the medical diagnosis. They help to individualize the client's care and to communicate what is different about each client's interventions. For instance, the hospitalized client may need assistance when ambulating. The nursing orders would describe specifically what assistance is needed—a cane, a walker, two nurses, and so forth.

Nursing orders promote accountability within the nursing profession. Once written, the orders should be followed by all nurses providing health care. In the hospital setting, this aspect is made easier by primary nursing. In primary nursing one professional nurse is responsible for planning and directing the client's 24-hour care. Other nurses are expected to implement the plan when the primary nurse is not on duty.

Nurses should consider nursing orders as important as medical orders and as such the orders should meet the same expectations. Nursing orders usually contain five components: date, specific action verb, prescribed activity or content area, time elements, and signature or initials.[13,17] Although the components of a nursing order are similar to those described for behavioral objectives, the two are not the same. Remember that the behavioral objective reflects the response or desired behavior of the client; the nursing order reflects the desired behavior of the nurse.

All nursing orders that are written should be **dated.** The date indicates when the order was initially written. Each order is reviewed regularly and discontinued, renewed, or revised. When the order is renewed or revised, the date will be changed to reflect the date this occurred.

The frequency for review and updating of nursing orders will depend on the situation. Although orders may be revised at any time, a maximum time limit between review periods should be set. In some instances—the hospital setting—the orders should be reviewed daily. In extended care facilities or in the home, the frequency of the review of orders may be weekly or monthly. When reviewing nursing orders in situations where changes occur slowly, for example, the community, longer time periods between reviews are acceptable.

Each nursing order contains a **specific action verb.** This verb communicates the specific behavior to be performed by the nurse. In addition to the action verb, a modifying word or phrase may be added to make the desired behavior more precise.

A **prescribed activity or content area** is also contained in the order. This component deals with the *what* and *where* of the nursing order. What information is to be taught? What foods is the client to avoid? What type of counseling is the client (family) to seek? What resources are available to the client?

The **time elements or time units** in the order indicate *when, how often,* or *how long.* Clock hours (8 – 12 – 4 – 8), days (every Wednesday and Saturday), dates (6/15), nursing actions (when you enter the room), or client response (when client complains of pain) may be used to denote time. The time element must be written in clear, precise terms.

The last component of a nursing order is the **signature or initial** of the person writing the order. This is another indication of accountability. By means of the signature, the nurse writing the order becomes identifiable and therefore accountable for what is written. When only initials are used instead of the complete signature, the record should contain a method for identifying each set of initials. The signature also provides information needed by colleagues who may want to contact the person who originally wrote the order for clarification or to give feedback on the effectiveness of the order.

Using these five components, a nursing order would appear as follows:

[6/15] [Demonstrated] to Mr. J. and his family [how to change eye dressing]
*Date      Action Verb*                                                    *Prescribed Activity*

[today at 4 PM and tomorrow at 9 AM.] Signature
         *Time Element*

The following example illustrates the relationship between the nursing diagnosis, goal, objectives, outcome criteria, and nursing order.

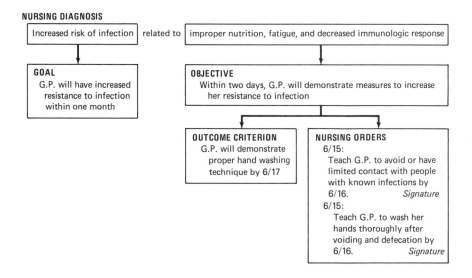

The following suggestions and examples should help you to write appropriate nursing orders.

1. The action verb, prescribed activity (content area), and time element should be stated in a clear, precise, and specific manner. If orders are not specific, each nurse must interpret what should be done.

Incorrect:   6/15 Encourage the client whenever he voices concern about his
             progress.
             *Signature*

The verb "encourage" is imprecise. Encouragement is generated by many forms
of behavior. Since most of the behavioral actions associated with this verb cannot be used interchangeably, the person writing the order must decide which
action is appropriate for this client.

Correct:   6/15 Stay with Mr. T. whenever he voices concern about his prog-
           ress.
           *Signature*

The verb "stay" describes a specific, precise action the nurse should take. The
order could even be more precise if it designated how long the nurse should stay
and what actions should be taken during the time spent with the client.

Other verbs that are imprecise and require further explanation include:[13]

|              |           |
|--------------|-----------|
| have         | force     |
| reassure     | provide   |
| teach        | reinforce |
| support      | ambulate  |
| counsel      | observe   |
| give         | recognize |

Incorrect:   6/15 Force fluids every 2 hours.
             *Signature*

The verb "force" is imprecise in that it doesn't indicate if the client will literally
be forced to drink the fluids or if the client will be offered fluids. The term
"fluids" is nonspecific. What type of fluids? How much fluid? Is the temperature
of the fluid important? These aspects must be considered before writing the order. The order is also not clear because it does not indicate what 2 hour cycle
is to be followed: 9–11–1–3, etc., or 8–10–12–2, etc.

Correct:   6/15 Offer J.B. 100cc of water every 2 hours, 8–10–12–2, etc.
           *Signature*

Incorrect:   6/15 Teach client about diabetes before discharge.
             *Signature*

This nursing order contains incomplete information regarding the content area
and the time element as well as an imprecise action verb. The verb "teach" is
open to many interpretations and does not indicate what techniques might be
most appropriate in this situation. The content area, "about diabetes," is so
broad that anything could be taught. "Before discharge" does not establish a
time schedule for the teaching.

Correct:   6/15 Demonstrate urine testing via test tape to Mr. D.G. today,
           6/16.
           *Signature*

2. Nursing orders must be realistic and achievable. The client's preferences were
   considered earlier when you selected appropriate interventions. At this point,
   you must be certain that you can achieve the behavior described in the order
   and that it is realistic for this particular client. You should take into consideration available resources. Make certain that facilities, material resources, and
   personnel are appropriate.

   Incorrect:   6/15 Arrange for lawn maintenance service for Mr. P. by tomor-
                row afternoon.
                *Signature*

   Although the idea of getting lawn care for a disabled client is appropriate, you
   would need to make certain that such an arrangement was within the financial
   scope of the client. Perhaps the following nursing order would be more realistic.

   Correct:   6/15 Discuss with Mr. P. possible solutions for his lawn care needs
              by this afternoon.
              *Signature*

3. The nursing order should not repeat orders written by other health care providers. For example, if the situation is addressed by a medical order, don't repeat
   that content in nursing orders unless specific clarification is needed.

   Incorrect:   6/15 Change Mr. T.'s dressing every AM.
                *Signature*
   Incorrect:   6/15 Ambulate Ms. S. twice a day.
                *Signature*

   Many institutions require written medical orders for dressing changes and client ambulation. These nursing orders would be duplications of information already provided. In addition, they are not specific or clear.

   Correct:   6/15 Change Mr. T.'s abdominal dressing using two 4 × 4's and one
              ABD every morning at 9AM
              *Signature*

   Correct:   6/15 Walk Ms. S. with the assistance of two people 10 meters in the
              hall at 9AM and 6PM each day.
              *Signature*

4. Some nursing orders relate to observations of the client's behavior, reactions,
   and responses. In respect to the steps in the nursing process, observation is primarily a function completed in the first step, assessing. Once the initial data
   base has been compiled, it is essential for you to decide what ongoing assess-

ment data are needed. Decisions regarding the type and frequency of ongoing assessment are part of planning and must be clearly stated within the nursing orders.[12]

Once determined, the nursing diagnosis, goals, objectives, outcome criteria, and nursing orders should be recorded on the plan of care.

## FORMULATE PLAN OF CARE

A plan is a detailed scheme or method worked out beforehand for the purpose of accomplishing or achieving an end result. Nurses have always had a plan in mind as they cared for clients. The written plan of care, however, is usually more explicit and effective. A **care plan** can be defined as a written source of client information that serves as a guide to client-centered nursing care.

From a historical perspective, the care plan, in some form, has been in use since the 1940s. Its use increased after World War II with the onset of the team approach to client care. In team nursing, several individuals were involved in the care of one client—it was important that each person giving care was aware of needed interventions and the progress of the client. The care plan provided the team members with a means of communicating. Although they were meant to be beneficial to the client and the nurse, the nurses found care plans difficult to use. They were uncertain what and how to record the information that they wanted to share with others.

The care plan was still being used primarily as a tool for improving communication in the late 1950s. The plan was usually labelled the nursing care plan or the nurse's plan of care, which implied that the client did not take part in its development. In the early 1960s, the nurse's ability to assess the client was being emphasized and the care plan became a central source for the assessed data. Goals and objectives were recorded as well as the approaches necessary to achieve them. In most instances, the goals and objectives were nurse-centered, not client-centered. Nurses continued to have difficulty using the care plans and complained that they were time consuming. It was not uncommon to find only notations of medical orders on the plans.[4,15]

During the late 1960s and early 1970s, the use of care plans expanded. The structure or format for the plans changed. One format that arose during that period was the circular care plan. This plan was initiated in the facility where the client was first seen. The same care plan was used at all three levels of care—primary, secondary, and tertiary—and went with the client from one health care facility to the next—clinic to hospital to community.[21] The concept of one plan of care spanning the different levels of health care added another dimension; the plan could now provide for (1) communication between health team members, (2) individualization of care, and (3) continuity of care.

Within nursing education, the care plan evolved as a teaching tool. Although the formats for the care plan used in the educational setting differ from those in the health care setting, some variation of the problem-solving approach is used in both. The primary purpose of the care plan in the educational setting is to provide students with a method for learning about the client's health needs and the rationales for the nursing actions needed to meet them. The primary purpose of the care plan in the health care setting is to communicate relevant data regarding client care. These differences are important and may cause confusion for the beginning practitioner who enters the health care field with only the educational model of care planning as a frame of reference.[17]

Care plans used within the health care setting remain in a state of evolution and flux even today. Every nurse at some point has learned about the functions and development of care plans. Health care facilities—hospitals as well as community agencies—require their staff to develop care plans. The Joint Commission on Accreditation of Hospitals (JCAH) upholds the use of care plans and requires a written, goal-directed plan for each client as evidence that appropriate nursing care is given. A scheduled JCAH visit is often the impetus that causes a health facility to bring their plans up to standard. Yet, with all of this support and pressure, care plans are not used effectively or consistently in many health care facilities.

What is the problem? Why don't nurses utilize care plans? Some of the reasons that have been given include: lack of time, work pressures, lack of administrative support, residual negative attitudes about care plans from nursing school days, inability to adapt educational care-plan model to health delivery model, failure to internalize purposes and values of care plans, inability of some nurses to view themselves as competent managers capable of directing care, lack of confidence about ability to write nursing orders, and anxiety about being accountable for what is written.

In order to be an effective professional care-provider, you must overcome all of these stumbling blocks. The development and use of a well-written care plan is one way of assuming accountability for your actions; you should view this as a step toward autonomy, not something to be feared. The care plan is the client's; it helps the client contribute to and receive high-quality, individualized care. Since it is the client's care plan, it is imperative that it be developed and used appropriately.

## Functions and Purposes of the Plan

Many functions and purposes for the care plan can be identified. Some of these include:

- Ensures a central source of information on the client.
- Provides a guide for client care and gives direction to health care providers.
- Gives details (in writing) of goals, objectives, and interventions.
- Promotes individualization of care. The plan of care provides a place for recording specific interventions that are unique to each client.
- Serves as a means of systematic communication. The plan of care provides a written means of conveying communication and serves as a point of reference to support the communication. Because the information is written, there will be less distortion of facts than when information is transferred verbally from one person to another. The plan also serves as a resource that can be checked at any time. It is possible for the plan to convey information to a variety of health team members: the client, family, nurse, physician, social worker, and so forth. A copy of the care plan can accompany the client should the client be transferred either within the health care facility or from one care facility to another. If the care plan is part of the permanent record, it can be checked on subsequent visits to the same health care facility for information.
- Provides for continuity of care. The care plan provides for an even progression of care from one nurse to another and from one discipline to another. Omissions, duplications, overlaps, gaps, and errors in care can be prevented. The transition difficulties that may occur when different nurses assume client care (change of shifts in the hospital, transfer of client) can be decreased or eliminated.
- Coordinates and provides an even flow of health care. All aspects of the client's

care, medical therapies, diagnostic tests, and nursing interventions, can be scheduled in a manner to preserve the client's energy and ensure continued comfort.

- Promotes comprehensive care that encompasses the whole person. Consideration of the client as a unique individual with roles, relations, coping abilities, and emotional, physical, spiritual, and cultural needs is easier to incorporate when planned.
- Provides a means of incorporating interventions for all three levels of health care—primary, secondary, and tertiary.
- Ensures adequate discharge planning.
- Assists in the evaluation of care. The efficiency of the plan and the achievement of goals, objectives, and outcome criteria can be determined more accurately with a written care plan.
- Serves as a key for care assignments. Assignments can be based on the complexity of the needs for nursing care and the personnel skills available.
- Provides a resource for client-centered conferences.

None of these functions can be fulfilled if the plan is not up to date or accurate—or not present.

## Initiation of the Plan

The written plan of care should be started as soon as possible. Delay in starting the plan can interfere with the quality of the nursing care given. Remember that the entire process started back when you first met the client and began gathering the data base. After the data base had been analyzed and nursing diagnoses established, the plan of care was developed. The entire process of assessing, diagnosing, and planning may take considerable time. Even then, the plan is not finished because it is constantly evaluated and updated.

The nurse responsible for the care of the client should be held accountable for developing the original plan of care and for revising the plan when necessary. In the hospital, if primary nursing is practiced, the client's primary nurse is responsible for the plan. In a community setting, the nurse is responsible for the plans of those clients in a particular case load. Although the professional nurse is responsible for developing and revising the plan, other health team members can and should contribute to it.

Some plans of care are developed and revised in nursing care conferences or multidisciplinary team conferences. The nursing care conferences include only the nursing staff responsible for client care; the multidisciplinary team conferences include any one contributing to the client's overall care—family members, physicians, dietitians, social workers, and other health care personnel. These conferences must be limited in time and scope, and the individual conducting the conference must direct the discussion to relevant content. Remember, the primary purpose of the conference is to plan care.

## Format for the Plan

Regardless of the format used, the plan of care should follow the steps in the nursing process as closely as possible. The plan should contain nursing diagnoses, goals, objectives, outcome criteria, and nursing orders. Assessment data are included in some plans. In addition, space must be provided for the evaluation data (Fig. 6–3 and Fig. 6–4).

The format used will vary with the health care facility and sometimes from division to division within the same facility. The plan should be easy to use and contain enough space to record everything that needs to be written down. It may not be possible to re-

181

CARE PLAN

Current diagnosis _____

Discharge plan _____

Addressograph

| DATE | NURSING DIAGNOSES GOALS | OBJECTIVES | EXPECTED OUTCOME | TARGET DATE | RESOLUTION DATE | NURSING ORDERS (DATE AND SIGNATURE) |
|---|---|---|---|---|---|---|
| | | | | | | |
| | | | | | | |

**Figure 6–3.** Example of a care plan form.

PLAN OF CARE

Client's name _____    Signature of primary nurse _____

_____ Room     __/__/__ Admission date

Social history

| DATE RECORDED | NURSING DIAGNOSES/ GOALS | OBJECTIVES/ NURSING ORDERS | OUTCOME CRITERIA | EVALUATION DATA |
|---|---|---|---|---|
| | | | | |
| | | | | |

Discharge planning:

**Figure 6–4.** Example of a care plan form with space for assessment data.

cord a written plan of care for every nursing diagnosis established. Those with high-priority rankings should be placed in the written plan. Kardex cards, loose-leaf notebooks, and computer printouts are formats frequently used.

Sometimes the plan of care is combined on the same form with the medical care plan. These kardex cards are divided into convenient sections that help the care providers to record data.

- Profile of Client. This section contains demographic data. The client's name, medical diagnosis, religion, marital status, occupation, and other identifying information are recorded.
- Assessment Data. In a brief form, pertinent information from the client's health history and physical assessment is included.
- Treatments, Medications, Diagnostic Procedures. This section varies greatly with the requirements of the agency. Medications will be itemized and the dosage, time, and method of administration noted. The types and times for treatments will be listed. Any adaptation of treatments or medication administration for this client should be recorded. The diagnostic procedures ordered for the client will be recorded with the date ordered and date completed.
- General or Routine Care. This section lists items of care common to many clients. What is included will vary with the type of clients cared for by the agency or by the unit within the agency. Some of the items which might be listed in the general care section for hospitalized clients are: bath, oral hygiene, diet, nourishments, activity level, mode of transportation, fluids, elimination, intake and output, rest and sleep, weight, and vital signs. A form used in an ambulatory setting might include: nutrition, prevention (immunization schedule, methods of preventing spread of communicable diseases), environmental control, health promotion (family planning, dental care, frequency and nature of screening tests), mental health, maternal–child health, and referrals.[12] (See Fig. 6–5A, B and Fig. 6–6A, B.)

Some forms are developed so that an interdisciplinary approach is possible. These forms allow each discipline involved in the client's care to record its plan so that it is accessible to the other disciplines. This approach promotes coordination of care (Fig. 6–7).

Although individuals have many differences, they also have common characteristics, needs, and responses. Because of these similarities, standard care plans are frequently used. A **standard care plan** is a protocol for care that is likely to be applicable to most clients with a certain nursing or medical diagnosis.[17] The plan is written in a format consistent with the facility's form for individualized care plans. The format should provide a space for the nurse's handwritten entries as well as the development of diagnoses specific to this particular client. The standard care plan must be carefully researched and written. Approval by an agency committee must occur before the plan is formally accepted for use (Fig. 6–8).

## Guidelines for Formulating the Plan

The following guidelines will help you to formulate a written plan of care.

1. The five steps of the nursing process—assessing, diagnosing, planning, implementing, and evaluating—should serve as the basis for the plan of care. For-

## ADMISSION DATA

| DATE OF ADMISSION | TIME OF ARRIVAL | | METHOD OF ARRIVAL | | | | ALLERGIES: |
|---|---|---|---|---|---|---|---|
| | | AMBU- LATORY | WHEEL CHAIR | STRETCHER | | | □ NKA |
| TEMPERATURE | PULSE | RESPIRATION | B.P. | HEIGHT | WEIGHT | | |

VALUABLES
WATCH  RINGS  MONEY  SENT HOME:
WITH PATIENT  □ YES  □ NO  WITH:

PATIENT COMPLAINS OF:

HOME MEDICATIONS
WITH PATIENT  □ YES  □ NO  □ NONE
□ UNKNOWN

SENT HOME WITH (NAME OF PERSON):

DENTURES
□ YES  □ NO  □ FULL  □ PARTIAL

### PATIENT HEALTH HISTORY

HISTORY OBTAINED FROM:
PATIENT  SPOUSE  PARENT  OTHER

| | | | DRUG, DOSE, FREQUENCY | LAST DOSE |
|---|---|---|---|---|
| HEART DISEASE | □ YES | □ NO | | |
| HYPERTENSION | □ YES | □ NO | | |
| RESPIRATORY DISEASE | □ YES | □ NO | | |
| CANCER | □ YES | □ NO | | |
| DIABETES | □ YES | □ NO | | |
| SEIZURES | □ YES | □ NO | | |
| SURGERY | □ YES | □ NO | | |

IF "YES" IS CHECKED, EXPLAIN:

ADDITIONAL COMMENTS:

## ADMISSION ASSESSMENT — REVIEW OF SYSTEMS

### I. SKIN
CONDITION  COLOR  TURGOR  DECUBITUS
COMMENTS:

### VII. GENITOURINARY
NO PROBLEMS  HEMATURIA  INCONTINENT  CATH
COMMENTS:

### II. NEUROLOGICAL
ALERT & ORIENTED  DISORIENTED  RESTLESS  LETHARGIC  COMATOSE  RESTRAINTS
COMMENTS:

### VIII. MUSCULOSKELETAL
NO PROBLEMS  APPLIANCES
MOBILITY
AMBULATORY  WITH ASSISTANCE  WHEELCHAIR  BEDRIDDEN
PAIN
COMMENTS:

### III. SENSORY
VISION  NORMAL  GLASSES  WITH PT.?  CONTACT LENSES  WITH PT.?
HEARING  NORMAL  DEAF  HARD OF HEARING  HEARING AID  WITH PT.?

### IX. PSYCHOSOCIAL
LIVES WITH:
SIGNIFICANT PROBLEMS

### IV. RESPIRATORY
NO PROBLEMS  SPUTUM  DYSPNEA  O₂  COUGH  USE OF TOBACCO
COMMENTS:

### V. CARDIOVASCULAR
NO PROBLEMS  CHEST PAIN  EDEMA  SYNCOPE  PALPITATIONS
COMMENTS:

### VI. GASTROINTESTINAL
DIET  APPETITE  FOOD ALLERGIES
ALCOHOL INTAKE  TYPE  FREQUENCY  AMT
NAUSEA/VOMITING  DYSPHAGIA  PAIN
NORMAL  IF NOT, DESCRIBE:  STOOLS
LAXATIVE OF CHOICE:  OSTOMY
COMMENTS:

ATTENDING PHYSICIAN NOTIFIED  TIMES NOTIFIED  ADMITTING NURSE'S SIGNATURE

**Figure 6–5A.** Example of care plan form combined with medical plan of care.

184

| DATE ORDERED | TREATMENTS | | DATE COMPL'TD | DATE ORDERED | X-RAY AND OTHER STUDIES | | DATE COMPL'TD | DATE ORDERED | LAB | | DATE COMPL'TD |
|---|---|---|---|---|---|---|---|---|---|---|---|
| DAILYS | | | | DAILYS | | | | DAILYS | | | |

| DATE | NURSING DX | DATE | PATIENT OBJECTIVE | DATE | PLAN OF CARE |
|---|---|---|---|---|---|

PATIENT AND FAMILY TEACHING

| DIET | Date | Measurements | | RESPIRATORY | Date | IV FLUIDS |
|---|---|---|---|---|---|---|
| | | V.S. | | | | |
| | | Temp | | O₂ | | |
| | | I & O | | | | |
| NOURISHMENTS | | SP. CKS | | TREATMENTS | | |
| | | Weights | | | | |
| | | LBM | | | | |
| Dentures | | OTHER | | | | |

ACTIVITY LEVEL — ASSIST ___ CATH ___  FEED ___ CHANGED ___  NPO ___ NG ___  HOLD ___ OTHER ___  T.F. ___

SPECIAL PROCEDURES (short form permit) — Date ___

SPECIAL FLUIDS (Blood, Hyperal, Dialysis) — Date ___

ANCILLIARY SERVICES: OT ___ PT ___ SPEECH ___ S. SERVICE ___ OTHER ___

SURGICAL PROCEDURES (long form permit) — Date ___

OTHER

Siderails ☐ UP ☐ DOWN
Release form signed ☐ Yes ☐ No
BATH ☐ SELF ☐ PARTIAL ☐ COMPLETE ☐ SHOWER
MODE OF TRANSPORTATION ☐ WHEELCHAIR ☐ STRETCHER ☐ BED ☐ OTHER

STATUS  M  W  D  S  SEP   CONSULTS
SMOKER ☐ YES ☐ NO
DIAGNOSIS

HOME PHONE    NEXT OF KIN    RELIGION    ANNOINTED

ADM. PHYSICIAN

| ADM. DATE | AGE | DOB | ACUITY | | CODE STATUS |
| ROOM NO. | NAME | | | | |

**Figure 6–5B.** Example of care plan form combined with medical plan of care.

186

| | | |
|---|---|---|
| | ACME #79412-8 | |

ADMISSION DATE

MEDICINES:-

TREATMENTS:-

PRN MEDICINES:-

PRN TREATMENTS:-

DIET

HISTORY NO

| ROOM | NAME | | AGE | DIAGNOSIS | | DOCTOR |
|---|---|---|---|---|---|---|

**BATH**
SELF     ASSIST
____COMPLETE ____
____TUB ____
____SHOWER ____
____BED ____

**GROOMING**
SELF     ASSIST
____HAIR ____
____NAILS ____
____FEET ____
____SHAVE ____

**MOUTH CARE**
INDEPENDENT    ASSIST
☐ BRUSH TEETH ☐
DENTURES
UPPER ____
LOWER ____
SPECIAL ____

**SKIN CARE**
_____ BACK RUB
_____ SPECIAL
_____ SKIN CONDITION
_____ POSITIONING
LOCATION _____
CARE _____

**PROSTHESIS**
DENTURES _____
GLASSES _____
CONTACTS _____
HEARING AID_____
LIMB _____
OTHER _____

**SAFETY**
SIDERAILS _____
RESTRAINTS _____
OTHER _____

**MENTAL ATTITUDE**
_____ ALERT
_____ NERVOUS
_____ DEPRESSED
_____ COMBATIVE
_____ CONFUSED
_____ OTHER

**SPEECH**
____ SPEAKS WELL
____ APHASIC
____ LANGUAGE BARRIER
LANGUAGE SPOKEN
_____
_____

**PHYSICAL LIMITATIONS**
      L. R.
PARALYSIS __ __
WHERE _____
DEAF __ __
HARD OF HEARING __ __
BLIND __ __
REDUCED VISION __ __

**DEXTERITY**
RIGHT HANDED _____
LEFT HANDED _____

**LOCOMOTION AIDS**
SELF     ASSIST
____ WALKS ____
____ CANE ____
____ WALKER ____
____ CRUTCHES ____
____ WHEEL CH. ____
____ NO. WT. BEARING____
____ UP & ABOUT ____
____ OOB / CHAIR ____
____ BEDREST ____

**RESTRICTIONS**
LOUNGE____ LOBBY____
HALL____ ROOM_____
PLAYROOM _____

**DIET**

**EATING HABITS**
INDEPENDENT   ASSIST
____ FEEDS SELF ____
____ PREPARE FOOD ____
____ OOB IN CHAIR ____
____ FEED ____

**BOWEL     BLADDER**
____ BEDPAN ____
____ BATHROOM ____
____ COMMODE ____
____ URINAL ____
____ TRAINED ____
____ INCONTINENT ____
CATHETER ____

**FLUIDS**
_____ FORCE
_____ RESTRICT
_____ INTAKE
_____ OUTPUT
_____ N. P. O.

| TPR | OD-WT | B/P |
|---|---|---|
| CLINITEST | | SLIDING SCALE |

PERTINENT PATIENT INFORMATION

**LONG RANGE GOALS**

____ ASSIST PATIENT TO REACH OPT-IMUM LEVEL OF HEALTH

____ ASSIST PATIENT TO REACH AND MAINTAIN HIGHEST LEVEL OF FUNCTIONING

____ ASSIST PATIENT TO PEACEFUL AND DIGNIFIED DEATH

GROWTH AND DEVELOPMENT

**Figure 6–6A.** Example of care plan form combined with medical plan of care.

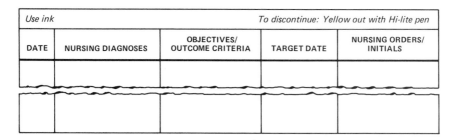

| | | | | |
|---|---|---|---|---|
| Use ink | | | | To discontinue: Yellow out with Hi-lite pen |
| DATE | NURSING DIAGNOSES | OBJECTIVES/<br>OUTCOME CRITERIA | TARGET DATE | NURSING ORDERS/<br>INITIALS |
| | | | | |
| | | | | |

**Figure 6–6B.** Example of care plan form combined with medical plan of care.

mats for the plan will vary according to the needs of the people using it. The more flexible the format the more useful it will be to a variety of clients and in a variety of situations. Nursing diagnoses, goals, objectives, outcome criteria, and nursing orders should appear on the plan. Space for evaluation and assessment data can also be provided.

2. The plan is dated and contains the signature of the responsible nurse. Revisions and additions to the original plan are also dated and signed.
3. Nursing diagnoses should be numbered in order of their priority. The rank order of the diagnoses are changed as the client's needs change.

DISCIPLINE CODES

N = Nursing
DS = Dietary Service
SS = Social Service
PT = Physical Therapist
AC = Activity Coordinator

Long Term Goal _____

_____

_____

Diagnosis _____

_____

Discharge Plan _____

_____

_____

Date Admitted __/ /__    Date of Birth __/ /__    Allergies _____

| DATE | RESPONSIBLE<br>DISCIPLINE | # | NURSING DIAGNOSES/<br>NEEDS/CONCERNS | OBJECTIVES | APPROACHES | *RRD<br>DATE |
|---|---|---|---|---|---|---|
| | | | | | | |
| | | | | | | |

*RRD = Resolution/Reassessment or Discontinue Date

| Last Name | First | Middle Initial | Identification # | Physician | Room # |
|---|---|---|---|---|---|

**Figure 6–7.** Interdisciplinary care plan form.

## CLIENT WITH IMPAIRED VENTILATION

| NURSING DIAGNOSIS | OBJECTIVES AND OUTCOME CRITERIA (individualize for client) | NURSING ORDERS: DATE AND INITIALS |
|---|---|---|
| Impaired ventilation related to increased pulmonary secretion.<br><br><br>GOAL<br>Client will have improved respiratory function within one week. | | 1. Increase oral fluid intake to 2000ml daily unless contraindicated.<br>Offer _____ ml of _____ (specific fluid) every two hours, 9–11–1–3, etc.<br><br>Date:<br><br>Initials:<br><br>2. Demonstrate proper deep breathing technique _____ (time and/or date)<br>Have client inhale deeply and slowly and exhale through pursed lips.<br><br>Date:<br><br>Initials:<br><br>3. Demonstrate technique for effective coughing _____ (time and/or date).<br>Have client cough in short bursts instead of vigorous prolonged coughs.<br><br>Date:<br><br>Initials:<br><br>4. Turn client every two hours, 9–11–1–3, etc.<br>Right side _____ (specify time)<br>Left side _____ (specify time)<br><br>Date:<br><br>Initials:<br><br>5.<br><br>Date:<br><br>Initials: |

**Figure 6–8.** Standard plan of care.

4. Nursing interventions directed at all three levels of care should be included when appropriate.
5. The plan of care should incorporate elements of the medical care plan (dependent interventions) so that the two plans complement rather than conflict with each other.
6. The plan of care should reflect the uniqueness and individuality of the client. A holistic approach should be used so that all needs are considered.
7. The plan should be written in a clear, concise manner. Specific terms that give direction to the behavior of the client and nurse should be used.
8. The plan should be written legibly in ink. Writing the plan of care in ink places more importance on what is being written. When the content of the plan can be erased, the nurse may not feel accountable. If the nursing diagnosis is resolved, write "discontinued" by it with a date. A line may also be drawn through any content of the plan that is not current. A yellow marker, a highlighter, can be used. This is a legal way of altering the plan because it allows you to see what was originally written.
9. The plan should become a permanent part of the health record. Keeping the plan as a legal part of the record will help nurses to place higher priority on care-plan development. This approach will promote accountability. In addition, should successive health problems arise, the old care plans can be used for supplementary data.
10. The plan of care must be accessible to all members of the health team. The kardex or folder containing the plan can be separate from the rest of the health record if this increases accessibility.
11. Plans must be revised and changed regularly. An out-of-date plan is meaningless and useless. Instead of helping the nursing staff, it may actually deter the nursing personnel from using the plan. The nurse responsible for developing the plan can set aside time each day or week for revision of the care plans. Plans can also be revised at change of shift report or care conferences.
12. Not all nursing care performed for the client is derived from orders written on the care plan. Many situations require you to assess, diagnose, plan, intervene, and evaluate on the spot. If actions are likely to be repeated for the client, they should be added to the care plan. If repeat occurrence is unlikely, do not add to the plan of care but record your actions and the client's response in the appropriate section of the permanent health record.

Once the plan has been developed, it must be implemented and the results evaluated.

## SUMMARY

This chapter has presented the third step in the nursing process—planning. Planning describes the nursing strategy or scheme designed to assure goal-directed care for the client.

In order to develop an appropriate plan of care, priorities must be established, prognoses determined, goals, objectives, and outcome criteria formulated, and nursing interventions identified. Each of these aspects requires input from the client, client's family or significant others, nurse, and other health care providers. Past experiences, intellectual levels, value systems, beliefs, attitudes, feelings, and cultural factors will influence contributions from these people. A comprehensive plan of care cannot be written quickly. Adequate time must be allowed for the development of a plan that meets the specific needs of the client. Although planning begins as a mental process, the completed care plan must ultimately be recorded to ensure continuity of care.

With the client's plan of care completed and recorded, we can move on to the fourth step, the implementation of the plan. In this step, you perform or direct the actions necessary to accomplish the goals and objectives and to resolve or support nursing diagnoses.

## STUDY GUIDE

1. Based on data in the nursing health history collected for Chapter 4, identify factors that might affect this client's priority setting and goal setting.
2. Using this same data base, write three nursing diagnoses appropriate for the client. Rank these diagnoses according to basic human needs.
3. Using one of the nursing diagnoses that you have developed, write a goal, two objectives, and two outcome criteria.
4. Write the following nursing interventions as nursing orders:

   Teach Mrs. S. about preoperative care.
   Ambulate Mr. P.
   Encourage Mrs. N. to eat.

5. Identify five functions or purposes of the care plan.
6. Compare two care-plan forms used within health care agencies in your area. Identify their similarities and differences. Which components of the nursing process are apparent within these plans of care?

## REFERENCES

1. Bailey, J., & Claus, K. *Decision making in nursing*. St. Louis: C. V. Mosby, 1975.
2. Bloom, B. S. (Ed.). *Taxonomy of educational objectives: The classification of educational goals—Handbook I: Cognitive domain*. New York: D. McKay, 1956.
3. Bower, F. *The process of planning nursing care: A model for practice* (3rd ed.). St. Louis: C.V. Mosby, 1982.
4. Ciuca, R. Over the years with the nursing care plan. *Nursing Outlook,* November 1972, *20* (11), 706–711.
5. Davies, I. *Objectives in curriculum design*. New York: McGraw-Hill, 1976.
6. Discharge planning: Good planning means fewer hospitalizations for the chronically ill. *Nursing '81,* May 1981, *11* (5), 70–75.
7. Duvall, E. M. *Marriage and family development* (5th ed.). Philadelphia: Lippincott, 1977.
8. Erikson, E. *Childhood and society*. New York: W. W. Norton & Co., Inc., 1963.
9. Havighurst, R. J. *Developmental tasks and education* (3rd ed.). New York: D. McKay, 1972.
10. Kibler, R. J., Cegala, D. J., Miles, D. T., & Barker, L. L. *Objectives for instruction and evaluation*. Boston: Allyn & Bacon, 1974.
11. Krathwohl, D. R., Bloom, B. S., & Masia, B. B. *Taxonomy of educational objectives: The classification of educational goals—Handbook 2: Affective domain*. New York: D. McKay, 1956.
12. Lewis, L. *Planning patient care* (2nd ed.). Dubuque, Iowa: Wm. C. Brown Company Publishers, 1976.
13. Little, D., & Carnevali, D. *Nursing care planning* (2nd ed.). Philadelphia: Lippincott, 1976.

14. Mager, R. *Preparing educational objectives*. Palo Alto, Calif.: Fearon Publishers, 1962.
15. Marriner, A. *The nursing process: A scientific approach to nursing care* (3rd ed.). St. Louis: C.V. Mosby, 1983.
16. Maslow, A. *Toward a psychology of being*. New York: D. Van Nostrand Co., 1962.
17. Mayers, M. G. *A systematic approach to the nursing care plan* (3rd ed.). New York: Appleton-Century-Crofts, 1983.
18. Reilly, D. E. *Behavioral objectives in nursing: Evaluation of learner attainment*. New York: Appleton-Century-Crofts, 1975.
19. Stanhope, M., & Lancaster, J. *Community health nursing: Process and practice for promoting health*. St. Louis: C.V. Mosby, 1984.
20. Stuart, M. The nursing care plan: A communication system that really works. *Nursing '79*, August 1979, *8* (8), 28–33.
21. Sweet, P. R., & Stark, I. The circular nursing care plan. *American Journal of Nursing*, June 1970, *70* (6), 1300.
22. Tyler, R. W. *Basic principles of curriculum instruction*. Chicago: University of Chicago Press, 1949.
23. Urdang, L., & Swallow, H. H. (Eds.). *Mosby's medical and nursing dictionary*. St. Louis: C. V. Mosby, 1983.
24. Whaley, L., & Wong, D. *Nursing care of infants and children*. St. Louis: C.V. Mosby, 1983.
25. Yura, H., & Walsh, M. B. *The nursing process: Assessing, planning, implementing, evaluating* (4th ed.). Norwalk, Conn.: Appleton-Century-Crofts, 1983.
26. Zimmer, M. J. Guidelines for development of outcome criteria. *Nursing Clinics of North America*, June 1974, *9* (2), 317–321.

# BIBLIOGRAPHY

Burgess, W. *Community health nursing: Philosophy, process, practice*. Norwalk, Conn.: Appleton-Century-Crofts, 1983.
Clemen, S. A., Eigsti, D. G., & McGuire, S. *Comprehensive family and community health nursing*. New York: McGraw-Hill, 1981.
Eigsti, D. G., Stein, K. Z., & Fortune, M. The community as client in planning for continuity of care. *Nursing & Health Care*, May 1982, *3* (5), 251–253.
Fletcher, S., & Mulligan, J. Care plans: Why should nursing care plans be made a permanent part of the medical record? *Nursing Management*, May 1982, *13* (5), 57–61.
Forman, M. Building a better nursing care plan. *American Journal of Nursing*, June 1979, *79* (6), 1086–1087.
Friedman, M. *Family nursing: Theory & assessment*. New York: Appleton-Century-Crofts, 1981.
Fromer, M. J. *Community health care and the nursing process*. St. Louis: C.V. Mosby, 1983.
Griffith, J. W., & Christensen, P. J. (Eds.). *Nursing process: Application of theories, frameworks, and models*. St. Louis: C.V. Mosby, 1982.
Hanlon, J. *Public health administration and practice*. St. Louis: C.V. Mosby, 1974.
Helvie, C. O. *Community health nursing: Theory and process*. Philadelphia: Harper & Row, 1981.
Kelly, N. Nursing care plans. *Nursing Outlook*, May 1966, *14* (5), 61–64.
Kibler, R. J., Barker, L. L., & Miles, D. *Behavioral objectives and instruction*. Boston: Allyn & Bacon, 1970.
Kurose, K. A standard care plan for alcoholism. *American Journal of Nursing*, May 1981, *81* (5), 1001–1006.
Leonard, B. J., & Redland, A. R. *Process in clinical nursing*. Englewood Cliffs, N.J.: Prentice-Hall, 1981.
McCarthy, M. M. The nursing process: Application of current thinking in clinical problem solving. *Journal of Advanced Nursing*, May 1981, *6* (3), 173–177.
McCloskey, J. C. Nurses' orders: The next professional breakthrough? *RN*, February 1980, *43* (2), 99+.

Moughton, M. The patient: A partner in the health care process. *Nursing Clinics of North America,* September 1982, *17* (3), 467–479.

Murray, M. *Fundamentals of nursing* (2nd ed.). Englewood Cliffs, N.J.: Prentice-Hall, 1980.

Narrow, B., & Buschle, K. B. *Fundamentals of nursing practice.* New York: Wiley, 1982.

Predd, C. How to stay efficient in hectic nursing situations: Setting priorities. *Nursing Life,* May/June 1982, *2* (3), 50–51.

Sanborn, C. W., & Blount, M. Standard care plans. *American Journal of Nursing,* November 1984, *84* (11), 1394–1396.

Shortridge, L., & McLain, B. Levels of intervention for a coexistence model. *Nurse Practitioner,* March 1983, 74–80.

Sorensen, K., & Luckmann, J. *Basic nursing: A psychophysiologic approach.* Philadelphia: Saunders, 1979.

Spradley, B. W. *Community health nursing: Concepts and practice.* Boston: Little, Brown, 1981.

Stone, M. Discharge planning guide. *American Journal of Nursing,* August 1979, *79* (8), 1446–1447.

Tinkham, C., Voorhies E., & McCarthy, N. *Community health nursing: Evolution and process in the family and community* (3rd ed.). New York: Appleton-Century-Crofts, 1984.

Vasey, E. Writing your patients care plan efficiently. *American Journal of Nursing,* April 1979, *79* (4), 67–71.

Wagner, B. Care plans—right, reasonable, and reachable. *American Journal of Nursing,* May 1969, *69* (5), 986–990.

Yura, H., Ozimek, D., & Walsh, M. B. *Nursing leadership: Theory & process* (2nd ed.). New York: Appleton-Century-Crofts, 1981.

# 7

# Nursing Process:
# Step IV. Implementing

The implementation step in the nursing process begins once the plan of care has been developed. To implement means to carry into effect a plan or procedure. In nursing, **implementing** describes the actual giving of nursing care. Implementing is the action-oriented phase of the nursing process. This step involves the initiation and completion of actions necessary to accomplish defined goals and objectives and to resolve or support the nursing diagnosis.

Since the implementing step involves the actual giving of nursing care, it is essential that you become familiar with some of the qualities, characteristics, and skills of a competent caregiver. In this chapter, we will discuss some of the intellectual, interpersonal, and technical skills that you will use. Your role as a leader and manager will be considered as well as methods and guidelines for enhancing your effectiveness during this step.

Study of this chapter will help you to:

1. Define implementing as it relates to the nursing process.
2. Discuss characteristics of effective nursing actions.
3. Identify intellectual, interpersonal, and technical skills used by the nurse during the implementing step.
4. Define the term leadership.
5. Describe leadership techniques used in nursing.
6. Define the term management.
7. Describe the role of the nurse–manager.
8. Discuss other roles assumed by the nurse during implementation of the plan of care.
9. Describe the role of decision making in the implementing step.
10. Describe the role of problem solving in the implementing step.
11. Discuss methods that will enhance effective implementation of the care plan.

If considered sequentially, implementing is the fourth step in the nursing process. It may also be concurrent with the other steps. While giving care, you may actually be evaluating the response to your current nursing actions and at the same time assessing, diagnosing, and planning future care. The time involved in completing this step will range from a few minutes to hours or even years. The actual time required depends on what is necessary to carry into effect the plan for that client.

## IMPLEMENTING THE PLAN OF CARE

Nursing actions are needed to implement the interventions identified during the planning step. In addition, you will need to respond to changes in the client's condition—actions that could not perhaps be anticipated and planned. Any action that you perform is aimed at protecting the client from harm and improving the client's mental, emotional, or physical functions.

### Types of Nursing Actions

Nursing actions can be grouped into three main clusters: physiologic, psychological, and socioeconomic.[8,51] **Physiologic nursing actions** are directed at meeting the client's basic needs: oxygen, food, water, elimination, sleep, and comfort. These actions are usually overt or highly visible; they are task-oriented and can be easily observed by another person. Physiologic nursing actions usually require the use of tools or pieces of equipment (stethoscope, thermometer, or hypodermic syringe) and some degree of manual skill. These high-visibility actions or functions require minimal verbal interaction with the client.

**Psychological nursing actions** include activities that affect the emotional well-being of the client. Some of the psychological nursing actions are visible, but most are low-visibility tasks that require cognitive or affective skills.

**Socioeconomic nursing actions** relate to those activities that consider the client from a holistic point of view. Discharge planning, health education, and referrals are examples of socioeconomic nursing actions. These are frequently low-visibility tasks and require more cognitive skills than psychomotor.

A nursing action may fall into more than one of the three groups. For example, almost any intervention may have a psychological effect on the client—a back rub (a physiologic nursing action) can reduce the client's anxiety.

In the past, high-visibility tasks that were more easily measured and validated were considered more important than low-visibility tasks. Gradually, nursing care has become a combination of low- and high-visibility tasks. Today, the nurse ministers to the client's physical, psychological, and socioeconomic needs.[6,8]

### Guidelines for Nursing Actions

Implementation of nursing interventions from a plan of care is only one aspect of this step. Just as important as *what* interventions are used is *how* they are implemented. Your actions should be directed by the following suggestions in order to increase their effectiveness.

1. Implementation is accomplished by or under the direction of a professional nurse. An infinite number of nursing actions may be involved in this step.
2. During this step in the nursing process, you are implementing the nursing orders and medical orders; therefore your actions must be consistent with the medical care plan and the client's plan of care.

3. Your actions must be supported by a scientific rationale. Do not implement a nursing order blindly. You should be aware of the physiologic or psychosocial reason for performing the action.
4. Each action should be goal-directed and purposeful.
5. Make certain that your actions are considered therapeutically safe. Is it possible that a particular nursing intervention might cause physical or mental harm to the client?
6. You should organize your care to coincide with the client's need for sleep, rest, activity, and food.
7. Your actions should contribute to comprehensive care for the client—physical, psychological, emotional, spiritual, social, cultural, economic, and rehabilitative.
8. Your actions should promote continuity of care.
9. Nursing orders are written to take into consideration the individuality of the client. Make certain that your approach also reflects the client's uniqueness.
10. Collaborate with the family and client in the implementation of the care plan.
11. Nursing orders are untested hypotheses—assumptions used as the basis for action. When you write a nursing order you cannot be absolutely certain of the client's reaction or response to it. You *assume* that it will be effective; therefore, you can consider your orders as untested hypotheses. As such, they require constant evaluating and updating.
12. Implementation is not completed until the actions taken, the results of the actions, and the client's reaction to them have been recorded in the client's health record.

To use these guidelines effectively and at the same time perform physiologic, psychological, and socioeconomic nursing actions, you must draw heavily on your intellectual, interpersonal, and technical skills.

## SKILLS USED DURING THE IMPLEMENTING STEP

At one time technical skills were the only skills associated with the process of nursing. The nurse was perceived as a "doer"—someone who performed manual tasks. Intellectual and interpersonal skills were in the domain of other disciplines. Emphasis on interpersonal skills developed next. In the Christian era, nurses were kind to those under their care because it was the appropriate Christian behavior. Later, because the emphasis was on the totality of the individual, nurses were expected to meet the physiologic and psychological needs of the client; nurses were to give "total patient care." During this same period, nurses were expected to know "what" to do in a situation, but they were not expected to know the scientific rationale for the action. Eventually, the scope of nursing responsibility broadened, and the educational expectations changed. Nurse educators and nursing service personnel recognized the importance of educating nurses in all three levels of knowledge—technical, intellectual, and interpersonal (Fig. 7–1).

All three levels are of equal importance; you cannot be a competent nurse unless you have mastered intellectual, interpersonal, and technical skills. Intellectual skills affect your ability to perform interpersonal and technical skills. The rationales for most of your technical skills are derived from your knowledge base—your cognitive storehouse. Several important intellectual skills are discussed in other chapters of this book

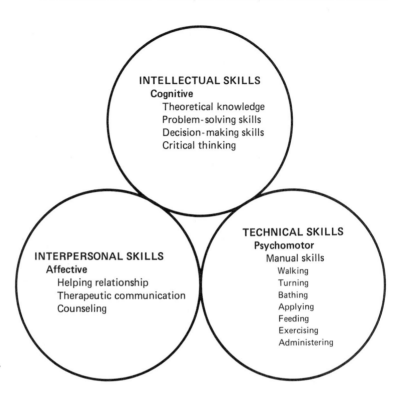

**Figure 7–1.** Skills used in implementing plan of care.

and are therefore not presented again in this chapter. (Refer to Chapters 2, 11, and 12.) Technical skills are equally important. A discussion of these skills is not found within the scope of this book. You may refer to books that are written specifically about technical or psychomotor skills for more information. Considering these factors, we will spend most of our time in this section discussing interpersonal skills.

## Intellectual Skills

Intellectual skills reflect cognitive learning—intellectual processes concerned with all aspects of perception, thinking, reasoning, and remembering. You will recall that six levels of cognitive behavior were identified: knowledge, comprehension, application, analysis, synthesis, and evaluation. Implementing intellectual skills represents the cognitive behavior of application—the ability to use what is learned in a new situation.

Intellectual skills are based on each nurse's personal knowledge base. The level of skill performance will therefore vary from nurse to nurse. Transfer of learning from classroom and previous clinical experiences to various client situations is required. Knowledge is not transferred in its "pure theoretical form" but should be adapted to the client so that the result is creative, innovative care.

It is important that you have a realistic understanding of your level of intellectual skills and your ability to apply them. You should be able to recognize and accept your own strengths and limitations—do not hesitate to indicate when your intellectual skills are not sufficient. It is also important that you keep your knowledge base current. How can you give safe, effective care if you have done nothing to add to your knowledge since graduation?

During implementation, you will constantly be using your assessment skills. Based on new data, you will determine if any modifications in the plan of care are needed. Even a slight change in the client's status might require reorganization of nursing actions and establishment of different priorities. The ability to recognize when to alter the original plan of care is important and requires the application of critical-thinking, problem-solving skills, and decision-making skills. All of these are cognitive intellectual processes.

Every clinical situation can be viewed as a problem or dilemma that needs to be resolved. In order to resolve these problems, you apply problem-solving skills. You will recall from your reading in Chapter 2 that the nursing process itself is a problem-solving mode of acting. The application of the nursing process in the clinical setting, therefore, requires problem-solving skills. Problem solving is an intellectual process that incorporates the skills of critical thinking and decision making. Experience, patience, understanding, and reflective thinking are required to apply problem-solving skills effectively. In addition, you must make a conscious effort to develop and improve your problem-solving skills. (Refer to Chapter 2 for more information on problem solving.)

Decision-making skills will also be used continuously as you implement the plan of care. You will judge the value of newly assessed data; decide when to communicate with the client; decide when to question nursing and medical orders; determine when procedural methods and the timing of technical procedures must be modified; decide when to consult with other health team members or when to seek assistance with the implementation of the plan. These are only a few of the nursing actions that require decision-making skills. As with problem solving, you must strive to develop and improve your skills in this area. (Refer to Chapter 11 for information on the decision-making process.)

## Interpersonal Skills

The term **interpersonal** refers to any transaction or contact between two or more individuals. Interpersonal skills reflect the affective domain of learning behaviors—aspects such as attitudes, beliefs, and values are considered. Almost every action that you will take when implementing the plan of care will require interpersonal contact—for example, bathing the client, teaching the family member about nutrition, talking with other health team members about the client's care. In order to make interpersonal transactions rewarding and beneficial to the people involved, definite skills and techniques must be employed. In this section, we will direct our attention to the interpersonal skills that are used in the helping relationship, in therapeutic communication, and in counseling.

*Therapeutic Communication.* Effective application of the communication process requires appropriate use of interpersonal skills. **Communication** is a transactional process that allows for the generation and transmission of information. Two types of communication occur—intrapersonal and interpersonal. **Intrapersonal communication** is the process that occurs within the individual. It represents the unique interpretation of stimuli by each person. The stimulus may originate internally, such as a headache or hunger pangs, or from external sources, such as a sound in the environment.

**Interpersonal communication** involves a transaction between two or more individuals. Thoughts, messages, feelings, attitudes, and ideas are exchanged with another person. Communication should elicit a response; if the stimulus is ignored and no response occurs, communication has not taken place. Examples of interpersonal communication are dyadic, triadic, intragroup, intergroup, and multigroup communication. The basic interpersonal form is the dyad—two people directly communicating with one another. Dyads compose a large portion of our professional relationships in health care. Although dyads occur frequently, the context of each dyad is different. Effective interpersonal communication requires an understanding of the meaning of the information shared; individual interpretation of the meaning can create problems.[3,26,36,40] In this section, we will focus on interpersonal rather than intrapersonal communication.

*Purpose of Communication.* Communication is meant to inform, persuade or influence, entertain, or provide for survival. When communication is used to **inform,** information is provided. This information should be transmitted in a manner that can be understood and retained. You use this type of communication when you do client teaching. When people share your attitudes but have not been moved to action or if they hold beliefs or attitudes that oppose yours, communication is used to **persuade** or **influence.** It is necessary that you give information if you expect to influence someone; the information must be communicated in such a manner that it stimulates the person to change. As a nurse, you will frequently resort to this approach when talking to a client about smoking or dieting. The client, however, ultimately decides how to respond to the communicated information. Communication may contain informative and persuasive elements and be meant to **entertain** or to bring pleasure. You want the receiver to enjoy the message. The message need not be funny or humorous to bring pleasure. Entertainment may come in the form of an anecdote or story that helps to make the receiver feel more comfortable. Another major purpose of communication is **survival.** Individuals, groups, and complex organizations require continuous communication input in order to survive. You include in your care measures that supply the client with sensory stimuli—music, radios, or voice contact. Since individuals cannot maintain emotional stability for prolonged periods of time without interpersonal communication, these sensory stimuli promote their survival and well-being.[36,40]

*Process of Communication.* Communication is a dynamic, circular, unpredictable series of actions. As a circular process it has no definite beginning or ending. Each individual simultaneously acts as sender and receiver of messages and as interpreter of meaning for the messages. The communication process is also continuous, irreversible, complex, and ever-changing. You cannot "uncommunicate". Once you have spoken, it is impossible to retrieve your words. Nonverbal messages that are sent are also considered irreversible. You may deny the importance or meaning of inappropriate communication—verbal or nonverbal—but it becomes a permanent part of future interactions with the individual or group involved. The communication process is a complex process which is influenced by many internal and external factors.[5,36]

*Models of Communication.* Numerous models have been used to explain the communication process. The purpose of these models is to break down the process of communication into components or elements. This enhances the understanding of the process.

In its simplest form, the communication process involves the sending and receiving of messages. Most models of the communication process contain four to six elements or components. Sender, receiver, message, and feedback are elements common to all the models. We will also discuss the elements *context* and *signal* (Fig. 7–2).

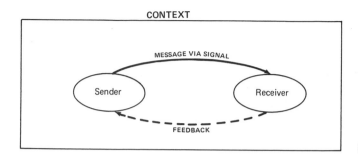

**Figure 7–2.** Communication process.

The **sender** (also called the source, producer, initiator, transmitter, informer, or encoder) is the person who generates or sends the communication transaction. This person is responsible for **encoding**—selecting specific signals, symbols, or codes by which to transmit the message.

The **message** consists of stimuli that are generated by the sender. It is what is said, written, or transmitted by way of body language. The message may be responded to or not responded to by the receiver.

Messages are transmitted through **signals,** codes, mediums, or channels. The sender changes, converts, or encodes the message to a form that can be sent or given to the receiver. The signal must be appropriate for the message. For example, written communication is more appropriate for a message that must be preserved. Three primary classifications of signals or channels have been identified: visual, auditory, and kinesthetic.

The **receiver** (also called the responder, recipient, consumer, listener, or decoder) is the person to whom the communication is directed. The message must be received, analyzed, and decoded. During decoding, the receiver relates the perceived message to a storehouse of knowledge and exposure. The receiver decides whether to respond to the message.

The response that each participant in the communication process makes to the message received results in **feedback.** Feedback can be negative or positive; it can be given by verbal or nonverbal responses. Feedback reflects the circular, continuous nature of the interpersonal communication process. The response of the receiver to the communication transaction is transmitted back as a signal to the original sender who in turn perceives and interprets it and responds.

**Context** represents the setting or situation in which communication takes place. It also includes the content or focus of communication.[5,6,22,26,36,40]

*Factors Influencing Communication.* Many factors or variables affect interpersonal communication. The sender and receiver are influenced by physiologic, psychological, and sociocultural variables. If participants in the communication process have sensory losses, or visual or auditory difficulties, they will have difficulty receiving messages. In addition to seeing and hearing problems, some people may have diminished perception to touch; this may interfere with nonverbal communication. Each participant's level of consciousness will affect the process. If the participant's alertness is impaired because of drugs, alcohol, or a disease process, not only will the person be unable to receive the message accurately but the interpretation of the message may be altered. In addition, the messages that the participant sends may be neither clear nor accurate. Motor impairments will also interfere with the participant's ability to form words. If one side of the face is paralyzed, words cannot be formed easily or spoken clearly; this will make it more difficult for the receiver. Another physical factor that will affect communication is the participant's level of language development. Growth in language development is affected by intelligence, sex, status in family, parental stimulation, and socioeconomic components.[22]

Among the sociocultural variables which will affect interpersonal communication are values, life experiences, language differences, and the concept of territory and personal space. Language differences, dialects, and cultural word connotations may interrupt both the sending and receiving of messages. Within the United States, regional dialects (Texan, Southern, and New York) and dialects reflecting various ethnic groups (Italian, German, and black) exist. Not only will the same word have different meanings for these groups but pronunciation will vary. You should listen carefully to the language spoken, be accepting of the dialect, and clarify the meanings of words when necessary. Personal values can also interfere with the decoding of a message. For example, if you as a nurse place strong values on men being "brave and not showing emotion," you may not interpret a message of anxiety or concern that is being sent by a male client.

The concept of territory and personal space affects interpersonal communication. **Territoriality** is a basic behavioral system characteristic of living organisms. The term describes the behavior by which a person lays claim to space and things and defends them against intruders. Each cultural group views territoriality differently. If the sender of a message intrudes upon the receiver's territory, it can cause a disruption in communication. The receiver can become angry and withdrawn; this will affect both receiving and interpreting the message.[2,4,15,28]

**Personal space** is an invisible area immediately surrounding an individual in which the majority of that person's interactions take place. This area does not have fixed or geographical reference points; the boundaries move, expanding and contracting as situations vary. Personal space is divided into four distance zones. Each zone differs in the type and quantity of sensory input.

| | |
|---|---|
| Intimate Distance: | 7.5 to 45.0 cm (3 to 18 inches) |
| Personal Distance: | 0.4 to 1.2 m (1.5 to 4.0 feet) |
| Social Distance: | 1.2 to 3.7 m (4 to 12 feet) |
| Public Distance: | beyond 3.7 m (12 feet) |

The *intimate distance* is characterized by body contact, increased sensations of body heat and smell, and vocalizations that are low. Visual distortion of the other person's features occurs. (Americans are especially uncomfortable with the visual distortion.) Many nursing actions require the nurse to communicate at this distance—comforting a child, turning and positioning a client, or assessing the client. Your invasion of the client's personal space may cause discomfort to you and the client. When possible, you should avoid intrusion into the intimate zone. If this is impossible, make certain that the client is informed in advance of the need for such contact. In *personal distance*, voice tones are moderate, and body heat and smell are less noticeable. Since you can see more of the person at a personal distance, body language is more apparent and less visual distortion occurs. Personal distance is frequently used by nurses. While you are collecting the health history or interviewing the client, you maintain personal distance. *Social distance* permits visual perception of the whole body. Body heat and odor are not perceptible; eye contact is increased, and voice levels are loud enough to be overheard by others. Social distance allows more activity; several people may participate in the process at the same time. When you smile and speak to a client as you pass in the hallway or greet several people when you enter the clinic waiting room, you are communicating at a social distance. *Public distance* requires voice projection and careful pronunciation. Individuals are involved in the communication process only impersonally—individuality is lost.[15,22,41,45] The client's feelings about your entering and altering the client's personal space will affect all aspects of interpersonal communication.

In addition to physiologic and sociocultural variables that affect communication, there are psychological factors that are important. Both the sender's and receiver's emotional state will govern what is said, what is heard, what is seen, and what meaning is given to the message. The participants' current moods or attitudes, plus feelings remaining from previous interactions, will influence the communication process. Intelligence and level of vocabulary usage will affect the participants' ability to understand and interpret messages. Even an individual's placement on Maslow's hierarchy of needs will affect communication. Those participants with high self-esteem will communicate honestly and with confidence while those with low self-esteem will lack confidence and send messages with double meanings. Individuals who have not met or who are struggling to meet low-level comfort needs may be unwilling or unable to communicate high-level concerns.[22] Roles that the sender and receiver fulfill—student, teacher, mother, child, wife, husband—will also alter the sending, receiving, and interpreting of messages.

Other variables such as the content of the message, the sender's knowledge of the receiver, and the external environment will affect communication. Some people may be so frightened by the health care setting that they cannot communicate anything but the briefest of messages regardless of their needs and concerns. Noise level, odors, and sights in an environment may hinder effective interpersonal communication. If background noise interferes with the receiver's hearing, the message is bound to be misunderstood or misinterpreted. Odors and sights in the environment might distract both the sender and receiver. For example, clients who have never been inside an emergency room may become so overwhelmed with the sights, sounds, and odors that the client cannot send a message effectively to the health care provider.[22,26]

Selective communication can also affect the total communication process. Refer to Chapter 4 for a discussion of selective exposure, selective attention, selective perception, and selective retention.

*Types of Communication.* Two main types of communication exist: **verbal** and **nonverbal.** Language is the symbolization process basic to verbal communication. Language contains words—"Words are tools or symbols used to express ideas and feeling or to indicate objects; . . ."[34] Words are assigned a particular meaning by the people who use them. Word meaning can change over time and in different situations. Health professions have created a language that changes the meaning of many common words. For example, in common usage the word "void" means empty, unoccupied, invalid, or to evacuate. According to nursing and medical usage, the word means to empty urine from the bladder—"You will need to void before the pelvic examination." This statement would not convey the correct message to a client unfamiliar with the nursing and medical use of the word. Another language barrier produced by health professionals is the liberal use of abbreviations. New abbreviations are developed daily. There is no way that members of the health team can remain informed, much less the clients. Use of professional jargon will increase the chance of misunderstanding and incorrect interpretation.

Verbal language includes both oral and written words. Oral use of words is the most common vehicle for communication. Written communication is more formal and permanent and requires more skill. You will be using both forms as a nurse. Many of your nursing actions—teaching, counseling, comforting, explaining—require oral communication. Written communication is used in compiling the health record—nurses' notes, health history, physical assessment.

Nonverbal communication consists of symbols and actions. Since nonverbal communication is culturally determined, it will vary from culture to culture and even from person to person within a culture. In your personal and professional life, you must make yourself aware of your own, and others', nonverbal behavior. In some instances, nonverbal behavior may actually express the intended meaning more clearly than verbal behavior. Some clients can only use nonverbal communication—the depressed client, an infant or toddler, a deaf client, or an aphasic client.

Many nonverbal behaviors can be observed. Facial expressions, gestures, body postures, muscle tension, body movements, breathing patterns, and general physical appearance send nonverbal messages. Facial expressions, gestures, and body postures may convey happiness, fatigue, sadness, anger, depression, disgust, or frustration. Gestures may convey aggression, enthusiasm, excitement, receptivity, rejection, or defensiveness (shaking a closed hand). Body movements—rocking, leg swinging, or foot tapping—can indicate nervousness or boredom. Interest, boredom, attraction to or repulsion from a person, object, or event, or relaxation can be indicated by the individual's body posture. Eye contact or the lack of eye contact during verbal–oral communication can indicate confidence, lack of confidence, trust, ease, or embarrassment. The general physical appearance of an individual or the environment conveys messages nonverbally. An individual who is unkempt in appearance may unintentionally and incorrectly be saying to others that all aspects of the person's life are sloppy—job performance as well as physical appearance.

Colors also send messages. The color white is perceived as an indication of cleanliness, a characteristic expected of health professionals. This is one of the reasons for the use of white uniforms in health care settings. Warm colors—yellow, red, orange—elicit warm, happy responses. These colors are used in play rooms in an attempt to stimulate activity. Cool colors—blue, gray, green—have a quieting effect and are frequently used in hospital rooms, waiting rooms, and examination rooms.

Some nonverbal behaviors are heard. Sighs, cries, changes in voice inflection and pitch, and hesitations in speech can indicate many of the feelings of the sender. Surprise, excitement, confusion, sarcasm, fear, uncertainty, and mistrust can all be conveyed by these nonverbal sounds. Silence can also convey feelings—boredom, anger, and contemplation can be conveyed through silence.

Touch is another means of nonverbal communication. For the sender to touch the receiver, the intimate zone of the receiver's personal space must be entered. As indicated earlier, this form of communication may be difficult for the client and health care provider. Touch may be viewed by some as an act of interest and kindness while others may interpret it as an invasion of privacy.[26,34,40]

Communication in nursing differs from communication in a social or business setting. A social or business conversation is usually unplanned and unstructured. Social conversations do not have a well-defined goal or task; they are usually satisfying to both the receiver and sender of messages. Business conversations are more purposeful with a well-defined goal to be accomplished—buying a car, contracting for repair work on a house, arranging for day care for an infant. The direction and flow of conversation is not planned and is determined by the goal and the progress being made toward its achievement. A business conversation is also usually satisfying to both people involved. In nursing, conversation is purposeful, structured, and planned. There is a well-defined task to be accomplished, usually within a time limit. The conversation in a nurse–client relationship is central to the interaction. The benefits to be derived are one-sided—the client should profit from the interaction. This type of interaction in which you consciously influence a client or assist the client to achieve a certain outcome through verbal and nonverbal communication is called therapeutic communication.[22,26,34] Therapeutic communication is an essential part of the nurse–client relationship and is used extensively when implementing the plan of care. In Chapter 4, we discussed attentive listening and therapeutic and nontherapeutic communication techniques when we described the assessment interview. Refer to this content as well as references by Book, Bradley, Carlson, Hays and Larson, Pluckhan, and Smith and Bass for more information on communication, communication patterns, and therapeutic communication.

***Helping Relationship.*** The helping relationship also requires the use of interpersonal skills. A **helping relationship** is an interpersonal transaction in which one individual helps to promote personal development, growth, maturity, and adaptability in another.[34,38] The nurse–client relationship is a helping relationship. This type of relationship is essential to the implementation of the plan of care.

Several authors have identified characteristics of an effective helper. An individual who functions effectively in the helping relationship is:[1,7,34,39,44]

- **Understanding.** Responds to the client's deeper feelings as well as superficial feelings.
- **Genuine.** Communicates in a constructive manner what is felt and thought; uses verbal and nonverbal communication methods.
- **Attentive.** Demonstrates an interest in people; listens to verbal and nonverbal messages.
- **Respectful.** Expresses concern for experiences, feelings, and potential of others; sees the client as unique.
- **Nonjudgmental.** Refrains from evaluating the worth of the client or the value of ideas and feelings.
- **Sensitive.** Is perceptive of the client's and the helper's own feelings; responds to social changes.
- **Knowledgeable.** Has a knowledge based on study and experience.

In addition to these characteristics, you must be willing to share with the client your own uniqueness as a person. You must accept the fact that as you help the client to develop you will also continue to expand your own personality—you are always in the process of becoming.[34]

Does everyone possess these qualities? Are we born with these characteristics? How do the knowledge and skills necessary for an effective helping relationship develop? The answers to the first two questions are obviously no. You must work to develop the qualities needed in a helping relationship. To a large extent, the helping relationship depends on your experiences and your attitude toward yourself and the client. There are no set techniques or rules which ensure an effective relationship. Review of the section in Chapter 4 that discusses behavior conducive to the development of an effective nurse–client relationship will be helpful. In addition, an understanding of rapport, trust, and empathy is important.

*Rapport* is a sense of mutuality and understanding; it is the feeling of harmony, accord, confidence, and respect that underlies a relationship between two individuals.[49] In order to establish rapport, you must offer an accepting, open attitude, and show interest in the client. Everything possible should be done to make the client feel comfortable.

*Trust* is a belief in the dependability, credibility, and reliability of another individual. Trust is central to a therapeutic nurse–client relationship. Without a sense of trust, the interaction between the client and nurse will be superficial with minimal personal involvement by either.

It usually takes an extended period of time for people to develop a sense of trust in each other. The initial period of time spent together is marked by uncertainty and exploration—nurse and client attempt to clarify their roles. It is during this time that you, as the nurse, should let the client know *your* goals. Client goals will be established later in the relationship. As the relationship grows, both the nurse and the client share feelings and concerns. Confidentiality is established. The client slowly moves from an external to an internal frame of reference, and the inner concerns of the client become the focus of the interaction. Termination or ending of the trust relationship should be done gradually so as not to produce distrust or separation anxiety in the client.[6]

The following strategies will help with the development of trust:[6,34,35,47]

- **Demonstrate Competence.** Indicate through your actions that you are capable or competent and that you have sufficient knowledge and experience to handle the situation. Convey a caring attitude; use a relaxed unhurried manner. Sloppiness in appearance or in implementing nursing actions may decrease the client's perception of your competence.
- **Demonstrate Concern.** Indicate your regard for or interest in the client. Frequently, nurses feel that not getting involved and not demonstrating sensitivity is the appropriate behavior—that it will prevent them from "overinvolvement." Only when involvement interferes with your ability to support the client, make objective judgments, or perform needed therapies, is it nontherapeutic. Do not try to hide your innate sensitivity; the client may interpret this as a lack of feeling on your part. Try to demonstrate compassion and sensitivity that is part of your own makeup. Be genuine in your interest and concern. Remember that your approach will reflect your own personal attitudes, values, and beliefs; it is therefore important that you have a clear understanding of yourself.
- **Offer Comfort.** Use measures that will produce physical and emotional comfort for the client. Initiate these actions on your own; do not wait for the client to ask.
- **Use Therapeutic Communication.** Verbal and nonverbal communication techniques can be used—eye contact, touch, silence, body movements, comforting sounds and words. Become sensitive to the client's messages so that you can respond appropriately. Be willing to clarify messages and seek clarification when needed.
- **Demonstrate Consistency.** Behaviors and responses exhibited toward the client should be consistent with each contact. When you do not receive positive strokes or reinforcement from the client, you must be tolerant and nondefensive. Do not

allow the client's behavior to stimulate inconsistent responses from you—accepting and warm on one occasion, and critical and judgmental on another.
- **Demonstrate Equanimity.** Be calm, even-tempered, and composed. Such behavior will do much to establish an environment or atmosphere of trust.

*Empathy* is the ability to recognize and to some extent share the current thoughts and feelings of another and to understand the meaning and significance of that individual's behavior.[20,37] It is not the same as sympathy, which is an expressed interest or concern regarding the problems or concerns of another.

Empathetic skills are enhanced by certain personal qualities and attributes. Some of the characteristics that will increase your ability to be empathetic are the ability to:

- Express warmth and spontaneity verbally and nonverbally.
- Time responses to match the client's feelings and needs at that moment.
- Abstract the essential meaning of the client's feelings and concerns.
- Interpret verbal and nonverbal messages correctly and avoid distortion of perceptions.
- Discuss the client's feelings and concerns in acceptable and understandable terms.
- Move the discussion in the direction of the client's feelings and concerns.
- Listen attentively.
- Use a variety of words, phrases, or statements that are expressive of emotion.
- Cope with egocentricity, anxiety, fears, or other feelings that might interfere with your sharing of feelings and thoughts of another.
- Become involved in another and lose self-consciousness.[9,20,34,53]

A variety of life experiences will help you to acquire a broader understanding of people and will promote flexibility and spontaneity in your use of empathetic skills. In addition, similarity with the client—values, beliefs, attitudes, religion, age, occupation, and experiences—will make it easier to empathize.[53]

The helping relationship is divided into four phases: orientation, identification, working, and termination. Some sources also identify a preinteraction phase.[8,14,34,47]

In the **preinteraction phase,** you are the sole participant. This is the time for you to prepare yourself for your interaction with the client. You should review pertinent theoretical information and past clinical experiences. You should focus on your feelings regarding your prospective client and plan for the first interaction with the client. The **orientation phase** (introductory, initial, or establishment phase) begins when you first meet the client. During this phase, you introduce yourself, explain your role and the purpose of the relationship. Depending on the clinical situation and the length of time spent with the client you should formulate a tentative care plan and develop a written or informal verbal contract. Aspects which are usually included in the contract are location, frequency, and length of meetings, overall purpose of the relationship, duration of the relationship, and manner in which confidential material will be handled. In the **identification phase,** you and the client become better acquainted. If the client perceives you as accepting and empathetic, you become the surrogate parent or identification figure. During the **working phase** (therapeutic or maintaining phase), the client and you work on the problems and needs which have been identified. The **termination phase** is important. Too often the time for termination arrives before adequate planning has been done. You should plan for this phase early in the helping relationship. Termination of the relationship occurs when the client is discharged, the mutually agreed-on goals have been attained, or the nurse leaves the clinical setting (transfer to another division, etc.). You and the client must work through feelings about separation.

***Counseling.*** Counseling is another nursing action that requires the use of interpersonal skills. Counseling skills can be used in the implementation of the plan of care, especially with the family and individual client. ***Counseling*** is "an interaction process that facilitates meaningful understanding of self and environment and results in the establishment and/or clarification of goals and values for future behavior."[39] Insight into problems, discovery of solutions, exploration of feelings, and decision making are encouraged.

As early as the 1940s, Dr. Hildegard Peplau saw the need for nurses to join the rank of other professionals providing counseling.[35] Most of Peplau's efforts were directed toward preparing nurses to counsel clients with mental and emotional problems that required hospitalization. It was not until 20 or 30 years later that the role of the professional nurse expanded to incorporate counseling. Today, as nurses become more active in this area, many situations have been identified in which counseling is appropriate. Counseling can be used to help the client in:

1. Identifying, stating, and reducing anxiety, stress, or uncomfortable feelings.
2. Clarifying conflicts.
3. Formulating decisions; sorting out alternatives; gaining different perspectives.
4. Clarifying and reinforcing values; determining consequences of values, decisions, and actions.
5. Adjusting to developmental or situational crises.
6. Changing behavior to problem solving instead of problem producing.
7. Achieving new self-understanding.
8. Reducing psychopathology and emotional illness.[27,34]

In counseling, there are at least two participants, the counselor and the counselee. As indicated earlier, the nurse–counselor role is most commonly applied with individuals and families. Counseling skills are also used with community groups. For example, a community health nurse may provide counseling sessions for a group of women whose husbands have recently died. An occupational health nurse may use counseling skills to help a group of workers adjust to organizational changes that are occurring in the industrial setting.

Before discussing some of the specific skills and techniques necessary for counseling, there are some general points that you should consider.

- **Understand Yourself.** Throughout our discussion of interpersonal skills we have indicated how essential it is to gain an understanding of yourself—your feelings and thoughts. In counseling, self-understanding is especially important. This does not mean that you should exhaustively search your mind, but it does mean that some introspection is needed. For example, if you are working with a teenager with venereal disease, give some thought to your feelings about sexual relations between teenagers. How do you feel about people who contract a venereal disease? If you were talking to a young adult who had been injured during an attempted robbery, you would need to determine how you felt about people who did not obey the law. Through introspection and an understanding of yourself, you will be better prepared to react in similar situations.

When you find yourself in sympathy with someone else, this also requires introspection. Why do I feel so sorry for this person? Perhaps you see a resemblance between yourself and the client. Being sympathetic is not therapeutic or is protectiveness. You cannot help the client if you feel that you must soothe the client's feelings and give assurance that everything is going to be all right.

- **Be Yourself.** When you are counseling, you cannot imitate the behavior, techniques, or words of others. You must learn to be yourself—the more natural the better. Use your personality to help you understand the client and the client's reactions to you. Use yourself to convey ideas and to help the client toward self-understanding.
- **Use Your "Self."** Note your reactions to the client—nonverbal communication by the client, what the client fails to say, and what can be read between the lines of the client's monologue can stimulate reactions in us as counselors. You may not be able to pinpoint why a certain reaction was produced, but you can learn to become aware of any unusual reactions. For example, if most people seem to like you and are comfortable talking with you, either socially or professionally, you begin to assume that everyone should respond to you in that manner. If you were interviewing a client and suddenly noticed that you were anxious, you should try to determine what stimulated this anxiety in you. Is the client sending a message above and beyond the verbal communication? Is he scared? Angry? Whenever you note a feeling or emotional tone rising in you, bring it to your conscious mind and respond to it.

With these general comments to guide us, we can look at some specific techniques. A variety of techniques and skills are essential in counseling. Peplau identified seven principles that can be used to direct effective client counseling. Although these principles were used originally in psychiatric hospitals, they can be adapted and applied in any clinical setting—clinic, physician's office, home, hospital, school.

1. Set an example for the client.
2. Maintain a professional attitude.
3. Respect the client.
4. Assess the client's intellectual competence.
5. Guide the client to reinterpret personal experiences rationally.
6. Ask sensible questions to aid description.
7. Study and apply theory in counseling.[35]

*Set an Example for the Client.* In counseling, it is important that you set an example for the client. You must appear confident and capable of meeting your own needs as well as focusing on the needs of others. You must demonstrate the ability to understand the difficulties of others and a competence for investigating and resolving problems.

You should approach the client in a serious manner; the client must feel that you want to understand and help. Give the client your full attention; use an attitude and posture of alertness. Listen carefully to what is said. Deal with each topic in a logical, orderly way that will serve as an example for the client.

*Maintain a Professional Attitude.* Approach the client in a professional manner. In counseling, do not behave toward the client as you would toward friends socially. Remember that different modes of behavior will have different effects on the client. For example, even a smile or a nod may be misunderstood. They may be interpreted as approval or an indication of disapproval or amusement at what is being said. Because you are not in counseling to establish friendships, it is not necessary to give the client biographical or personal data about yourself. Information about you will not help the client.

Avoid giving verbal or nonverbal approval or disapproval of the client's actions or words. You should maintain strict neutrality toward all client behavior. Being neutral, however, does not mean being indifferent. Indifference reflects a lack of interest and concern. Although indicating approval or disapproval may meet the immediate need of the client, or even of yourself, this action will do nothing to enhance the long-range counselor–client relationship.

*Respect the Client.* Each client is an unique individual. Clients should not be stereotyped. For example, responding to all clients in a developmental crisis in the same manner fails to recognize their individuality. There may be times when you will care for a client who has broken a social standard or a law. While you cannot approve of the behavior, you can assure the client that as a person, the client is liked by you and deserves your respect—who the client is and what the client does are two different things.

*Assess the Client's Intellectual Competence.* Your initial assessment included subjective and objective data on the client's mental capacity and competence. This information helps you to focus on the client's assets and limitations. However, it is not enough just to rely on the initial data. As your contact with the client continues, make certain that you keep the data base up to date. Because we tend to become less aware as we become more familiar with a person, place, or thing, this need to update the assessed data will keep us on our guard and more perceptive of changes.

*Guide the Client to Reinterpret Personal Experiences Rationally.* Counseling tries to eliminate or modify behavior patterns by the examination of experiences which gave rise to the behavior. Therefore, one of the first things that you seek to do is to elicit a description of the experiences from the client. Make certain that your approach encourages the client to *describe* experiences, not classify or give conclusions about events. If a client says, "The kids at school hate me," the client is not describing experiences. Instead, the client is giving you a conclusion about events that the client has already evaluated and classified. You want to hear about the experiences on which the conclusions are based—"There was this after-school party and everyone was invited but me," or "I walked into the classroom and Mike said to me. . . . "

Clients more often than not do not start talking about the concerns that are uppermost in their minds. When they have attained enough courage and when they trust you, they will discuss their major concerns more freely. There may also be a tendency for the client to get off the main subject or to start talking about irrelevant subjects. You can attempt to return the client to the desired subject by stating, "Earlier in the conversation you were talking about. . . . " You may also point out to the client the change in subjects or the wandering away from the main focus.

*Ask Sensible Questions to Aid Description.* To be effective, you must develop an awareness of your verbal and nonverbal communication patterns. Nondirective questions while useful in other forms of interviews may create undesired responses in counseling. Gestures and nodding can cause misunderstanding; the client might interpret these actions as approval or disapproval.

To gain direct answers, it is best to restrict your questions to who, what, where, and when. To explain how or why something happens is too difficult for most clients. Make each question simple and direct. Avoid two questions in the same statement: "Where do you live; how long have you lived there?"

*Study and Apply Theory in Counseling.* You should use concepts from theories of personality development and from other sources to understand the behavior of clients and yourself and to guide you in identifying deficiencies in the client's development.[35]

Most of the techniques and principles discussed earlier in this section under communication and the helping relationship are applicable to counseling. In addition, the section on attentive listening and interviewing skills in Chapter 4 will be of help to you.

## Technical Skills

Most technical skills are task oriented and contain some activity requiring direct client contact—turning, feeding, applying, supporting, walking, exercising, folding, giving, and so forth. Technical skills reflect the psychomotor domain of learning behaviors—ability to perform manual or motor skills. Performing technical skills also includes cognitive and affective behaviors as well as psychomotor.

Technical skills should not be performed in a routine, mechanical fashion. Critical thinking and judgment are required to determine if the activity is appropriate for the client at this time. For example, the nursing order, *Walk the client 6 meters (20 feet) three times a day, at 9:00, 1:00, 5:00,* would need to be altered if the client complained of dizziness after dangling at the bedside.

Intellectual skills are also needed to determine the priority of the planned activities. We spoke of priorities earlier in relation to listing nursing diagnoses in order of importance and nursing orders according to the one best suited for the situation. At this time you are actually implementing your plan and you may need to modify the plan to reflect new priorities. For example, with the prior nursing order to walk the client, ambulation or activity would not be your highest priority at this point. Client safety would have priority over activity until the client's condition stabilized again.

The individuality of the client must also be considered. Adaptation of the activity to meet the need of each client is essential. In addition, the client is entitled to an explanation of the activity to be performed. This explanation should include the role of the client, the expected results from the action, any special equipment that might be used, and any discomfort the client might experience. Giving clients an adequate explanation will elicit their cooperation and increase their feelings of trust and confidence in the nurse.

***Implementing the Family Care Plan.*** Implementation of the plan of care for the family or community also requires intellectual, interpersonal, and technical skills. It is important when working with a family that you adapt your activities so that they are appropriate to the family's level of functioning. In Chapter 5, we discussed a tool devised by Tapia and Meister that could be used to derive conclusions about the family's health status and need for nursing care. This same tool can now direct your implementation of the plan of care. A family functioning at Level I, the infancy level, will require you to function in a mother role. Your major focus while implementing the plan of care will be to develop a trusting relationship. This task will require maturity, patience, limit setting, and repeated clarification of your role. Once the family's need for security has been met, you can move the family into Level II activities. With the Level II family, the childhood level, your functions are directed at forming a counseling relationship. Your goal is to help the family grow to where they can resolve some of their problems. Working with a Level III family, the adolescent level, requires a variety of technical, intellectual, and interpersonal skills. You will provide teaching, information, coordination, referral, or specific technical skills. The main nursing activity with a Level IV family, the adulthood level, is preventive health teaching. The family views the nurse as an expert teacher. The Level V family, the maturity level, does not require nursing activities unless there is a crisis. When nursing assistance is needed, you would use nursing activities appropriate to the level of functioning at that time.[48]

*Implementing Community Care Plan.* Within the community, implementation is viewed somewhat differently. It is not just nursing action or nursing intervention but collaborative implementation. The nurse is a primary resource, catalyst, and facilitator in activating the nurse–client action plan. Because a primary goal in community health is to help the client (the community) learn to help itself, the nurse must involve the client.[42]

As with the individual and family client, individualization of the implementation step must occur at the community level. Implementation of a plan for improved community health is shaped by the nurse's preferred mode of practice, the type of health problem involved, the community's readiness to participate in the plan, and the characteristics of the social change process. Because the factors that shape implementation at a community level are multiple and the force of their impact complex, the nurse in the community setting must be adaptable and flexible. The nurse cannot implement a community plan alone—change on behalf of the community client requires multiple implementation mechanisms. (Stanhope and Lancaster define implementation mechanisms as the vehicles or modes by which proposed innovations are transferred from the planners to the units of service.) The nurse must decide which mechanism(s) to use—small interacting groups, lay advisors, mass media, or public policy.[43]

Thus far in this chapter the physiologic, psychological, and socioeconomic actions that are used during the implementing step have been discussed. Intellectual, interpersonal, and technical skills needed for effective performance of these actions have also been presented. We now need to focus our attention on your role as a leader and manager.

## ROLES ASSUMED IN THE IMPLEMENTING STEP

Leadership and management skills will help you to implement the plan of care effectively. These skills will help you to organize and plan your own actions and to direct the actions of others.

## Role as a Leader

**Leadership** is the interpersonal process of influencing a person, group, family, or community toward goal-setting and goal-achievement. Leadership involves directive influence upon others and is considered a social transaction and interaction. The person who controls or commands the social transaction and interaction is identified as the leader.

Where there is leadership, authority, and power struggles exist. Within the structure of nursing, capable nurse–leaders frequently do not have the authority and power proportionate with their responsibility for planning and decision making. Traditional management practices reflect the belief that nurses at the operational level require close supervision and control. Because of this divestment of authority, power struggles occur.[10]

To better understand your role as a leader, it is important for you to have a clear understanding of the terms *authority, power,* and *influence.* All three are forms of interpersonal relationships. **Authority** is an interpersonal relationship in which a person is given the right to make selected decisions that affect another's behavior. This person is given the right to give commands, enforce laws, or exact obedience. Generally, the person who has the authority is considered to have the knowledge and expertise necessary to make decisions and direct others. In the formal organizational structure, authority is viewed as originating at the top of the organizational hierarchy and moving downward by delegation.[10,11,52]

**Power** is an interpersonal relationship that is reciprocal in nature. Within this interpersonal relationship, a person is capable of satisfying or not satisfying the needs of another. As a result, the other's behavior can be affected. Power implies an interdependent relationship.[10,11,50,52]

It is difficult to think objectively about power; subjective and emotionally laden ideas such as good, evil, justice, and freedom are closely intermingled with the concept of power. Power has both a positive and a negative connotation. It can be used to resolve problems, but improper use of power can create problems.[12,18,31,50]

**Influence** is an interpersonal relationship that lacks power and authority. Through influence, the behavior of a person or group is affected by another person or group. Influence can come from direct or indirect sources. Role expectations associated with a position—nurse–client, counselor–client, nurse–physician—are direct sources of influence. With indirect influence, the relationship is subtly based upon mutual trust and respect. Influencing techniques used by the leader may consist of advice, suggestion, persuasion, or role modeling.[10,11,52]

Authority, power, and influence are interdependent and vital to the leadership role. As a professional nurse, you will use all three in order to fulfill your role as a leader. As you grow in your leadership knowledge and skills, you will assume a leadership style that will determine how you use authority, power, and influence.

*Leadership Patterns.* Different styles of leadership patterns exist. Three generally accepted styles are: autocratic, democratic, and laissez-faire.[17,23,24,29,32,44]

**Autocratic** or **directive leadership** emphasizes commanding and order giving. The leader makes most of the decisions, entrusting little authority to subordinates. Autocratic leadership is something in which nursing has traditionally excelled. With this type of leadership, communication is in one direction, from the leader downwards.

In contrast to autocratic leadership, **democratic** or **participative leadership** is employed with the consent and support of those who are led. Rather than constantly telling other people what to do, the leader frequently asks them. Communication flows in both directions. The ideas and suggestions of subordinates are valued, and consultation with them may be used to secure their contributions. In democratic leadership, the leader plays an active role in stimulating group thinking to develop a solution or reach a decision.

The **laissez-faire** or free-rein leader goes a step farther and turns an entire problem or project over to subordinates. Subordinates may be asked to set their own objectives and to develop plans for achieving them. In one sense, this approach is characterized by the absence of any active leadership by the formally designated leader. Although laissez-faire leadership may be effective occasionally when the group is capable of constructive response, chaos may result in some situations.

In addition to these three traditional leadership styles, management theorists have described two behavior styles: task behavior and relationship behavior. In **task behavior,** the leader organizes and defines the roles of each group member and explains the activities of each. The leader will also describe when, where, and how the tasks are to be accomplished. This leadership style has also been labeled production-oriented, goal achievement, or autocratic. In **relationship behavior,** the leader engages in personal relationships with a person or members of the group. Socio-emotional support and interpersonal communication are part of the leader's function. This leadership style has also been labeled employee-oriented, group maintenance, or democratic.[16,46]

One style of leadership is rarely practiced alone. Combinations of different styles are used based on the situation, the need of the group, and characteristics of the leader. Two of the most common variations seen in nursing are benevolent–autocratic and manipulative–autocratic. The **benevolent–autocratic** leader wants to use the democratic style of leadership but actually practices the autocratic style. Nurse–leaders who follow this style attempt to secure acceptance of their decisions without really considering the requested input from other people. The **manipulative–autocratic** leader attempts to make people feel that they are participating in decision making when in fact the leader is making the decisions. The leader directs discussions so that the predetermined decision that the leader wants is reached by the group.[44]

It is important for you to become aware of your preferred style and to be able to adjust your style so it is more effective. Since you will probably use a combination of leadership styles, it is also important that you understand the advantages and difficulties inherent in each style (Table 7–1).

*Effective Leadership.* Effectiveness in leadership is based on the interrelationships among personality traits, characteristics, and behaviors of the leader and follower. In addition, leadership effectiveness is affected by the situation in which leadership occurs. Some of the desired traits, characteristics, and behaviors of a leader are:

1. Leaders tend to be more intelligent than the group they lead.
2. Leaders possess initiative and are able to perceive and start actions not considered by others.
3. Leaders are creative.
4. Leaders possess emotional maturity—integrity, a sense of purpose and direction, persistency, dependability, and objectivity.
5. Leaders are risk takers and willing to accept success or failure gracefully.
6. Leaders possess self-respect, self-confidence, and self-assurance.

**TABLE 7–1. LEADERSHIP STYLES**[10,13,16,18,21,29]

| Characteristics of Style | Characteristics of Followers |
|---|---|
| **Autocratic or Directive** | |
| Leader has complete power | Some are leader dependent |
| Leader makes all the decisions | Unwilling to ask questions |
| Emphasis on adherence to policy and rules | Comply with demands but retreat personally |
| Minimal emphasis on respect, warmth, consideration, and mutual trust | Unwilling to exercise initiative for fear of punitive measures |
| Low degree of participation from others | Lower feelings of self-worth |
| High degree of punitiveness | Interest or needs elsewhere take precedence |
| Leader firmly entrenched in position | May have lowered morale and productivity (poor client care) |
| **Democratic or Participative** | |
| Consultative type situation | Expect to have some control over methods used |
| Leader has limited power | Feel their own feelings and thoughts are important |
| Conducive to exploration and discovery of the individual | Possess successful experiences in having needs and expectations met |
| Authority invested in leader by individuals or group | Can express controversial beliefs and give feedback |
| Leader can be stripped of power | |
| Leader confident in ability to work with people | |
| **Laissez-Faire** | |
| Leader passes decision making on to others | Have more power than leader |
| Leader has no power to compel action | View guidelines, rules, and limit setting as infringements on their rights |
| Open and permissive attitude | |
| May develop in rebellion to autocratic leader or when leader too weak to exercise functions | Loosely organized |
| | Will rebel successfully if they so choose |

7. Leaders are interested in and have concern for others. They are sincere and willing to share themselves with others.

8. Leaders accept responsibility for their actions and do not seek scapegoats.

9. Leaders are interested in accomplishments and are usually involved in several projects at one time. They are, however, realistic about how far they can extend themselves.

10. Leaders enjoy work and have intrinsic motivation. They do not intentionally seek external rewards.

11. Leaders possess a sense of humor and enthusiasm. They have the ability to instill their enthusiasm in their followers.

12. Leaders use communication effectively.

13. Leaders possess social maturity—the ability to socialize with all kinds of people and adapt to various groups.

14. Leaders are effective problem solvers.[10,16,23,44,52]

Now that we have looked at the various leadership styles and identified some of the qualities of an effective leader, we will discuss these aspects in relationship to nursing—the nursing leadership process.

Leadership is inherent in nursing. It is the unifying force that brings people in nursing together to strive to achieve the mutual goal—quality client care. **Nursing leadership** has been defined by Yura, Ozimek, and Walsh as "a process whereby a person who is a nurse effects [sic] the actions of others in goal determination and achievement."[52]

Leadership is not solely the responsibility of those in hierarchical positions of authority within health care settings. Leadership occurs whenever there is interaction between people. Nurses, regardless of their position, should exert leadership: nurse practitioners should be leading their clients toward optimal health; nurse administrators should be leading their faculty and staff to higher levels of performance; and nurse educators should be leading nursing students at all levels to become future leaders in the nursing profession.[32]

Leadership may occur within the formal or informal organizational structure of the health care setting. Formal organizational structure is typified by administration, management, and supervision—hospital administrator, unit manager, and clinical supervisor. People in these positions are guided by a plan that relates them and their tasks to the work environment. The plan may include formal rules, policies, procedures, and control mechanisms that govern their actions in addition to job descriptions and organizational charts that indicate the lines of authority and communication. Informal organizational structure is seen as a network of social and personal relationships. These relationships arise spontaneously and do not follow position lines. Both types of organizational structure are needed to assure effective implementation of the plan of care.

Regardless of the clinical setting there will be some form of formal organizational structure. Within the hospital, the hierarchical structure of authority may be primary nurse, charge nurse, division supervisor, assistant director of nursing service, director of nursing service, and hospital administrator. Although the only individual who is actually functioning at the level of direct client contact is the primary nurse, other people are also involved with the client's care. Through their leadership role they can affect the type and quality of nursing care given.

The nurse who is directly responsible for client care is actually part of both the formal and informal organizational structure at a health care setting. The informal organizational structure exists in association with the other professional nurses in the setting, health team members, clients, and families. Leadership in the informal organizational structure is usually assumed by one person or unofficially delegated to someone. The nurse who appears the most competent, organized, and confident often becomes the leader.

Nursing leadership has been identified as an **interactional process** with four key components—deciding, relating, influencing, and facilitating. Interpersonal communication and interaction pervade all four components. The participants in the nursing leadership process are the leader and follower(s). The desired result of the process is the achievement of predetermined goals. Variables external to both the leader and follower(s) will affect goal setting and achievement.

The nursing leadership process is viewed as dynamic, not static, which means there is movement within the process from one state to another. This movement from one state to another denotes change which is inherent in the leadership process. To proceed from data base to goal setting to goal achievement constitutes a change. To determine the effectiveness of the leadership and the degree of goal achievement, constant feedback is necessary. Once feedback has been received and interpreted, the process must adapt—thus change occurs again (Fig. 7–3). The nursing leadership process is applicable to clients, families, communities, peers, and colleagues. It is also applicable to the nurse–leader's immediate surroundings and to local, state, and national groups.[10,24,32,52]

Leadership behavior is shown throughout the nursing process. It is not isolated to the implementing step only. Leadership behavior is demonstrated when you decide to

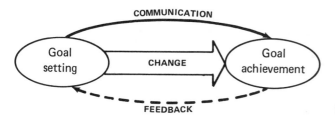

**Figure 7–3.** Nursing leadership process.

collect the health history and physical assessment; when you use communication skills to determine if the client–nurse perceptions are similar; when you determine how the needs of the client will be met; when you decide how and by whom the plan of care will be implemented; and when you establish a method of evaluating the effectiveness of your care. Combining nursing leadership with the nursing process improves the effectiveness of your care.

You will find yourself in a leadership role at some level each day. As a professional nurse, you will assume the lead in defining and planning care. In addition, you will be responsible for coordinating and directing the activities of other health team members. In order to accomplish these tasks, you will need to adopt a leadership style that is flexible, adaptable, and effective. You will need to use the power and authority delegated to you and develop your own style of influencing action. Perhaps the most important aspect of your nurse–leader role is the development and display of intellectual skills— critical thinking, problem solving, validating inferences, and making sound judgments.

## Role as a Manager

To manage means to direct, control, or supervise. In nursing, **management** is seen as the process whereby human and physical resources are manipulated or changed in order to accomplish specific predetermined results.

The dual role of nurse and manager applies at every level in nursing—staff nurse, head nurse, or administrator. The professional nurse is both nurse and manager— *nurse*–manager or nurse–*manager*—with the emphasis shifting according to the situation. As *nurse*–manager, the emphasis is on the nurse implementing the skills associated with the nursing profession. The nurse may be functioning as a primary-care nurse, team leader, public health nurse, school nurse, or clinic nurse. The nurse–*manager* role emphasizes the role of the nurse as a professional manager. Nursing knowledge and skills are still essential but the clinical skills are practiced less as management skills are assumed. The nurse–*manager* may be seen in the role of charge nurse, supervisor, coordinator, director of nursing, vice president for client care services, director of nursing education, staff development director, and so forth.[13]

Management and leadership are not synonymous. It is possible to be a leader without a management position and to be a manager without leadership abilities. Management involves many of the same skills as leadership, but has a wider range of functions with a wider variety of roles and more legitimate power and authority.

When management is viewed as a process, it is possible to identify four basic management functions. The four functions that provide the framework for analyzing management activities are planning, organizing, directing and motivating, and controlling.

**Planning** involves thought and decisions concerning a proposed course of action. The plan may include, in addition to the decision to take action, such aspects as "who," "when," and "how." Planning anticipates and precedes action; it is a proactive approach. **Organizing** includes the provision of physical facilities, capital, and personnel. It is also concerned with the determination of relationships among functions, jobs, and personnel. Organizing involves an integration of resources. **Directing and motivating** involve stimulating a person or a group to carry out the management plans. Any organized effort requires some centralized planning and decision making. The process of communicating these choices may be thought of as the function of directing. **Controlling** refers to the regulation of the organizational structure to insure the achievement of objectives and the completion of plans.[16,44]

There are at least three areas of skill necessary to implement the process of management: technical, human, and conceptual. Technical skills include the ability to use knowledge and equipment to perform specific tasks acquired from experience and education. Ability and judgment in working with and through people are included in human skills. Conceptual skills include the ability to understand and function within the overall organization. To be effective, less technical skills are needed as advancement from lower to higher levels in the organization occurs. At the same time, more complex conceptual skills are needed. Human skills are essential at all levels of the organization. Skills such as communicating effectively, conceptualizing, decision making, discussion leading, instructing, motivating, managing time, and problem solving are included in these three areas.[13,16]

Various attributes and characteristics of an effective nurse–manager can be identified. Some of these attributes and characteristics are summarized in Table 7–2.[18,21] These qualities will help you to function in the dual role of nurse–manager.

Some of the specific nurse–manager functions that you may be performing during the implementing step might include:

- Planning strategies for implementing the plan of care with other members of the nursing team. Be certain to use all available resources.
- Organizing planned activities as to time and location. Decide "when" and "where" certain nursing interventions will be performed.
- Assigning and delegating activities. You can delegate activities that can be performed safely by other members of the nursing team. Make certain that you know the capabilities of each member of the team as well as the responsibilities that accompany their title and role. Check their job description.
- Directing the counseling of the client, family, or nursing team member. (You should be aware when nursing team members are in need of personal counseling.)

**TABLE 7–2. CHARACTERISTICS AND ATTRIBUTES OF EFFECTIVE NURSE–MANAGERS[18,21]**

1. Views management as primarily a human process.
2. Has a positive view of self.
3. Has favorable opinions of others.
4. Is well informed.
5. Is able to communicate knowledge effectively.
6. Has ability to cope with change.
7. Possesses ability to motivate others.
8. Is sensitive to values, feelings, and attitudes of others.
9. Encourages growth in others.

- Scheduling activities for maximum nurse efficiency and client benefits.
- Controlling the implementing process by developing and using evaluation procedures.
- Supervising performance of ancillary nursing personnel.

We have identified the skills used by the nurse while implementing the plan of care: intellectual, interpersonal, and technical. In addition, we have described the roles that are assumed during this action-oriented phase of the nursing process. Now, let us consider some suggestions on how to improve your overall performance during this step.

## METHODS OF INCREASING YOUR EFFECTIVENESS

Managing your time, monitoring your professional image, and evaluating your performance are important in the implementing step of the nursing process. It is during this step that you usually have the most direct and prolonged client contact. This is the time for you to help the client resolve concerns, needs, and problems and achieve goals and objectives. You want your actions to be effective and to reflect your professional competence.

### Managing Your Time
The ability to manage your own time productively and effectively is important. Activities that will help you to manage your time include:

1. Planning and organizing your activities
2. Setting goals
3. Setting deadlines
4. Concentrating on critical, high-priority activities
5. Eliminating trivial activities
6. Learning to concentrate
7. Delegating responsibilities and authority
8. Thinking before acting
9. Monitoring your actions
10. Analyzing your use of time[19,30,33]

Every nurse–manager needs a plan. This is not necessarily the client's plan of care. In fact, your plan as *nurse*–manager might include how to implement the plans of care for six clients effectively. Planning will help you to determine priorities and to generate alternative actions. Planning also creates goals and therefore standards for you to follow. One way to help you to achieve your goals is to make a list of the things you need to accomplish. Look at each item on the list and decide if it will help you to achieve your goals and objectives—if not, eliminate it from your list. Now, divide the tasks into three groups—must be done, should be done, and routine. Within each group establish priorities for the tasks in order of importance. Try to accomplish the "must be done" tasks first.

Concentrate your efforts on a few critical, high-priority activities. You should respond only to those urgent problems that affect the immediate situation. Some problems will go away if left alone. By selectively ignoring these problems, you may conserve time and effort. You should also avoid unnecessary detail and selectively neglect all but essential information. Think back—probably at some point you were told by a parent or teacher that they would be better off not knowing the details regarding some event—this was selective neglect on their part.

Eliminate trivial activities. Everything cannot be completed; the most important tasks or activities must come first. Time should be allocated to tasks in order of their priority. You should avoid overcompletion (stretching out familiar tasks to avoid new tougher undertakings), procrastination, and perfectionism.

You should think before acting; don't let impulse or habit dominate your actions. You should act consciously. Do not treat every situation as if it were a crisis. Overreaction causes anxiety, impaired judgment, hasty decisions, and stress.

All of your activities should be ranked and organized. To know what needs to be done and to be able to do it within a reasonable time are two different things. If you are in a hospital, you may have an 8- or 10-hour shift in which to implement your clients' plans of care. As you read your care plans and receive reports on your clients, make a list of the things you need to do. Assign each of the items a time period within your shift. Make certain that you discuss with your clients their preferences when possible. Within each time period, rank your list of items. You can then place this information on a grid with the clients' names across the top and the hours of your shift on the left (Fig. 7–4). Check off your tasks as you accomplish them; this will help direct your actions.

Another method of enhancing your effectiveness in implementing is to keep a time log. The time log is important in helping you to identify unimportant, routine activities that are consuming your time. You will also be able to identify how much actual time is spent with your high-priority items. To begin a time log, list ten activities that are the core of your job. Next, rank them according to their importance in achieving desired results. Finally, assign a percentage to each activity to indicate the percentage of time you think you spend at each activity. One hundred percent (100%) should represent the total amount of work time available for the period of time you selected—day, week, month, quarter. At the end of each day, write down what you did and the time involved. At the end of the time period—day, week, month, quarter—look at the actual percentage of time spent on each activity. If your actual time allocation is far from the ideal time allocation, work to bring these activities into desired time allocation. Determine why you spend so much time on activities that do not achieve results. Why does it take so long to perform certain functions? Can portions of the most time-consuming but least

| TIME | K.J. | N.L. | G.E. | T.H. |
|---|---|---|---|---|
| 8 A.M. | Vital signs Set up for breakfast | Vital signs Set up for breakfast | Vital signs NPO Set up for bath | Vital signs Set up for breakfast |
| 9 A.M. | Medications | Medications | Administer 9:30a.m. preoperative medication | Set up for bath |

**Figure 7–4.** Time grid.

productive activities be reduced? Check your list of priorities. You may need to reorder them.[19,30,33]

## Monitoring Your Professional Image

Consider the message that your appearance is giving. The clothing and accessories that you wear are statements to others with whom you come in contact. Clothing has a variety of meanings. It can denote status, occupation, sex, or age. Some people select clothing for comfort or economy; others seek conformity or self-expression. In health care settings, uniforms are usually worn for covering and protection. Make certain that you dress appropriately and observe the dress code of your agency.

Like clothing, your shoes, nails, hair, and makeup can reflect your personal habits and attitudes. For example, shoes that are dirty, scuffed, or worn down at the heels are not attractive. Unfortunately, clients sometimes draw conclusions from the appearance of shoes about the quality of care a facility offers. Unattractive shoes may be interpreted by the client and client's family as an indication of unprofessional or poor quality care.

You will need to keep your knowledge base current. This gives you the basis for implementing a plan that is both safe and creative. You can participate in self-directed learning activities or formal educational programs—either way, you must consider yourself an independent life-long learner. Self-directed learning activities can take several forms. It is helpful to subscribe to at least one monthly professional journal and set aside time each month to read it. Take the opportunity to share ideas with your co-workers and to discuss with them the latest literature in your clinical setting. An example of an activity that serves both as a social outlet and as a means of keeping current is a journal club. This type of club is informal and composed of a group of nurses who meet once a month to share articles or current literature.

Formal educational programs can take the form of continuing education workshops and conferences, formal courses and programs for credit which are offered by local colleges and universities, or in-service education programs. Formal education is meant to keep nurses current with the developments within the profession, to teach new skills, to review appropriate methods of implementing current skills, or to prepare the nurse to assume a new role, for example, clinical specialist or nurse practitioner.

You will need to continue your socialization process in the profession. Socialization can occur through casual interactions with other people within the health care system. This form of socialization helps to establish attitudes and beliefs concerning the nurse's role. Socialization can also occur through formalized educational experiences and membership in professional organizations. It is important that you join and participate in the local chapter of your professional organization. Contact with nurses outside your immediate surrounding will help to establish further your attitudes and beliefs concerning the nurse's role. In addition, the professional organization will keep you informed concerning local, state, and national developments within the nursing profession.

## Evaluating Your Performance

It is important that you continually evaluate your performance. Performance evaluation does not end when you graduate from your nursing program. It should continue throughout your professional life.

Look at the quality of care you give. Could it be improved? If so, how? Monitor yourself so that you do not fall into a routine that prevents you from implementing the plan according to the individuality of the client. Keeping a diary or a journal will give you the opportunity to reflect on the actions taken in a particular situation. The process-recording will help you to analyze your communication patterns.

The process-recording is a written account of the responses (verbal and nonverbal) of client and nurse and an analysis of these responses. The process-recording may be written during the conversation with the client or from recollection. Review of the recording will allow you to examine your responses carefully to determine inconsistent or inappropriate responses. The process-recording can improve your communication techniques and make you focus more accurately on the client's needs.

## SUMMARY

The implementing step in the nursing process is action oriented. It is during this step that you implement the plan of care. You will use a variety of intellectual, interpersonal, and technical skills. These skills will help you to give individualized, competent, and effective care.

As you implement the plan, you will assume the roles of leader and manager. Managing your time, monitoring your professional image, and evaluating your performance will increase your effectiveness in these roles.

The last step in the nursing process, evaluating, looks at the degree of success of the plan of care and at the overall quality of care given in a particular health care setting. Chapter 8 is devoted to the evaluating step.

## STUDY GUIDE

1. List all of the nursing actions that you performed during your last clinical experience. Label them as to their type—psychological, physiologic, socioeconomic.
2. Name five suggestions for improving the implementations of these actions.
3. Compare and contrast intellectual, interpersonal, and technical skills. How are they related to cognitive, affective, and psychomotor skills?
4. Analyze your performance in the clinical setting. Identify what leadership qualities you demonstrate.
5. Prepare a time grid to incorporate the activities that you must accomplish during your next clinical day.

## REFERENCES

1. Aiken, L., & Aiken, J. A systematic approach to the evaluation of interpersonal relationships. *American Journal of Nursing,* May 1973, *73* (5), 863–867.
2. Allekian, C. I. Intrusions of territory and personal space: An anxiety-inducing factor for hospitalized patients—an exploratory study. *Nursing Research,* May–June 1973, *22,* 236–241.
3. Almore, M. G. Dyadic communication. *American Journal of Nursing,* June 1979, *79* (6), 1076–1078.
4. Ardrey, R. *The territorial imperative.* New York: Atheneum, 1966.
5. Book, C. *Human communication: Principles, contexts, and skills.* New York: St. Martin's Press, 1980.

6. Bradley, J. *Communication in the nursing context*. New York: Appleton-Century-Crofts, 1982.
7. Brammer, L. M. *The helping relationship: Process and skills*. Englewood Cliffs, N.J.: Prentice-Hall, 1973.
8. Brown, M., & Fowler, G. R. *Psychodynamic nursing*. Philadelphia: Saunders, 1971.
9. Buckheimer, A. The development of ideas about empathy. *Journal of Counseling Psychology*, 1963, *10* (1), 61–71.
10. Douglass, L. M. *Nursing management and leadership in action* (3rd ed.). St. Louis: C.V. Mosby, 1979.
11. Duncan, J. The curriculum director in curriculum change. *Education Forum*, November 1973, *38* (1), 51–77.
12. Edmunds, M. Concepts of power. *Nurse Practitioner*, July–August 1981, 45–49.
13. Ganong, J., & Ganong, W. *Nursing management* (2nd ed.). Rockville, Md.: Aspen Systems Corporation, 1980.
14. Grace, H. K., Layton, J., & Camilleri, D. *Mental health nursing: A socio-psychological approach*. Dubuque, Iowa: Wm. C. Brown, 1977.
15. Hall, E. T. *The hidden dimension*. Garden City, N.Y.: Doubleday, 1966.
16. Hersey, P., & Blanchard, K. *Management of organizational behavior: Utilizing human resources*. Englewood Cliffs, N.J.: Prentice-Hall, 1977.
17. Hersey, P., Blanchard, K., & LaMonica, E. A situational approach to supervision: Leadership theory and the supervising nurse. *Supervisor Nurse*, May 1976, *7* (5), 17–20.
18. Hicks, H., & Gullet, C. R. *Management* (4th ed.). New York: McGraw-Hill, 1981.
19. Hutelmyer, C. Managing your time. *Nursing '81*, May 1981, *11* (5), 97–107.
20. Kalisch, B. What is empathy? *American Journal of Nursing*, September 1973, *73* (9), 1548–1552.
21. Keane, C. B. *Management essentials in nursing*. Reston, Va.: Reston, 1981.
22. Kozier, B., & Erb, G. *Fundamentals of nursing* (2nd ed.). Menlo Park, Calif.: Addison-Wesley, 1983.
23. Kron, T. How to become a better leader. *Nursing '76*, October 1976, *6* (10), 67–72.
24. Kron, T. *The management of patient care: Putting leadership skills to work*. Philadelphia: Saunders, 1981.
25. Kyes, J. J., & Davies, M. A. Pseudocommunication is the nurse–patient game. *Nursing Life*, January/February 1982, *2* (1), 50–54.
26. Lindberg, J., Hunter, M., & Kruszewski, A. *Introduction to person-centered nursing*. Philadelphia: Lippincott, 1983.
27. Litwick, L., Litwick, J., & Ballou, M. *Health counseling*. New York: Appleton-Century-Crofts, 1980.
28. Lyman, S. M., & Scott, M. B. Territoriality: A neglected sociological dimension. *Social Problems*, 1967, *15* (2), 236–237.
29. Marriner, A. Theories of leadership. *Nursing Leadership*, December 1978, *1* (3), 13–17.
30. McCarthy, M. Managing your own time: The most important management task. *Journal of Nursing Administration*, November–December 1981, *11* (11 & 12), 61–65.
31. McFarland, D. *Management: Foundations and practices* (5th ed.). New York: Macmillan, 1979.
32. Moloney, M. *Leadership in nursing: Theory, strategies, action*. St. Louis: C.V. Mosby, 1979.
33. Moskowitz, R. How to make the most of your time with simple techniques that work. *Nursing Life*, January/February 1982, *2* (1), 21–24.
34. Murray, R. B., & Huelskoetter, M. W. (Eds.). *Psychiatric mental health nursing: Giving emotional care*. Englewood Cliffs, N.J.: Prentice-Hall, 1983.
35. Peplau, H. *Basic principles of patient counseling*. New Braunfels, Tex.: P. S. F. Productions, 1975.
36. Pluckhan, M. *Human communication: The matrix of nursing*. New York: McGraw-Hill, 1978.
37. Rogers, C. *Client-centered therapy*. Boston: Houghton-Mifflin, 1961.
38. Rogers, C. *On becoming a person*. Boston: Houghton-Mifflin, 1961.

39. Shertzer, B., & Stone, S. C. *Fundamentals of counseling* (3rd ed.). Boston: Houghton-Mifflin, 1980.
40. Smith, V., & Bass, T. *Communication for health professionals.* New York: Lippincott, 1979.
41. Sommer, R. *Personal space: The behavioral basis of design.* Englewood Cliffs, N.J.: Prentice-Hall, 1969.
42. Spradley, B. W. *Community health nursing: Concepts and practice.* Boston: Little, Brown, 1981.
43. Stanhope, M., & Lancaster, J. *Community health nursing: Process and practice for promoting health.* St. Louis: C.V. Mosby, 1984.
44. Stevens, W. *Management and leadership in nursing.* New York: McGraw-Hill, 1978.
45. Stillmann, M. Territoriality and personal space. *American Journal of Nursing,* October 1978, *78* (10), 1670–1672.
46. Stogdill, R., & Coons, A. (Eds.). *Leader behavior: Its description and measurement.* Research Monograph No. 88. Columbus, Ohio: Bureau of Business Research, Ohio State University, 1957.
47. Sundeen, S. J., Start, G. W., Rankin, E. D., & Cohen, S. P. *Nurse–client interaction: Implementing the nursing process.* St. Louis: C.V. Mosby, 1976.
48. Tapia, J. A. The nursing process in family health. *Nursing Outlook,* April 1972, *20* (4), 267–270.
49. Urdang, L., & Swallow, H. H. (Eds.). *Mosby's medical & nursing dictionary.* St. Louis: C.V. Mosby, 1983.
50. Votaw, D. What do we believe about power? *Nursing Dimensions,* Summer, 1979, *7,* 50–63.
51. Weiss, J. (Ed.). *Nurses, patients, and social systems.* Columbia, Mo.: University of Missouri Press, 1968.
52. Yura, H., Ozimek, D., & Walsh, M. *Nursing leadership: Theory and process* (2nd ed.). New York: Appleton-Century-Crofts, 1981.
53. Zderad, L. Empathetic realization of a human capacity. *Nursing Clinics of North America,* 1969, *4* (4), 655–662.

# BIBLIOGRAPHY

Belkin, G. *An introduction to counseling.* Dubuque, Iowa: Wm. C. Brown, 1980.
Blake, J., & Towell, D. Developing effective management for the general nursing service. *Journal of Advanced Nursing,* July 1982, 7 (4), 309–317.
Blocher, D., & Biggs, D. *Counseling psychology in community settings.* New York: Springer-Verlag, 1983.
Carlson, R. *The nurse's guide to better communication.* Glenview, Ill.: Scott, Foresman, 1984.
Ceccio, J., & Ceccio, C. *Effective communication in nursing: Theory and practice,* New York: Wiley, 1982.
Ceronsky, C. Family/staff conferences open to communication, resolve problems. *Hospital Progress,* August 1983, *64* (8), 58–59.
Collins, M. *Communication in health care: Understanding and implementing effective human relationships.* St. Louis: C.V. Mosby, 1977.
Cronenwett, L. R. Helping and nursing models. *Nursing Research,* November/December 1983, *32* (6), 342–346.
DeVillers, L. What to do when you just can't communicate. *Nursing Life,* March/April 1982, *2* (2), 34–39.
Dillon, A. Congratulations! you're in charge. *Nursing Life,* March/April 1982, *2* (2), 21–28.
Duldt, B. W., Giffin, K., & Patton, B. *Interpersonal communication in nursing,* Philadelphia: F.A. Davis, 1984.

Griffith, J., & Christensen, P. *Nursing process: Application of theories, frameworks, and models.* St. Louis: C.V. Mosby, 1982.

Hays, J. S., & Larson, K. *Interacting with patients.* New York: Macmillan, 1963.

Hein, E. *Communication in nursing practice* (2nd ed.). Boston: Little, Brown, 1980.

Huttmann, B. All about hectic situations. *Nursing '84,* July 1984, *14* (7), 34–35.

Krieger, D., Peper, E., & Ancoli, S. Therapeutic touch: Searching for evidence of physiological change. *American Journal of Nursing,* April 1979, *79* (4), 660–662.

Kroner, K. How to take charge—when you're put in charge. *Nursing '85,* January 1985, *15* (1), 97–99.

Lees, S. Developing effective institutional managers in the 1980s—Part 1: A current analysis. *Journal of Advanced Nursing,* March, 1980, *5* (2), 209–220.

Marriner, A. Time management. *Journal of Nursing Administration,* October 1979, *9* (10), 16–18.

Narrow, B., & Buschle, K. B. *Fundamentals of nursing practice.* New York: Wiley, 1982.

Nugent, P. Management and modes of thought. *Journal of Nursing Administration,* February 1982, 11 (2), 19–25.

O'Brien, M. *Communication and relationships in nursing* (2nd ed.). St. Louis: C.V. Mosby, 1978.

Rogers, C. The characteristics of a helping relationship. In D. Avila, A. Combs, and W. Purkey (Eds.), *The Helping Relationship Sourcebook.* Boston: Allyn & Bacon, 1977, pp. 3–18.

Schwartz, E. B., & Mackenzie, R. A. Time management strategy for women. *Journal of Nursing Administration,* March 1979, *9* (3), 22–26.

Schweiger, J. L. *The nurse as manager.* New York: Wiley, 1980.

Wlody, G. S. Effective communication techniques. *Nursing Management,* October 1981, *12* (10), 19–23.

# 8

# Nursing Process:
# Step V. Evaluating

Evaluation can be viewed as the final step in the nursing process or as a separate process within itself. This chapter will emphasize evaluation within the context of the nursing process. To help you understand and apply the evaluating step, it will be divided into five separate but interrelated steps: (1) establish criteria, standards, and evaluative questions, (2) collect data about the current situation, (3) analyze data and compare data to criteria and standards, (4) summarize findings and reach conclusions, and (5) take appropriate action(s) based on conclusions. Purposes and types of evaluation will be identified and discussed. In addition, application of evaluation on a professional level will be presented.

Study of this chapter will help you to:

1. Define evaluating as it relates to the nursing process.
2. Name three aspects of quality care that should be evaluated.
3. Discuss the purpose of evaluation.
4. Define the terms concurrent and retrospective.
5. Identify those people responsible for evaluating client care.
6. State the steps in evaluation.
7. Identify possible conclusions of evaluation.
8. Describe three concurrent methods of evaluating client care.
9. Describe three retrospective methods of evaluating client care.
10. Describe the application of the evaluation process at the professional level.

To evaluate means to judge and examine, to appraise or estimate the value or worth of something. Evaluating is the fifth sequential step in the nursing process, but it is an integral part of each of the preceding steps. Activities within each step can be evaluated, as can the outcome of the nursing process as a whole. In this context, *evaluating* can be defined as the process of assessing the client's progress toward the attainment of established goals and objectives in order to determine the value or worth of the plan of care. Inherent in this process is the determination of the quality of care given to the client.

Three aspects of quality care can be considered: structure, process, and outcome. **Structure** is the setting in which care is given. This can be an ambulatory-care setting, acute-care institution, or an extended-care facility. Evaluation would be concerned with such items as physical aspects, equipment, expertise of personnel, administrative processes, communication processes, and staff development processes.

**Process** is the events and the sequence of those events that enter into the actual care. Process reflects the practice of the health care providers—the actual performance of care in relation to client needs. **Outcome** is the end result of client care. Outcome is usually determined by comparing the client's response to the care given to preestablished standards and criteria.[3,13,24,25] In the evaluating step of the nursing process, process and outcome are the primary concern.


# FRAMEWORK FOR EVALUATION

Evaluation is a planned, ongoing, deliberate activity that involves the client, nurse, family, significant others, and other health care providers.

## Purpose of Evaluation

In the planning step, nursing interventions were identified. During the implementing step, nursing interventions were tested as hypotheses. The client's response to the nursing interventions are now examined to determine their effectiveness. Evidence gathered during the evaluation process is used to support or reject the hypothesis that a prescribed nursing intervention is capable of producing a desired outcome. Without evaluation, you do not know if the care given met the client's needs. In addition, data needed to continue the nursing process will be missing—data needed to replan the client's care.

Within this context, evaluation is used to determine the:

1. Response of the client to the overall plan of care.
2. Appropriateness of specific nursing interventions.
3. Appropriateness of nursing diagnoses, goals, and objectives.
4. Progress of the client toward established goals and objectives.
5. Omissions during the assessing, diagnosing, planning, and implementing steps.
6. Effectiveness of the care given.

A well-planned, systematic evaluation will determine the status of each of these aspects.

## Types of Evaluation

Various methods exist for classifying or categorizing the types of evaluation. Evaluation as it relates to a time frame (concurrent and retrospective) and to a level (client and institution) will be discussed.

*Concurrent Evaluation.* Concurrent or formative evaluation is concerned with the process and outcome of quality care. This type of evaluation occurs while the client is still receiving care; it can be ongoing or intermittent. Ongoing evaluation should be done immediately after an intervention has been implemented to help you to determine the effectiveness of that particular nursing action. Are the sustaining factors which caused the situation reduced, resolved, or unchanged? Intermittent or periodic evaluation which is instituted at specified times throughout the care process will show progress—or the lack of progress—toward goal achievement. If data reveal progress, this information may serve as a motivating force for the client. Intermittent evaluation will also help you to correct any inadequacies that currently exist within the client's care. Evaluation at the time of discharge (terminal, final, or summative evaluation) will indicate the client's current situation.[6,25] The status of specific nursing diagnoses can be evaluated. Is the diagnosis still stated correctly? Does the nursing diagnosis still exist? Goals and objectives are also reviewed to determine to what extent they have been met. Data from concurrent evaluation should appear in the client's health record. This information can be used not only during the client's present care but for future admissions or follow-up visits in the clinic or home.

Concurrent evaluation continues until goal achievement is at the highest level of fulfillment possible. For example, if sleep for the individual client is to be expected as the result of implementing the nursing intervention, the response would be apparent within a short period of time. You could compare the client's current status to the behavior prior to the nursing action—noting amount of body movement, posture, and pulse and respiratory rates. Eventually the client's verbal indication of the effectiveness of the measure would be gathered. These data may be collected within a matter of hours. If the client was a family and the nursing diagnosis was, *Impaired family development related to ineffective communication patterns,* the evaluation process may take weeks or months before resolution of the situation is achieved.

Methods of collecting concurrent evaluation data consist of analysis of care plans, open-chart audit, group care conferences, interview with and observation of the client, and use of evaluative assessment tools. Each of these methods will be discussed in the section of this chapter—Collect Data about the Current Situation.

*Retrospective Evaluation.* Retrospective evaluation is concerned with the outcome of quality care. This type of evaluation occurs when the client is no longer receiving care from a particular agency. Retrospective evaluation poses minimal personal threat to care givers because it is conducted after their contact with the client is terminated.

Retrospective evaluation is objective, flexible, and efficient. It becomes more valuable when predetermined criteria of care are used. The individual or group conducting the evaluation seeks documentation to compare with criteria.[4,11,22,23]

Methods of conducting retrospective evaluation consist of closed-chart audit, postcare client interviews, postcare staff conferences, and client/client family questionnaires. Although information gathered by these methods cannot directly affect the client being evaluated, retrospective evaluation remains an effective method of monitoring the quality and efficiency of care given. Since retrospective evaluation will not be discussed in later sections of this chapter, we will discuss this evaluation method at this point.

The most common retrospective evaluation method is the **closed-chart audit**. Auditing is a method of evaluating the quality of care received by the client by examining or verifying the data in the client's health records. The closed-chart audit is concerned with the outcome of care and can be used in any care setting in which a record is an integral part of the care process.[4,19]

The health record can be reviewed for evidence of the client's progress toward the achievement of goals and objectives and the response to nursing interventions. (Determination of the client's goals and objectives must be made from documentation within the records. If goals and objectives are only recorded on the care plan and the care plan is destroyed at the time care terminates, this part of the closed-chart audit is ineffective. Maintaining the care plan as a permanent part of the health record helps to increase the usefulness of this evaluation method.) Notations such as, client walked the length of the hall, client administered own eye drops without assistance, or client changed incisional dressing, can be used to determine the effectiveness of interventions *and* the client's progress toward goal achievement.

Retrospective closed-chart audit can also be used with criteria of care. For example, an ambulatory-care setting might establish criteria of care for the client with the medical diagnosis of "simple fracture with cast application." One criterion might be—Able to verbalize cast care measures at time of discharge from facility. You would look in the health records for notations which described the teaching of cast care and the ability of the client to verbalize the cast care measures. If no notations were found, the criterion was not met. This is not to say that the teaching did not occur. However, the closed-chart audit is based only on what information is or is not found in the records.

**Postcare client interviews** are conferences conducted after an episode of care. As in any type of evaluation, predetermined criteria must be established. Interview questions or observation guides can be used to assess desired postcare client and family outcomes. This form of evaluation can be done over the telephone or during a conference at home or at the health agency.[13]

The telephone interview is sometimes the easiest and most appropriate method for data collection. This type of interview is less expensive than in-person interviews and still provides you with the opportunity for exploring answers to questions that you and the client might have. You must be careful to give the client an appropriate preliminary explanation so that the purpose of the interview is clearly understood.

The face-to-face conference at the client's home or at the health care agency may be conducted by members of the staff at the agency or by a special evaluation team. The home visit interview can also be conducted by public health nurses.

Regardless of the type of postcare interview format used, this form of evaluation is valuable in assessing the quality of care. It provides a mechanism for final validation of the care provided in the original health care setting. For example, if the client had been given instructions in the hospital as to how to administer daily insulin, the postcare interview can be used to assess the effectiveness of the original teaching program.[13]

**Postcare staff conferences** can be used to analyze all aspects of the care in relation to predetermined criteria. Predetermined criteria similar to those developed for the retrospective chart audit are used. Members of the health team who were involved in the client's care should participate in the conference.

The chart and care plan initially should be reviewed. This will give background information and provide the opportunity for the client's care to be reviewed from many perspectives by various members of the health team. The group should then analyze the answers to such questions as: When was the client assessed? What assessment tools were used? What plan of care was developed? What was the client's response to the plan? Were there circumstances requiring revisions of the plan of care? Were any communication difficulties encountered? Were there factors in the health care system that enhanced or inhibited the giving of care?[13]

**Questionnaires** which are answered by the client after care has been completed can also be used. This form of evaluation supplies subjective information and general indications of client satisfaction. If constructed properly, questionnaires can also provide a basis for determining the effectiveness of care and outcomes of care.

Questionnaire responses are often influenced by the "halo effect." This phenomenon causes the client to respond to all items on the questionnaire based on feelings regarding one experience; the experience could be either positive or negative. For instance, the client may have been unhappy with the manner in which follow-up appointments were arranged. The response to this event may overshadow all responses on the questionnaire.

Since retrospective questionnaires are given after care has been terminated, they also serve as memory testers. The client will respond from the client's most recent frame of reference. Responses may not reflect completely the admission and interim phases of care, but, instead, reflect only the time immediately preceding discharge—a time when the client is more self-sufficient and receiving less intensive nursing care.[13]

Questionnaires are fairly economical and can be distributed to a large number of clients. In addition, they provide anonymity and thus are less threatening to the client.

*Institutional Level.* Evaluation at the institutional level is done to determine if nursing care within the health agency meets legal and professional standards. As a professional nurse, you are concerned with quality of care. The information provided by most institutional evaluation tools, however, will not assist you during the evaluating step. These tools provide general evaluation information which will not help you identify if a *particular* client achieved the goals. Instead, these tools usually focus on the structural aspect of quality care.

*Client Level.* Evaluation at the client level is concerned with the process and outcome of quality care. It is designed to determine the effectiveness of the overall plan of care; the appropriateness of specific nursing interventions, nursing diagnoses, goals, and objectives; the progress of the client toward established goals and objectives; and the effectiveness of the care given. In other words, evaluation at the client level can meet all of the purposes of evaluation previously identified.

Now that the purposes and types of evaluation have been identified and discussed, we will focus our attention on the components of evaluation.

## COMPONENTS OF EVALUATION

All steps in the nursing process are interdependent; each step builds on the actions and happenings of the other steps. Since the nursing process is cyclic (Fig. 8–1), the evaluating step is not the end of the process. Instead, the evaluating step provides you with information that is needed to begin another cycle. The type of evaluative information that you need is gained from concurrent, client evaluation. You will want to determine if the plan of care was effective. If not, why wasn't it? What portion of the plan was ineffective? Does the plan of care need revisions or does a totally new plan need to be developed? Only through careful evaluation of the client's current situation can you determine the answer to these questions. The evaluating step can be divided into five components or substeps:

1. Establish criteria, standards, and evaluative questions.
2. Collect data about the current situation.

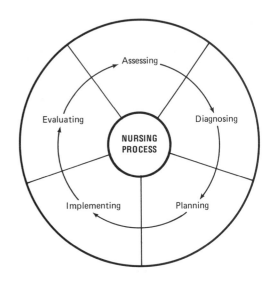

**Figure 8–1.** Overview of the nursing process.

3. Analyze data and compare data to criteria and standards.
4. Summarize findings and reach conclusions.
5. Take appropriate action(s) based on conclusions.

## Establish Criteria, Standards, and Evaluative Questions

You may use criteria, standards, and evaluative questions to determine the client's response to the plan of care. Each of these formats will elicit different information, and in some instances, a combination of the three will be beneficial.

*Criteria.* Criteria serve as observational guides for data collection and as means of judging the value of the data collected.[12] Most criteria used in the evaluating step are written as outcome criteria. Outcomes represent the end result of activities performed by the nurse. Outcome criteria are related to the objectives that you developed in the planning step. Objectives are oriented to the future—what the client *wants* to achieve or accomplish. Outcome criteria are oriented to the past—evidence of what the client *has* achieved or accomplished.

Some references use outcome criteria and standards of care interchangeably. Within this text, the two terms are not used interchangeably. Standards of care are more general and are used as the basis for evaluating broad areas of nursing practice. Outcome criteria are a type of standard and are used in evaluating specific nursing interventions.

**Outcome criteria** were defined in Chapter 6 as standards used to describe responses to or results of nursing interventions. These outcomes describe how the client will look, feel, or be after nursing action has been implemented. Outcome criteria are stated in behavioral terms so that they can be observed or measured and then described in unambiguous terms. Ideally, desired outcomes should be recognizable by everyone evaluating the care.[8,11,12]

In Chapter 6, we indicated that outcome criteria may contain:

1. A description of the change, specific behavior, or response that must be evident as a result of the nursing action.
2. A statement of the conditions under which the behavior, change, or response occurs.
3. A statement defining the limits of acceptable performance or behavior.

Remember that it is not necessary to include all three items in each evaluative criterion as long as the criterion communicates the expected outcome of the nursing intervention. (Refer to Chapter 6 for a discussion of the specific characteristics of criteria.)

***Standards of Care.*** Standards of care can be used to evaluate broad areas of nursing practice. A standard states what should be done and is used as a model for quality care. Standards must be based on research findings, theoretical concepts, and currently accepted nursing practice. They must be carefully formulated and tested to determine their appropriateness.

The ANA (American Nurses' Association) developed a set of broad standards that are used to evaluate the extent to which the nursing process is being used. These eight generic (general) standards were published in 1973. They can be used within any health care setting and for an individual client or a group of clients.

The ANA Standards of Nursing Practice are:

1. The collection of data about the health status of the client/patient is systematic and continuous. The data are accessible, communicated, and recorded.
2. Nursing diagnoses are derived from health status data.
3. The plan of nursing care includes goals derived from the nursing diagnosis.
4. The plan of nursing care includes priorities and the prescribed nursing approaches or measures to achieve the goals derived from the nursing diagnoses.
5. Nursing actions provide for client/patient participation in health promotion, maintenance, and restoration.
6. Nursing actions assist the client/patient to maximize his health capabilities.
7. The client's/patient's progress or lack of progress toward goal achievement is determined by the client/patient and the nurse.
8. The client's/patient's progress or lack of progress toward goal achievement directs reassessment, reordering of priorities, new goal setting, and revision of the plan of nursing care.[1]

To use these standards in the evaluating step, you develop specific criteria for each standard. Criteria provide the means of determining if the standard has been met. For example, look at Standard 1: *The collection of data about the health status of the client/ patient is systematic and continuous. The data are accessible, communicated, and recorded.* Criteria such as: Nursing health history collected by professional nurse within 1 hour of admission; Health history written legibly in ink; Health history contained within client's health record; Physical assessment collected by professional nurse within 1 hour of admission; and Additional assessment data collected daily, would provide the needed information to determine if this standard had been met.

In addition to the eight generic standards, specific standards for various individual clinical areas—for example, maternal and child health nursing, medical–surgical nursing, geriatric nursing, and community health nursing—have been developed by the ANA. Standards have also been identified and published by the National League for Nursing and the Joint Commission for Accreditation of Hospitals. These standards are also stated in broad terms and require specific criteria to increase their effectiveness in the evaluating step.

*Evaluative Questions.* In addition to or in place of criteria and standards, you may decide to use evaluative questions as the basis for evaluating the quality of care and the client's response to the care.[20,21] Examples of questions which might be used to evaluate the client's involvement in the nursing process are summarized in Table 8–1. Answers to these questions may be gathered from the client, the client's family or significant others, and health care providers. Information gathered by this format is useful in the evaluating step. The questions give you an indication of the client's involvement in the development of the plan of care. This format cannot, however, be used to determine the effectiveness of specific nursing interventions.

### TABLE 8–1. EXAMPLES OF EVALUATIVE QUESTIONS

**Assessing**
1. Was an initial assessment done on the client?
2. Was the initial assessment done within 2 hours of admission?
3. Was the assessment done by a registered nurse?
4. Does the assessment provide the basis for a plan of care?
5. Does the assessment contain client's perception of own health needs?

**Diagnosing**
1. Do the diagnoses contain diagnostic labels?
2. Do the diagnoses contain sustaining factors?
3. Are the diagnoses arranged in order of importance?
4. Are the client's concerns reflected in the diagnoses?
5. Are the diagnoses shared with the client?

**Planning**
1. Are goals identified on the plan of care?
2. Are objectives identified on the plan of care?
3. Are outcome criteria identified on the plan of care?
4. Are nursing orders clear and precise?
5. Are nursing orders initialed?
6. Is the care plan developed from the assessment data?
7. Was an initial care plan developed within 2 hours of admission?
8. Were goals and objectives developed with the client?
9. Was the client involved in developing the overall plan?

**Implementing**
1. Is psychological support provided the client?
2. Is the client informed of what is being done?
3. Are needs for other services identified?
4. Does the chart reflect the client's condition?
5. Has a discharge plan been started?

**Evaluating**
1. Are modifications of the care plan needed?
2. Are modifications of the care plan made routinely?
3. Is the client included in the evaluation process?
4. Are family members included in the evaluation process?
5. Is the client progressing toward achievement of established goals?

Once you have decided what evaluation format you want to use—criteria, outcome criteria, standards, evaluative questions—you need to collect data about the current situation.

## Collect Data about the Current Situation

In this step you need to consider some important questions: Who is responsible for gathering data? When will data be collected? and What tools will be used to collect the information?

*Persons Responsible for Evaluating.* The professional nurse who originally assessed the client and developed the plan is responsible for evaluating the client's response to the care given. Other nurses and health care personnel who assisted in implementing the plan should participate in the evaluation process whenever possible. It is not feasible for one nurse to gather all data necessary for an accurate evaluation. The validity of the information increases when more than one person evaluates the situation. Other health team members can help to supply new data and to validate information collected by the primary evaluator. Physicians can also be of help in evaluating the effectiveness of dependent and some interdependent nursing interventions. In addition, the recipients of the care must be involved in evaluating its effectiveness.

The individual client is best qualified to know when subjective symptoms such as pain, nausea, anxiety, or fear are relieved. In a hospital setting, observations can be made during actual care or during rounds made to determine the client's status. The individual client or the client's family are the main source of evaluation data concerning teaching. They are the ones to give you the feedback needed to determine the success or failure of a teaching plan. The family input is especially important in ambulatory care settings where the nurse may not be present to observe the client's responses. A nurse in a clinic, school, industry, or community health setting can watch for subtle responses, for example, behavioral changes resulting from previous teaching or counseling, but the family will probably be the one to offer the most descriptive evaluative data.

For other people to participate in the evaluation process effectively, you will need to assist them by establishing guidelines. The client, family, and other health care personnel need to be informed concerning: what should be assessed; how to collect evaluative data; how to describe or report what is experienced or observed; and when and how to report data.[11,12]

It is difficult to discuss exactly what the observer (a term used to indicate the individual who collects the evaluative data) should be told to assess. This assessment will differ with each client and may vary from side effects associated with drug therapies to desired or undesired responses to a diet and exercise program. Regardless of the situation, remember that you must make your explanations as clear and specific as possible. You must establish clearly how the data are to be collected. Are verbal and nonverbal responses to be noted? Is the observer to use all five senses to aid in data collection—hearing, touch, smell, taste, and sight? The observer may need assistance in selecting correct terms to describe color, location, odors, and so forth. Do not confuse the observer with complex terms; a sophisticated medical vocabulary is not necessary to convey responses to care. Make certain that you clarify to whom the data should be reported—nurse, physician, physical therapist—and when—at the time of the occurrence, at the next clinic visit, etc. To complete your instructions, you should indicate if the data should be reported face to face, by the telephone, or in writing.

*Methods for Collecting Data.* The evaluation format that you use will help you to determine the type of data to be collected and the method of collection. Some of the methods that are available to you are open-chart audit, interview and observation of the client, analysis of the written care plan, group care conferences, and evaluative assessment tools. All of these methods are concerned with the process and outcome of quality care.

The **open-chart audit** is a review of the client's record while the client is still receiving care. Information in the record is compared to predetermined standards or criteria.[11,13] For example, for a client 1 week postoperative from a repair of a fractured hip, a criterion might be—Nurses' notes document absence or presence of drainage from the incision site. At the time of the audit, it would be necessary to determine if the records contained information about the condition of the operative site. As with the closed-chart audit, documentation within the chart can provide evidence that the client has achieved or is progressing toward the achievement of goals and objectives.

Open-chart auditing provides immediate feedback to the staff in the health care setting. Although the immediate feedback is one of the primary advantages of this form of concurrent evaluation, it may be perceived as a threat by some nurses.[12,13]

**Client interview and observation** can be used to collect information needed during the evaluating step. This method is used by most nurses to evaluate the effectiveness of the care they are giving. The interview and observation of the client can be planned or unplanned.

The unplanned approach is used for ongoing evaluation which is done immediately after an intervention has been implemented. Did the back rub decrease the client's discomfort? Was the client able to assist with the bed-to-chair transfer after being given instructions? Although the approach is unplanned, you must be constantly gathering information so that conclusions regarding the effectiveness of care may be reached.

The planned approach may be used for intermittent or periodic evaluation which is done at specified times throughout the care process. Predetermined criteria or standards are used as the basis for specific interview questions and for physical assessment. Direct contact with the client provides you with the opportunity to see what is occurring regardless of what is or is not charted.[13]

Criteria that are developed are used to guide your observations at the time of client contact. For example, if the criterion was, Skin moist and supple after one week, you would need to observe and feel the client's skin to determine if the desired outcome had been achieved.

Besides observing the client, you may also choose to have the client respond verbally to a set of preestablished questions. These questions can be developed to elicit the client's perception of the quality of nursing care being provided and the client's involvement in the nursing process.

Examples of questions that might be used would include:[20]

- Is your call light answered promptly?
- If you need medicine for pain, do you receive it promptly?
- Are other measures (changing your position, fluffing your pillows, smoothing your bedding) used to reduce your discomfort?
- Which of these measures make you comfortable?
- Does your nurse explain treatments and tests to you?
- Is your family kept well-informed?
- Are you taught how to care for yourself?

- Are your family members included in your care?
- Are your health concerns being met?
- What goals did you and the nurse establish for your care?
- Which nursing measures do you feel are contributing to your goal achievement?

It is important that the client and staff understand why these questions are being asked. Because questions are asked concerning the current quality of care and the client's perception of response to the care, the staff may perceive it as a threat. In addition, the client may feel embarrassed or uncomfortable about giving such information. These responses from the client and staff must be anticipated and measures taken to prevent their interference with the evaluative process. A clear explanation prior to the interview and observation period will help to alleviate the client's discomfort. In-service education programs and unit conferences to discuss this method of evaluation will help to gain the cooperation of the health care team.

**Group care conferences** can be conducted to evaluate the client's level of satisfaction with current care and to determine if the client is progressing toward the goals. You can analyze the results of these conferences and use the findings as the basis for future nursing care.[5,13]

These conferences can be structured or unstructured. The structured conference may be developed around a set of questions similar to those in Table 8–1. Because the group conference can include the client, client's family, significant others, and health care providers, the information that you collect will be more extensive and varied. An unstructured conference would allow the participants of the conference to determine the content and scope of the discussion. The *topic* of the conference has been preestablished—effectiveness of client care. But what aspects of this care are discussed would be determined by the group. You would serve as the group leader and provide the guidance needed to keep the discussion focused on the topic.

**Analysis of the care plan** will help you to identify components of the nursing process that are not used properly. Perhaps the staff has difficulty identifying goals and objectives with the client, writing appropriate outcome criteria, or including the client's preferences in the nursing orders. Any or all of these aspects could indicate difficulty with Step 3 of the nursing process, the planning step. Again, the questions in Table 8–1 would provide a basis for this method of evaluation.

**Evaluative assessment tools** have been developed that will assess specific psychological and physiologic responses of the client. Many of these tools can be used to determine how the client responded to a specific intervention or group of interventions. For example, if the client is experiencing anxiety related to the new, unfamiliar hospital environment, your interventions would be directed toward reducing the anxiety by familiarizing the client with the environment. You may use a variety of interventions to achieve the desired result. After implementation of these interventions has occurred, an assessment tool that determines the client's level of anxiety could be used to determine the effectiveness of the interventions. Several assessment tools that could be adapted to evaluate the effectiveness of nursing are mentioned in the reference list.[2,9,10,14,15,16]

Once you have gathered your evaluation data, you should organize the data and determine if they are meaningful and of sufficient quantity. If any omissions are apparent, collect the needed information at this time. Using a variety of methods to collect the information will increase the validity, quality, and completeness of the data.

## Analyze Data and Compare Data to Criteria and Standards

You will need to use critical thinking, problem solving, sound judgment, and decision making to determine what are essential data and the significance of data. Remember that you are trying to determine the effectiveness of the overall plan of care; the appropriateness of specific nursing interventions, nursing diagnoses, goals, and objectives; the progress of the client toward established goals and objectives; and the quality of the care given.

Comparison of evaluative data with preestablished criteria and standards is essential. Unless this comparison is made, evaluation has not occurred. As a result of the comparison, you will be able to determine some of the factors mentioned above, for example, appropriateness of specific nursing interventions.

Actual comparison of data with criteria and standards does not occur if evaluative questions are used. You may, however, choose to compare your *conclusions* concerning the information with criteria or standards.

The type of information received from evaluative questions differs from the information received by other methods of evaluation. Many of the questions may have received only a negative or a positive response instead of a quantitative reply. Nevertheless, even this form of information can be analyzed. Did all of the positive replies occur in response to questions about the quality of care? Did the staff's and client's response differ on a particular question? Was the client or staff hesitant to answer some questions?

During the analysis of evaluative data, you should also be identifying factors that might have prevented or impeded the effectiveness of the plan of care. Nurses, the client, significant others (to the client), and health team members could have contributed to an ineffective plan.

The client might have shared inaccurate or insufficient information about self and situation, causing the data base to be incomplete or inaccurate. An increase in physical and emotional stress factors might have produced a drain on the client's expected ability to cope. Other reasons might include unrealistic expectations of one's self and predicament, a lack of or insufficient participation in the diagnosing and planning steps, and a lack of interest in or inability to comply with the planned nursing interventions.[25]

As the nurse, you may have gathered an insufficient amount of or overlooked significant data, assigned inappropriate priorities and prognoses, failed to recognize your intellectual, interpersonal, and technical strengths and limitations, delegated nursing actions inappropriately, or failed to have involved the client, significant others, or health team adequately in the planning or implementing steps.

Significant others may lack understanding of or interest in the client's plan of care. They may fail to see or not want to acknowledge that a problem exists; they may not want assistance from "outsiders." In addition, significant others may have limited physical, financial, emotional, or intellectual resources. Other health team members may contribute to the failure of the plan by maintaining conflicting goals for the client, failing to view the client holistically, failing to convey important data about the client to the nurse, and failing to see the value of a plan of care. In addition, other health care personnel may lack necessary intellectual, interpersonal, or technical skills for implementing the plan effectively.

## Summarize Findings and Reach Conclusions

Once you have analyzed evaluative data, inferences are made and conclusions regarding outcomes of evaluation are reached. Conclusions regarding the effectiveness of the *overall* plan of care are made first. Next, you want to reach conclusions that reflect the effectiveness of the plan developed for each nursing diagnosis. Remember, it is almost impossible to have a plan of care that is 100 percent successful for each nursing diagnosis and that requires no alterations or revisions. Likewise, it is almost impossible to have a plan of care that is totally incorrect for each nursing diagnosis. Look carefully at the client's plan and responses and be as objective as possible.

The conclusions that are reached during evaluation are similar in format to those conclusions reached during the diagnosing step. The outcomes for the individual client or family client may be any one or a combination of the following:

1. Only healthy responses are evident; the client responded as expected to the plan of care and achieved the established goals and objectives. No further nursing actions are needed—neither supportive nor preventive.
2. Only healthy responses are evident; supportive action from the nurse is needed to assist the client to sustain these responses. A health maintenance plan should be developed jointly by the client and nurse.
3. Healthy and potentially unhealthy responses are evident; present coping mechanisms are effective, and no supportive action is needed from the nurse. Reevaluation will continue.
4. Healthy and potentially unhealthy responses are evident; present coping mechanisms are not effective, and supportive action is needed from the nurse. Measures to prevent possible problems will be introduced into the plan, and reevaluation will continue.
5. Healthy and unhealthy responses are evident; present coping mechanisms are not effective, and supportive action is needed from the nurse. Reassessment and replanning are needed.
6. Only unhealthy responses are evident. Some of the nursing diagnoses are in error; either the diagnostic labels or sustaining factors were incorrectly identified. Reassessment, rediagnosing, and replanning are needed. Supportive action from the nurse must continue.

The outcome for the community client will also follow the format used during the original diagnosing process. General outcomes that might be made are:

1. Health care services are comprehensive; care is available and accessible to all individuals in the community.
2. Health care is continuous and coordinated; primary, secondary, and tertiary settings are available and used.
3. Health care facilities, personnel, and finances are used.

   (For each of these three outcomes further nursing actions are not really indicated. The health status of a community can change quickly and constant evaluation of the situation is recommended.)

4. Health care facilities, personnel, and finances remain inadequate. Reassessment and replanning are needed.
5. Health care is not continuous or coordinated; care remains focused at the secondary level. Reassessment and replanning are needed.
6. Health care services are not comprehensive; care remains unavailable or inaccessible to portions of the community population. Reassessment and replanning are needed.
7. Major health concerns are still identifiable; methods for resolving the concerns

have not been effective. Nursing diagnoses are in error; either diagnostic labels or sustaining factors were not identified correctly. Reassessment, rediagnosing, and replanning are needed. Supportive action from the nurse must continue.

Immediate concurrent evaluation is usually not employed at the community level. Periodic and final concurrent evaluations are more effective.

## Take Appropriate Action(s) Based on Conclusions

Your actions are guided by the conclusions just discussed. In some instances, no further actions are required. In other situations, replanning must occur—goals, objectives, outcome criteria, and interventions must be revised. Although assessment occurs constantly, specific aspects may need to be reassessed for more data. If after reassessment, new concerns or problems are identified or new light is shed on existing concerns, revisions in the plan of care are required. New nursing diagnoses may be needed or existing ones revised if they contain incorrect diagnostic labels or sustaining factors. You will then need to develop goals, objectives, outcome criteria, and interventions for these new or altered nursing diagnoses.

At this point, you are continuing the cycle of activities that is characteristic of the nursing process—determine priorities and prognoses, establish goals and objectives, update and implement nursing orders, and then once again, evaluate the results. This cycle continues until the client achieves the goals and objectives and is no longer in need of nursing actions.

## APPLICATION OF EVALUATION—PROFESSIONAL LEVEL

In Chapter 7, we spoke of the need for you to evaluate the effectiveness and quality of the care that you provide. It was suggested that a journal or log and a process-recording would provide you with data needed for an analysis of your care. In addition, you should evaluate all your nursing actions in light of the following: safety, appropriateness, effectiveness, comfort, efficiency, economy, and legality.[7,18]

One aspect of evaluation at the professional level involves the **appropriateness** of your interventions. Were your actions appropriate at this time? Did they interfere with unmet needs of the client? Did they conflict with any of the client's personal values and beliefs? You would need to determine if the client's **safety** was jeopardized in any way at any time by your actions. If the client's physical or psychological safety was jeopardized, the intervention cannot be considered effective regardless of the quality of other aspects of the performance. Was your technique correct or do you need to review a procedure manual or a text to refresh your knowledge base?

A third aspect involves the **effectiveness** of your actions. Your intervention must accomplish whatever it is supposed to accomplish. Was your intervention based on scientific principles and theories? Were your actions modified as needed in response to feedback from the client? Were your actions consistent with the overall health team's plan of therapy? You must also consider the physical and psychological **comfort** of the client. Did you take into account the client's psychological comfort? Did the client know what to expect? Was the client's privacy maintained? Were your actions individualized to meet the needs of the client? Did you consider the client's physical comfort? Did you perform physical skills with gentleness and competence?

Evaluating the **efficiency** of your actions is determined by the amount of time and energy used to accomplish a task. Did you waste time and energy for yourself and the client because of missing or forgotten supplies? Was your performance enhanced by prior organization and planning? Efficient use of time and energy will be economic for you and the client. The conservation of resources and the prevention of waste during implementation of the plan of care affects the **economy** of health care. During your self-evaluation you will need to consider this aspect. When possible, did you use the least expensive and yet the most effective materials? Did you teach the client to use household materials rather than expensive, commercially prepared supplies whenever possible?

Another aspect to be considered is the **legality** of your actions. Obviously, legality was considered when you first formulated your plan. Now, you must consider if your behavior met the necessary legal statutes. Were there valid, signed physician's orders for dependent nursing actions? Were all your independent nursing actions within the legal boundaries of nursing?[17]

Awareness of these aspects and how care is affected by them will improve the evaluation of your actions. None of the other evaluative methods will affect your performance if you cannot and do not look at your own care carefully and honestly.

## SUMMARY

Evaluating the effectiveness of your care is an important professional action. Your willingness to look at the results of your actions indicates that you are willing to accept the responsibility for them. Evaluation provides for personal and professional growth as well as ensuring efficiency of care for the client.

The evaluating step is the last of the five steps in the nursing process. It provides a means of reflecting on the events that occurred in the other steps and of thinking ahead about future nursing actions. Evaluating is not the end of the process but the beginning of another cycle.

## STUDY GUIDE

1. Determine the types of evaluation used within your clinical facility. How frequently are these evaluations conducted?
2. Using the following ANA Standard—Nursing actions assist the client/patient to maximize his health capabilities—develop two criteria that could be used to evaluate its achievement.
3. Describe three aspects of quality that can be evaluated.
4. Compare and contrast two concurrent and retrospective methods of evaluating client care.
5. Recall your last clinical experience and evaluate your actions as to appropriateness, safety, effectiveness, comfort, efficiency, economy, and legality.

## REFERENCES

1. American Nurses' Association. *Standards of nursing practice.* Kansas City, Mo.: The American Nurses' Association, 1973.
2. Clough, D. A behavior checklist to measure dependence and independence. *Nursing Research,* January/February 1980, *29* (1), 55–58.

3. Donabedian, A. Promoting quality through evaluating the process of patient care. *Medical Care,* May/June 1968, *6* (3), 181–202.
4. Eddy, L., & Westbrook, L. Multidisciplinary retrospective patient care audit. *American Journal of Nursing,* June 1975, *75* (6), 961–963.
5. Froebe, D., & Bain, R. J. *Quality assurance programs and controls in nursing.* St. Louis: C. V. Mosby, 1976.
6. Griffith, J., & Christensen, P. *Nursing process: Application of theories, frameworks and models.* St. Louis: C. V. Mosby, 1982.
7. Helvie, C. *Community health nursing: Theory and process.* Philadelphia: Harper & Row, 1981.
8. Inzer, F., & Aspinall, M. J. Evaluating patient outcomes. *Nursing Outlook,* March 1981, *29* (3), 178–181.
9. Johnson, M. Outcome criteria to evaluate postoperative respiratory status. *American Journal of Nursing,* September 1975, *75* (9), 1474–1475.
10. Jones, C. Glasgow coma scale. *American Journal of Nursing,* September 1979, *79* (9), 1515–1553.
11. Lewis, L. *Planning patient care* (2nd ed.). Dubuque, Iowa: Wm. C. Brown, 1976.
12. Little, D., & Carnevali, D. *Nursing care planning* (2nd ed.). Philadephia: Lippincott, 1976.
13. Mayers, M., Norby, R., & Watson, A. *Quality assurance for patient care.* New York: Appleton-Century-Crofts, 1977.
14. Meissner, J. Evaluate your patient's level of independence. *Nursing '80,* September 1980, *10* (9), 72–73.
15. Meissner, J. Measuring patient stress with the hospital stress rating scale. *Nursing '80,* August 1980, *10* (8), 70–71.
16. Meissner, J. Predicting a patient's anxiety level during labor: A two part assessment tool. *Nursing '80,* July 1980, *10* (7), 50–51.
17. Mullins, A., Colarecchio, R., & Tescher, B. Peer review: A model for professional accountability. *Journal of Nursing Administration,* December 1979, *9* (12), 25–30.
18. Narrow, B., & Buschle, K. B. *Fundamentals of nursing practice.* New York: Wiley, 1982.
19. Phaneuf, M. *The nursing audit: Self-regulation in nursing practice* (2nd ed.). New York: Appleton-Century-Crofts, 1976.
20. Ramey, I. Setting nursing standards and evaluating care. In M. Berger, et al. (Eds.), *Management for nurses: A multidisciplinary approach* (2nd ed.). St. Louis: C. V. Mosby, 1980.
21. Ryan, B. J. Nursing care plans: A systems approach to developing criteria for planning and evaluation. *Journal of Nursing Administration,* May–June 1983, *3* (3), 50–58.
22. Shortridge, L., & Lee, E. J. *Introduction to nursing practice.* New York: McGraw-Hill, 1980.
23. Sorensen, K., & Luckmann, J. *Basic nursing: A psychophysiologic approach.* Philadelphia: Saunders, 1979.
24. VanMaanen, H. M. Improvement of quality of nursing care: A goal to challenge in the eighties. *Journal of Advanced Nursing,* January 1981, *6* (1), 3–9.
25. Yura, H., & Walsh, M. B. *The nursing process: Assessing, planning, implementing, evaluating* (4th ed.). Norwalk, Conn.: Appleton-Century-Crofts, 1983.

## BIBLIOGRAPHY

Berger, M. S., et al. (Eds.). *Management for nurses* (2nd ed.). St. Louis: C. V. Mosby, 1980.
Blake, B. L. K. Quality assurance: An ethical responsibility. *Supervisor Nurse,* February 1981, *12* (2), 32–33.
Bloch, D. Evaluation of nursing care in terms of process and outcome: Issues in research and quality assurance. *Nursing Research,* July–August 1975, *24* (4), 256–263.
Bower, F. L. *The process of planning nursing care* (3rd ed.). St. Louis: C. V. Mosby, 1982.
Burgess, W., & Ragland, E. *Community health nursing: Philosophy, process, practice.* Norwalk, Conn.: Appleton-Century-Crofts, 1983.

Clemen, S. A., Eigsti, D. G., & McGuire, S. *Comprehensive family and community health nursing.* New York: McGraw-Hill, 1981.

Donabedian, A. Some issues in evaluating the quality of nursing care. *American Journal of Public Health,* October 1969, *59* (10), 1833–1836.

Egelston, E. M. New JCAH standard on quality assurance. *Nursing Research,* March–April 1980, *29* (2), 113–114.

Gallant, B., & McLane, A. Outcome criteria: A process for validation at the unit level. *Journal of Nursing Administration,* January 1979, *9* (1), 14–21.

Geoffrey, L. Professional standards review organizations: What are they and how they affect nursing and other health care professions. In M. Nicholls, & V. Wessels (Eds.), *Nursing standards & nursing process.* Wakefield, Mass.: Contemporary Publishing, 1977.

Goody-Koontz, L. Performance evaluation of staff nurses. *Supervisor Nurse,* August 1981, *12* (8), 39–43.

Hilger, E. Developing nursing outcome criteria. *Nursing Clinics of North America,* June 1974, *9* (2), 323–330.

Horn, B. Establishing valid and reliable criteria: A researcher's perspective. *Nursing Research,* March–April 1980, *29* (2), 88–90.

Jacobs, C. M. *JCAH retrospective patient care audit, nursing adaptation.* Chicago: Joint Commission on Accreditation of Hospitals, 1973.

Joint Commission on Accreditation of Hospitals. *Accreditation manual for hospitals.* Chicago: The Commission, 1970.

Lesnik, M. J., & Anderson, B. E. *Nursing practice and the law* (2nd ed.). Philadelphia: Lippincott, 1955.

Marriner, A. The research process in quality assurance. *American Journal of Nursing,* December 1979, *79* (12), 2158–2161.

Moore, K. What nurses learn from nursing audit. *Nursing Outlook,* April 1979, *27* (4), 254–258.

Nicholls, M., & Wessels, V. (Eds.). *Nursing standards & nursing process.* Wakefield, Mass.: Contemporary Publishing, 1977.

O'Loughlin, E., & Kaulback, D. Peer review: A perspective for performance appraisal. *Journal of Nursing Administration,* September 1981, *11* (9), 22–27.

Safford, B., & Schlotfeldt, R. Nursing service staffing and quality of nursing care. *Nursing Research,* Summer 1960, *9* (3), 149–154.

Schneider, H. *Evaluation of nursing competence.* Boston: Little, Brown, 1979.

Stanhope, M., & Lancaster, J. *Community health nursing: Process and practice for promoting health.* St. Louis: C. V. Mosby, 1984.

Taylor, J. W. Outcome criteria: As a measurement of nurse performance. *Nursing Digest,* September–October 1975, *3* (5), 41–45.

Wandelt, M., & Phaneuf, M. Three instruments for measuring the quality of nursing care. In M. Berger, D. Elhart, S. Firsich, et al. (Eds.), *Management for nurses: A multidisciplinary approach* (2nd ed.). St. Louis: C. V. Mosby, 1980.

Wandelt, M., & Stewart, D. S. *Slater nursing competencies rating scale.* New York: Appleton-Century-Crofts, 1975.

Zimmer, M. J. Guidelines for development of outcome criteria. *Nursing Clinics of North America,* June 1974, *9* (2), 317–321.

# 9

# Research Process: Method of Validating the Nursing Process

An expectation of professional nurses is to base their practice on current knowledge that has been validated by research. Even in the 1920s, nursing research articles began appearing in the literature. Most of these articles were not practice-based. Most nurses are not prepared to take on the role of primary researcher, but they are in a position to read about the latest advances in the nursing research literature and to apply validated interventions to their own practice. This chapter will enable you to understand how new knowledge is acquired. We will review each step of the research process, and then examine how these steps relate to problem solving and the nursing process.

Study of this chapter will help you to:

1. Describe ways in which a research problem can be identified.
2. Discuss the importance of the review of literature.
3. Identify the functions of a research hypothesis.
4. Explain the differences among the various types of research.
5. Describe data-gathering instruments that can be used in research.
6. Identify ways to disseminate research findings.
7. Identify similarities between the steps of the research process and problem solving.
8. Correlate the steps of the research process with the steps of the nursing process.
9. Explain the importance of cultivating a proper attitude toward research.
10. State the importance of research to nursing practice.

Before we discuss the research process, we will examine the ways in which we acquire new knowledge.

## METHODS OF ACQUIRING KNOWLEDGE

Throughout history people have sought answers to their questions. Sources of knowledge include: (1) experience, (2) authority, (3) deductive reasoning, (4) inductive reasoning, and (5) the scientific approach.

## Experience

By personal experience we find the answers to many of the questions we face. Much of the wisdom that is passed from generation to generation results from experience. For all its usefulness, experience has limitations as a source of truth. For example, individuals may have very different experiences in the same situation. Two persons observing the same incident at the same time could truthfully compile very different reports if one focused on the things that went right and the other focused on the things that went wrong.

## Authority

For the things that are impossible to know by personal experience, individuals frequently turn to authority. In other words, they seek the answers to questions from someone who has experienced the problem or has some source of expertise. They accept as truth the word of recognized authorities.

During the Middle Ages, one can find examples of reliance upon authority for truth because of threats, punishment, and torture. Ancient scholars, such as Aristotle and Plato, and the early Fathers of the Church were the preferred sources of truth—even over direct observation or experience. Today, however, individuals are reluctant to rely upon another as an authority simply because of position. For the most part, they are inclined to accept the assumptions of an authority only when the authority bases its assertion on experience or other recognized sources of knowledge.

Related very closely to authority are custom and tradition, which are depended on for answers to many questions related to personal as well as professional problems. Individuals often ask themselves, "How has this been done in the past?" and then use the answer as a guide for their actions.

As a source of truth, authority has shortcomings. First of all, authorities can be wrong; they are not infallible. Additionally, authorities may be in disagreement among themselves on issues, which may indicate that their statements are often more personal opinion than fact.

## Deductive Reasoning

Aristotle introduced the use of **deductive reasoning,** which can be thought of as a thinking process in which one proceeds from general to specific statements using prescribed rules of logic. (See Chapter 2 for more information on deductive reasoning.) This system organizes known facts in order to reach a conclusion.

Deductive reasoning enables you to organize data into patterns that provide conclusive evidence for the validity of a conclusion. Deductive reasoning is useful in the research process. It provides the link between theory and observation. It enables the researcher to deduce from existing theory what phenomena should be observed. Deductions from theory can provide hypotheses, which are a vital part of scientific inquiry. Deductive reasoning, however, has its limitations. You must begin with factual information in order to arrive at accurate conclusions. Since deductive conclusions are elaborations on previously existing knowledge, scientific inquiry cannot be conducted through deductive reasoning alone. It is difficult to establish the accuracy of many statements dealing with scientific phenomena. Deductive reasoning can organize what is already known and can point out new relationships as one proceeds from the general to the specific, but it is insufficient as a source of new truth.

## Inductive Reasoning

Francis Bacon[7] believed that thinkers should not accept information handed down by authority as absolute truth. He held that a researcher should establish general conclusions on the basis of facts gathered through direct observation. For Bacon, obtaining knowledge required that one observe nature itself, gather specific facts, and formulate generalizations from these findings. For Bacon, observations were made on particular events in a class, and then, on the basis of the observed events, inferences were made about the entire class. This approach is known as **inductive reasoning,** which is the reverse of the processes employed in the deductive method. (See Chapter 2 for more information on inductive reasoning.) These examples illustrate the difference between deductive and inductive reasoning:

> Deductive:
> > Every mammal has lungs.
> > All men are mammals.
> > Therefore, every man has lungs.
>
> Inductive:
> > Every man that has ever been observed has lungs.
> > Therefore, every man has lungs.

In deductive reasoning the factual information must be known before a conclusion can be reached. However, in inductive reasoning a conclusion is reached by observing samples and generalizing from the samples to the whole class.

## The Scientific Approach

Scholars learned to integrate the most important aspects of inductive and deductive reasoning into the inductive–deductive method or the scientific approach. The use of both inductive and deductive reasoning is characteristic of contemporary scientific inquiry—the most reliable method for obtaining knowledge.

The **scientific approach** may be described as a process in which researchers move inductively from their observations to hypotheses and then deductively from the hypotheses to the logical implications of the hypotheses. (See Chapter 2 for more information on the scientific approach.) Researchers deduce the consequences that would follow if a hypothesized relationship is true. If these deductions are compatible with the body of accepted knowledge, they are further tested by gathering empirical data. On the basis of the evidence, the hypotheses are accepted or rejected.

The use of the hypothesis is a principal difference between inductive reasoning and the scientific approach. In inductive reasoning one makes observations first and then organizes the information gained. In the scientific approach one reasons what one would find if a hypothesis is true, and then makes systematic observations in order to confirm or fail to confirm the hypothesis.

The scientific approach will be presented as a series of steps to be followed. This approach to research is a systematic process of inquiry involving interdependent parts. It is a method of inquiry that has been maintained over time because it has proved to be a successful method.

## STEPS IN THE RESEARCH PROCESS

The research process is composed of six steps. Each step and action involved in that step will be discussed in this section.

## Identifying the Problem

Systematic research begins with a problem. Selecting and formulating a problem is one of the most important aspects of doing research in any field. The researcher must decide on the general subject of investigation. The researcher's personal knowledge, experience, and circumstances usually determine these choices. Once chosen, the general subject is narrowed down to a very specific research problem. The researcher must decide on a specific question to be answered and must state precisely what is to be done to reach an answer.

***Sources of Problems.*** There are no set rules for locating a problem. Three important sources of problems are: (1) experience, (2) deductions from theory, and (3) related literature.

Among the best sources are the researcher's own *experiences*. Everyday experiences can yield worthwhile problems for investigation. The researcher may have hunches about new relationships or about alternative ways of accomplishing certain objectives. These can be developed into ideas for research. Observations of certain relationships for which no satisfactory explanations exist are another source of problems for investigation.

*Deductions* that can be made from various theories provide an excellent source of problems. From a particular theory the researcher hypothesizes the expected outcome in a particular situation. In other words, the researcher asks, "What relationship between variables will I observe if the theory correctly summarizes the events I am observing?" The researcher then conducts a systematic inquiry to determine whether the empirical data support the hypothesis and thus the theory.

Another valuable source of problems is *literature*. By reading about previous research, you become aware of examples of research problems and the way in which research is conducted. The conclusion of many research articles suggests further research that is needed to follow up the published work.

One of the characteristics of a scientific research study is that it should be replicable, so that the results can be validated. By repeating a study, the extent to which the research findings can be generalized are increased, and additional evidence of the validity of the results is available. It is likely that one can detect contradictions and inconsistencies in the published studies or may be dissatisfied with the findings.

***Significance of a Problem.*** The researcher must ensure that the problem area is important enough to spend time investigating it. Although some subjectivity enters into judging the worth of the problem area, criteria aid in determining the significance of the problem (Table 9–1).

The solution to the problem should make a contribution to the existing body of knowledge, either in the area of theory or practice. To show the significance of the problem, the researcher shows how the study is likely to fill in the gaps in present knowledge, resolve inconsistencies discovered in a review of the literature, or confirm that earlier studies were reliable.

***Statement of the Problem.*** After determining what the problem is and in what way it is significant, it must be formulated in such a way that it can be investigated. A problem statement clarifies what is to be solved and restricts the scope of the study to a particular question. It is important that the question be stated as clearly and concisely as possible.

**TABLE 9–1. CRITERIA FOR EVALUATING THE SIGNIFICANCE OF A PROBLEM**

1. The problem studied should lead to further research. The study generates other questions as well as answers the one under investigation.
2. The problem must be researchable. To be researchable, the problem must be concerned with the relation existing between two or more variables that can be defined and measured.
3. The problem must be suited to the researcher. In other words, the problem should be one in which the researcher has a genuine interest. The researcher should feel that the solution to the problem is personally important and will contribute to one's own knowledge and skills as a professional nurse.
4. The problem should be one in which the researcher is both knowledgeable and experienced. The researcher must be familiar with the existing theories and facts in order to identify the problem as worthy of research. The researcher must have the necessary skills and competencies to carry out the study to completion.
5. The problem must be one that is practical and possible to conduct. It must be determined if the data required to answer the question will be available and obtainable.
6. The problem must be one that can be completed in the allotted time. Adequate time should be allowed not only for collecting the data but also for analyzing the data and writing the report.

*Characteristics of the Problem Statement.* An essential step in the statement of the problem is the definition of the terms involved. The researcher does not, however, look up the definitions in the dictionary—the terms must be operationally defined. To define the terms operationally, one must designate some type of overt behavior that is directly observable and measurable by others. In other words, the definitions are in terms of the procedures that will be used to measure the variable. A **variable** is a concept (or a collection of ideas expressed by a single word) that is also operationally defined.

In stating the problem, there should be a balance between generality and specificity. If the problem is too broad, there is no clear indication of the direction the research will take. By including the subjects, the variables, and the type of data to be gathered, the problem statement is made more precise. By the same token, the problem should not be so narrow that it becomes meaningless.

It is suggested that the problem be presented as a question rather than a statement. The question form is more straightforward and simple. The research question should ask the relationship between two or more variables.

In order to be subject to research, a question must have one essential characteristic: It must be possible to formulate it in such a way that observation or experimentation in the real world can provide an answer. Questions that involve values cannot be answered on the basis of factual information alone. The following example illustrates this point: Do student nurses who are introduced to problem solving through special classes score higher on the licensing examinations after they graduate than student nurses who are introduced to problem solving through the independent study method? This could be investigated empirically by comparing scores on the licensing examinations for two groups who are equivalent except that one group was introduced to problem solving through special classes and the other through independent study. The question, "Is problem solving taught in special classes good for student nurses?" could not be investigated scientifically without knowing what "good for students" means or how to observe or measure "goodness." Words that imply value judgments should not be included in the definition of a problem.

*Narrowing the Focus of the Problem.* One way to sharpen the focus of the problem statement is to think in terms of the target population and variables. The **target population** is the persons about whom the researcher wants to learn. The variables are referred to as independent and dependent. The **independent variable** is the cause, stimulus, or treatment that the researcher manipulates in order to study its effect on the dependent variable. The **dependent variable** is the outcome or behavior resulting from the action of the independent variable or treatment.

*Review of Related Literature.* Once the topic has been selected, the investigator makes a thorough search of what is already known. This search is important for several reasons. The research topic must be related to relevant knowledge in the field being researched, and the related literature must define the scope of the field. The researcher is saying, "These authors have discovered this much about my research question. I am going to go beyond these studies in the following ways." The literature should show what is known and what remains to be investigated in the area of concern.

A review of literature gives the researcher an understanding of theories. This enables the investigator to place the research question in perspective and to interpret its significance. Investigators need to determine if their efforts will add to existing knowledge in a meaningful way. Generally speaking, studies that attempt to determine if the hypotheses generated by a particular theory can be confirmed are more useful than studies that are completely independent of theory.

A thorough search of the literature can also avoid unintentional replication of previous research. Often researchers find that the idea they want to study has already been investigated by others. In this case, the investigator must decide whether to deliberately replicate the work of another or to change the original focus and investigate a different aspect of the same problem.

## Formulating the Hypothesis

After finding and stating the problem and examining the literature, the researcher structures a hypothesis if the type of study calls for one. A **hypothesis** may be defined as a tentative proposition suggested as a solution to a problem or an explanation of some phenomenon. It presents a statement of the researcher's expectations concerning the relationship between variables within the problem. The hypothesis is then tested in a research study. It is, therefore, presented only as a suggested solution to the problem. The investigation will lead to its acceptance or rejection.

For example, suppose the question is: What is the role of beginning nursing students' perceptions of themselves in the process of learning to give an injection? One could hypothesize that there is a positive relationship between beginning nursing students' perceptions of themselves and their achievement in giving an injection for the first time. It can be seen that the hypothesis is a proposition relating two variables. The variables are self-perception and giving an injection.

The hypothesis serves several purposes (Table 9–2). It gives a tentative explanation of the events (phenomena) that occur within a particular discipline and facilitates an

**TABLE 9–2. PURPOSES OF HYPOTHESES**[1,5,7,9]

1. Explain events
2. Facilitate an increase in body of knowledge
3. Provide a relation statement
4. Give direction to the research
5. Establish basis for selecting the sample, research procedures, and statistical methods
6. Provide a framework for reporting the results of the study

increase in the body of knowledge. To arrive at reliable knowledge on which practice can be based, researchers must do more than gather isolated facts. In addition, generalizations and interrelations that exist among these facts must be obtained. This is what provides an understanding of the problem. Well-planned hypotheses give the researcher the necessary direction to propose explanations.

Since the research question cannot be tested directly, a hypothesis is needed to provide researchers with a relation statement that can be directly tested in their studies. An example would be the following:

Research question:     Does instructors' written feedback on papers cause a significant improvement in students' achievement?

Hypothesis:     The achievement scores of students who have had written feedback from their instructors on previous papers will be greater than those of students who have not had instructors' comments on previous papers.

By stating the research question as a hypothesis, the researcher can proceed to investigate the relationship between the variable of instructors' comments and student achievement.

Remember, it is the hypothesis that gives direction to the research. It determines the type of data needed to test the proposition. In other words, the hypothesis tells the researcher what to do. It acts as a screening device that narrows the scope of the study. Only those observations and facts that have relevance to the research question should be selected. Additionally, the hypothesis establishes the basis for selecting the sample and the research procedures to be used, as well as the statistical analysis needed and the relationship to be tested. After hypotheses are formulated, they are subjected to testing. A *pilot study* may be helpful to try out the proposed hypotheses, which may need to be refined further.

## Developing a Plan to Test the Hypothesis

In this step of the research process, we will discuss the research proposal, methods of research, instruments used for measurement, reliability and validity, sampling, and research ethics. After the question and the hypothesis have been formulated, you are ready to prepare the research proposal—the tentative research plan.

***Research Proposal.*** In most instances, researchers present their projects in written form on two occasions: in the planning stage which requires a research proposal and in the last stage which requires a finished report of the results of the research. The proposal stage is one of the most important aspects of the research process because it is at this time that the ideas of the project are crystallized into a substantive form. The research proposal generally includes the following: the problem, the hypothesis, the research design, the sample, and the statistical analysis. The following outline is suggested in writing a research proposal and contains the necessary steps for planning the study:

    Introduction
        Statement of the Problem
        Review of the Literature
        Questions and Hypotheses

Methodology
   Subjects
   Instruments
   Procedures
Analysis of Data
   Presentation of Data
   Statistical Procedures
Significance of the Study

*The introduction* to the proposed study is very important. Ideally, a clear and direct statement of the problem should appear in the very first paragraph followed by a description of the background of the study, including such elements as the significance of the study—why is this problem worthy of study, what impact will it have? Although the background of the problem will be more fully developed in the review of the literature, it is appropriate to mention those studies that directly led to the problem. If the problem arose from your experience, you can explain this briefly in the introduction. Any terms that may be unfamiliar or have specific meaning should be defined. This section should be concluded with the specific limitations of the scope of the study as well as a foreshadowing of the hypothesis.

In the review of the literature, the researcher presents what is known to date about the problem. This provides a setting for the hypotheses of the proposed study. In some way, the researcher should tie the relevant literature to the purpose of the study. Even though the review of literature does not have to be exhaustive, it should contain the most pertinent studies. The researcher should also include studies that are contrary to the stated hypothesis as well as those in agreement with it.

The conclusion of the literature review section should discuss the findings and their implications. Gaps can be pointed out in what is presently known about the topic, and then the researcher can lead into the research question posed for the study.

The generally stated problems should now be more specifically stated—as questions or hypotheses. If the research study is a survey, the problem will be stated in the form of a question. It is best if the hypothesis is stated concisely in operational form. If this is not possible, the general statement of the hypothesis should be followed by the definitions and information necessary to define it in operational terms. For example, what percentage of nursing students have taken physics in high school? On the other hand, if the research project is for the purpose of testing a theory, the problem will be stated in hypothesis form. For example, the pharmacologic achievement of nursing students who have used a programmed text will be superior to the achievement of those students who have taken a more traditional course in pharmacology.

In the *methodology* part of the proposal, the researcher shows how the study will be set up. The appropriate research design should be designated as well as all the steps that will be taken to investigate the question. The proposed sampling procedures, method of collecting data, and the instruments to be used should be described.

The population of interest should be described. In addition, the procedure for selecting the sample from the population should be stated. If random sampling is not going to be used, the reason for the particular procedure chosen should be explained. It is important to describe the subjects carefully so that the reader can determine if the results of the study can be generalized to the extent intended.

Because the instruments used will provide the operational definition of the variables, their use must be justified as being appropriate for that purpose. In this section you should explain why the instrument was selected. If the instrument is an established one, the proposal should include reported evidence of its reliability and validity for the purpose of the study. In the event instruments are developed by the researcher, it is necessary to outline the procedure to be followed in developing them. This outline should include the steps that will be taken to obtain reliability and validity data on these instruments.

*Analysis of data* is the next part of the research proposal. This section describes how data should be presented and statistical procedures used. A specific description of the plans for administering the instruments and collecting the data should be given. These plans should include the time schedule, procedure for replacing subjects who drop out of the study, and other necessary details. You must plan the presentation of the data in advance, as well as how the research results will be arranged. Tables, figures, and charts are ways in which a whole set of data can be organized and summarized. It is possible for the researcher to picture the way in which the data will be presented in tabular form. The design selected for the study will determine the statistical procedures that should be used.

The *significance of the study* can either be discussed in the introduction or later. If you choose to discuss the significance later, it can be related to the background and design of the study. The researcher needs to discuss to what extent these results will be useful in solving problems. You can also show how the present study will lay a foundation for future research in the area of interest.

In some instances, it may also be necessary for the researcher to list the personnel, equipment, space, and time required for the project. You should also make out a realistic schedule for completing the research project.

***Methods of Research.*** The way in which the researcher collects data is referred to as **research method**. The research method is related to the problem under study and to the design of the study. The **research design,** on the other hand, is the specified plan and structure of the research. Each design differs in the method of data collection, degree of control, target population, setting, and purpose.

The **experimental research design** is usually regarded as the most sophisticated research design for testing hypotheses. The experiment is the event planned and carried out by the researcher to gather evidence relevant to the hypotheses. The researcher deliberately introduces changes and then observes the results of these changes. In conducting an experiment, the researcher takes great care to manipulate and control the variables and to observe and measure the results. Through this research method, the researcher can obtain the most convincing evidence of the effect that one variable has upon another.

For the simplest experiment two groups are required—the experimental group and the control group. Each group is subjected to a different treatment. Sometimes nothing is done to the control group. Most often the control group is subjected to the usual treatment, while the experimental group is subjected to the unusual or innovative treatment. In an experiment investigating the effect of a new commercial protein supplement on increasing weight, the group of people receiving the routine supplement would serve as the control group. Both groups should be equal in all factors that may affect the dependent variable (weight gain). After the researcher has administered the new product for weight gain to the experimental group, each subject is measured on the dependent variable (amount of weight gain). Measurement is followed by evaluation. Is there a difference between the two groups? Is the effect of the new product different from that of the routine supplement? This question requires a comparison of the measures of the dependent variable in the control group with the measures of responses in the experimental group. The comparison should tell the researcher whether or not the differences in the dependent variables are associated with differences in the independent variable as represented by the two treatments (routine and innovative).

The **ex-post-facto design** can answer questions not answered by experimental research. If the researcher wants to investigate the influence of attributes such as motivation, habits, intelligence, environment, and so forth, the researcher cannot randomly assign subjects to different groups of these variables. These attribute variables are possessed by the subjects before a study begins. Ex-post-facto research is that which is conducted "after the fact"—at a time when the researcher has no direct control over the independent variables because the changes have already occurred or because they cannot be manipulated. The researcher achieves the variation desired by selecting subjects in which the variable is present but in different degrees.

An example is the hypothesis that all students possess problem-solving ability, but they possess it in varying degrees. One could compare the performance of successful problem solvers and unsuccessful problem solvers on the same measure of anxiety. Ex-post-facto research is similar to experimental research in that both aim to compare two groups, similar in all relevant characteristics but one, in order to measure the effects of that characteristic. The evidence obtained from experimental research is much more convincing than that obtained from ex-post-facto research. Because of the lack of control, it is more questionable to infer that there is indeed a genuine relationship between two variables in an ex-post-facto study.

Ex-post-facto research provides a method that can be useful in instances where experimental research cannot be conducted. It must be remembered that it is difficult in this type of research for the researcher to infer causal relationships. An example of an ex-post-facto study is the Surgeon General's study of the relationship between smoking and lung cancer. It would not be humane for a researcher to randomly assign a group of human subjects who are to smoke and a group who are not to smoke for a number of years so that this type of study could be done. The reversed causality hypothesis that lung cancer causes people to smoke is not plausible. None of the common cause hypotheses offered seem very likely—nervous people are prone to both smoking and lung cancer, some genetic predisposition leads to both, and so forth. Needless to say, caution must be exercised when interpreting ex-post-facto research studies.

**Descriptive research design** is not usually aimed at hypothesis testing. It is designed to obtain information concerning the current status of phenomena. This type of study is directed toward what is going on at the time of the study. There is no control or administering of a treatment as in experimental research. Several types of studies are categorized as descriptive research—case studies, surveys, developmental studies, follow-up studies, documentary studies, trend analyses, and correlation studies. Some of these methods may be used for hypothesis testing even though they are still classified as descriptive methods.

*Case studies* are usually an intensive investigation of one person or a single unit (family, social group). The researcher tries to discover all the variables that are important in the history or development of the subject. The focus is on understanding why the subject does what he does or what changes are made in behavior as the person interacts with the environment. Most case studies are directed toward solving a certain problem.

A *survey* generally gathers relatively limited data from a large number of cases. Its purpose is to gather information about certain variables. Most surveys are inquiries into what presently exists. Surveys do not question why something exists. The U.S. census is a good example of a survey.

*Developmental studies* investigate the characteristics of people and the ways in which these characteristics change with growth. The longitudinal method studies individuals—usually children—over an extended period of time. Since the researcher deals with the same group of people, certain factors remain constant. One practical difficulty is obtaining the commitment to remain with such a project over a period of years. The cross-sectional method is more practical than the longitudinal method of studying development. This approach studies people who are at various stages of development at the same point in time. The primary disadvantage of this method is that chance differences may bias the results of the study.

Similar to the longitudinal study is the *follow-up study,* which is concerned with investigating the subsequent development of subjects after a prescribed treatment. An example would be the follow-up study of graduates from a nursing school. The school of nursing wishes to "follow-up" and see if the curriculum prepared graduates for their role in nursing practice. In this example, the follow-up study is conducted to evaluate the success of a particular program.

*Documentary analysis* is often referred to as content analysis. It refers to obtaining information from records and documents. An example is an experienced nurse serving as an expert witness in a malpractice legal case. To prepare for the deposition, the nurse may do a content analysis of the client's hospital record to see if standards of nursing practice have been maintained. In the case of a fracture, the analysis would be made using the criteria of the Five P's: pain, paralysis, paresthesia, pallor, and pulselessness. The nurse would determine if these assessments were observed by the staff in the care of the client.

*Trend analyses* are used to project the demands that will be made on services in the future. This type of research is conducted through documentary analyses and surveys repeated at intervals. It is possible to study the rate and direction of changes and use these trends to predict future status.

*Correlation studies* are frequently used to determine the extent of relationship between variables. This type of study makes it possible to predict the extent to which variations in one variable are associated with variations in another variable. Generally speaking, correlation studies do not require a large sample. The sample, however, should be representative of the population. It is important that the instruments used have reliability and validity to measure the variables under study.

In **historical research design,** the researcher attempts to establish facts and arrive at conclusions concerning the past. The researcher systematically and objectively locates, evaluates, and interprets evidence from what can be learned about the past. As in descriptive and ex-post-facto research, the independent variable is not controlled by the researcher. The researcher has no choice in what documents, records, or artifacts made it through the passing of time. The researcher does not have control over the questions asked when witnesses were interviewed in the past.

***Instruments for Measurement.*** Dependable tools are used for quantifying the behaviors under study. A way of obtaining information is to ask questions. Both the interview and the questionnaire use this approach. Although both use the same approach, they are different.

**Interviewing** is a widely used method that is quite flexible. (Refer to Chapter 4 for discussion on interview techniques.) Remember that interviews can be either structured or unstructured. In structured interviews the researcher predetermines the questions and the alternative responses. This structure is rigidly adhered to with all subjects. The unstructured interview is less formal and can be adapted to the attitudes and values of the subjects. The subjects can determine how they wish to respond. Unstructured interviews require that the researcher be skillful and alert. Unstructured interviews do not lend themselves very well to quantification but are helpful in some types of research. Many times this type of interviewing is done in the preliminary stages of a study to determine which variables will be studied. The case study makes use of the unstructured interview.

**Written questionnaires** are more efficient and more practical than the interview. They also allow the researcher to use a larger sample. Much of the same information can be gathered by questionnaire as by interviewing. Questionnaires are of two types also—structured (closed form) and unstructured (open form). The structured questionnaire contains the questions and alternative responses. An unstructured questionnaire does not include the suggested responses. It is relatively easy to administer and score a structured questionnaire. The information gathered from the unstructured questionnaire is harder to process and analyze. Most researchers prefer the structured form.

There are also **tests** available as measuring tools. The tests are usually a statement of some type to which the subject responds. Some form of numerical scoring is assigned to the alternative responses. This score indicates the extent to which the subject possesses the characteristic being measured. It is necessary that the tests used as measuring devices be reliable, valid, and objective.

An **inventory** is an extensive collection of statements describing behavior patterns. Subjects are asked to indicate whether the statement is characteristic of their behavior. The responses are computed by counting the number of responses that agree with the trait being measured.

**Rating scales** are one of the most widely used measuring tools. One person usually assesses the behavior of another person. The rater–researcher places the subject at some point on a continuum or in a category that describes the subject's characteristic behavior. A numerical value is assigned to each category. An example of a rating scale would be a reference for a student wishing to enter nursing:

How would you rate the applicant's ability to get along with others?
1  2  3  4  5  6  7  8  9  10
very poor                    the best

There are several different types of **attitude scales**. Only the Likert summated rating scale will be discussed. Likert-type scales present a number of negative and positive statements regarding an object. The subjects respond whether they strongly agree, are undecided, disagree, or strongly disagree with each statement. A numerical value is assigned to each response. To arrive at the subject's score, values of the subject's responses are summed.

**Direct observation** is sometimes the most desirable method of measurement. The researcher determines the behavior to be studied, and then devises a plan for identifying, categorizing, and recording the behavior in either a natural or simulated situation.

*Reliability and Validity.* Every measuring instrument possesses two important attributes—reliability and validity. **Reliability** is the extent to which a measuring device is consistent in what it is measuring. You would not like it if every time you got on a scale, it weighed you differently—sometimes underestimating your weight and at other times overestimating your weight. The same holds true for a measuring device—you want it to yield the same results each time you use it on the same subject. It is very important to know how reliable or consistent the measuring instruments are that you use in conducting research. A test is reliable when the scores made by a subject remain nearly the same in repeated measures.

**Validity** refers to the extent to which an instrument measures what it is supposed to measure. Since not all the things you want to measure can be measured directly, you must rely on indirect methods, such as tests and scales. One never knows for sure whether these indirect methods measure what they are supposed to measure. It is extremely important to know what the specific purpose of the measuring device is before it is used.


*Sampling.* Since whole populations cannot be studied, it is a common practice to "sample" a population of interest. The purpose of drawing a sample from a population is to obtain information about the larger population. It is, therefore, extremely important that subjects in the sample are a representative cross-section of individuals in the population. If these conditions are met, the researcher will be able to generalize with confidence from the sample to the population. If the sample is biased, the findings cannot be legitimately generalized to the population from which it was taken.

The best known type of sampling procedure is **random sampling**. In this type of sampling every member of the population has an equal and independent chance of being included in the sample. The usual way of obtaining a random sample is to refer to a table of random numbers. This is a table containing columns of numbers that have been mechanically generated—sometimes by a computer—to insure a random order.

There is no rule about the size of the sample. The researcher uses as large a sample as possible to be representative of the population. Larger samples assure more accuracy and precision. Representativeness is the most important consideration in selecting a sample.


*Research Ethics.* Researchers have an obligation to plan and conduct their research in an ethical manner. There are several areas of concern. First, subjects involved in a research study must be protected from potential or actual harm of any nature. The guidelines of the U.S. Department of Health and Human Services, formerly the Department of Health, Education and Welfare (DHEW)[4] are the basis for the ethical standards of research. These guidelines define a "subject at risk" as a person who might suffer physical, psychological, or social injury as a consequence of participation in research.

Another area of concern is that every potential research subject is due the right of informed consent. The guidelines state that "informed consent" means the knowing consent of an individual or a legally authorized representative so situated as to be able to exercise free power of choice without any element of force or undue inducement, fraud, deceit, duress, or other form of constraint or coercion.[4]

A third and final concern is that the researcher must ensure the privacy of the subjects. Often the subjects are not required to identify themselves when it is possible to use anonymous responses. When the nature of the research mandates that the identity of the subjects be known to the researcher, the necessary consent is obtained and then precautions are taken to protect the confidentiality of the subjects.

Not only are researchers responsible to their subjects, but they are also responsible to the profession of nursing. Most research studies are published in journals, books, and other media, and are referred to and read by professional nurses. The researcher is under moral obligation to plan a study so that the findings obtained will not result in misleading information. The researcher is obligated to report exactly and honestly what the findings are.

## Testing the Hypothesis

The actual testing step of the research process includes the collection of the data, organizing the data for analysis, and implementing data analysis procedures.

***Collecting the Research Data.*** The procedures that are described in the research proposal are followed to collect data. For example, if the study is survey research, the steps would involve administering a questionnaire, conducting an interview, and so forth.

***Organizing Research Data.*** It is very difficult to describe data that have not been arranged in some type of order. Organizing research data is therefore an important step in the research process. Two ways of organizing data are arranging the measures into a frequency distribution and presenting them in graphic form. A **frequency distribution** can be defined as a systematic arrangement of individual measures from lowest to highest. Organizing the data into frequency distributions facilitates the computation of additional statistics.

***Implementing Data Analysis.*** It is beyond the scope of this book to discuss in detail descriptive and inferential statistical measures, which are used to describe data. Statistical methods are used in research to make the quantitative information more meaningful. These procedures enable you to describe and summarize observations. These particular methods are called descriptive statistics. Statistical methods also help you to infer that the events observed in the sample will also occur in the unobserved larger population of concern from which the sample was drawn. In other words, one can use inductive reasoning to infer that what was observed in a part will be observed in the whole. For these types of problems the researcher would use inferential statistics.

If you are going to read research, you must have a knowledge of basic statistical procedures. This skill will allow you to analyze and interpret the findings. A knowledge of basic statistics is also necessary to understand and evaluate research studies conducted by others.

## Analyzing Research Data

The first step in analyzing data is for the researcher to check the original proposal for the plans for presenting data and performing the statistical procedures. After this check is made, the researcher develops a strategy for organizing the raw data and proceeding with necessary computations.

Many researchers use electronic computing facilities for their data analysis. One of the advantages of using a computer for analyzing data is that you do not have to be concerned about the number of variables in the study.

After the data have been analyzed, the next step is interpreting the results. This is the stage in which the researcher shows to others what has been learned and how this knowledge fits into the existing body of knowledge. The original plan laid down in the proposal should facilitate the interpretation of the results. If the study has been thought out carefully, the results that have been generated will be easier to interpret. Interpretations should not be made beyond data that have been collected. At times, researchers are so pleased with getting the results they had anticipated that they start drawing conclusions on the basis of invalid data. There should not be more interpretations than data warrant.

Earlier, the researcher stated certain limitations of the study. These limitations should not be forgotten when it comes time to interpret the results. There might be limitations inherent in the restricted sampling, problems with internal validity, and so forth. The interpretations should take into consideration these limitations.

What if the results of the study are negative? It may be that the negative results obtained from a study are correct, and that previous studies have been wrong in their results. A difference in results indicates that the question has not been settled.

There may be several relationships that were not hypothesized but were observed during the course of the study. These relationships should not be ignored. They should be noted and interpreted as though they were part of the original plan.

## Disseminating Research Findings

Unless the results of research are communicated to others, it has little value. There are several ways to disseminate research: written reports and oral and poster presentations. In a research report, you communicate both procedures and findings, as well as implications of the findings and their relationship to the existing body of knowledge. The report should be succinct and logically organized. Since the purpose of the report is to present the research, the tone is usually formal. Some common errors in preparing reports are found in Table 9–3.

In practice, a formal and uniform method of presenting research reports serves a useful purpose. It is important that the research reports be arranged so that the readers know exactly where to find the specific parts of the report they seek. The presence of an established format eliminates the need for devising one's own. Most often, the established format follows the steps of the research process. The research report may take the form of a thesis or dissertation, a conference paper, or a journal article. A different approach is required for each of these cases. Most universities have a preferred style manual that describes the format to use. In preparing a research article for publication in a journal, the procedure for submission of manuscripts is found on the inside of the cover. If a manual of style is not specified, the preferred style and method of referencing can be determined by reading the articles included in a recent issue of the journal. A

---

**TABLE 9–3. COMMON ERRORS IN PREPARING REPORTS**

1. The titles of research reports are often very long and do not accurately reflect the problem under study.
2. The statement of the problem is too long, too vague, too complex, and not in keeping with the findings of the report.
3. Definition of terms is omitted.
4. Some of the literature reviewed is not related to the purpose of the study.
5. The methods and procedures of research are not reported.
6. Statistical devices are used incorrectly.
7. Findings of a secondary nature are overemphasized.
8. No generalizations are made even though the basis for making them is clear.
9. Researcher bias is obvious when reporting the results of the study.

major difference between writing a thesis or dissertation and a journal article is the length—an article is much shorter.

Papers presented at professional meetings are prepared similarly to journal articles. They are not necessarily reports of completed research but may be progress reports of ongoing projects. The presented paper is less formal and can be geared to the particular audience. The advantage of this type of presentation is that there is no lapse of time between the completion of a research project and the sharing of the findings (for example, the publication of a journal article). Many researchers find that presenting and hearing papers is a good way to keep up to date in their field.

Poster sessions are another alternative way of disseminating research. Announcements of meetings or conferences having a poster session appear in professional journals; directions are given for submissions. At the meeting or conference, a space is allocated for visual display, usually a table is available on which to place handouts.

We have explored the steps involved in the actual research process. How does this information relate to the nursing process? How does the research process relate to the problem-solving method? How do attitudes and socialization into the research role affect efforts? These aspects will be considered in the following section.

## APPLICATION OF THE RESEARCH PROCESS

From the previous discussion, it is clear that research involves collecting and analyzing data so that conclusions can be derived. In 1970, Lysaught[8] indicated the need for increased research in nursing practice. His report supported the thesis that nursing interventions require validation. Presently, research is conducted to validate every step of the nursing process. The challenge for professional nurses is to use this clinical research as the basis for practice. When this challenge is met, quality in client care is maximized.

There is a difference between nursing research and research in nursing. Nursing research studies the care process and the concerns that are encountered in the practice of nursing (for example, how pain is relieved, how nutrition is maintained). In contrast, research in nursing focuses on the profession, nurses, and characteristics of nursing. Today we are seeing more published clinical research articles, which makes it possible to base nursing practice on research.

Before establishing the link between research and problem solving and the nursing process, it is essential that the attitude toward research be addressed.

### Attitude toward Nursing Research

Anyone who registers for a research course soon becomes aware of preexisting feelings toward this subject. These same nebulous feelings prevail among persons conducting research and those who participate in clinical research.

Authors[3,11] have identified the need to consider professional socialization toward research in educating beginning professional nursing students. Rather than providing an environment where students are free to experience a creative and systematic exploration of potentially effective nursing interventions, students are expected to accept untested traditional comfort measures offered by textbooks and procedure manuals. Another common practice in schools of nursing is to place courses in clinical research toward the end of the curriculum because students are more likely to appreciate the content. Clinical research might find its rightful place within the role of each professional nurse more quickly if research content were integrated into every clinical nursing course.

You can begin your socialization into the research role by enhancing your ability to think critically. An example would be to ask yourself as you read and observe, "Has the rationale behind this nursing action been derived from other's experiences and observations or has it been experimentally tested in a systematic manner?" You may be thinking, "But my job is to care for clients. I'm not going to be a researcher." That may be true, but a positive attitude regarding research fosters cooperation and facilitation in allowing researchers to conduct their studies on your unit. You may even be involved in collecting data. It also motivates you to read research articles and incorporate them into the plan of care for clients.

Your particular cognitive style, values, responsibilities, and work environment may influence your socialization into the researcher role. Your cognitive style may be global rather than detailed in nature. Research tends to involve details and may not be motivating for some persons. Your values determine how you spend your time and money. If you do not hold certain values toward research, you will not assume the research role easily. You may have other responsibilities that hinder research efforts. Nurses must be committed to this role before they schedule their time for reading and participating in research activities.

Your work environment is an important influencing factor. Nurses need a supportive environment that will value and reward their interest and participation in research. Management and administrative personnel vary in their efforts to facilitate research activity. There are hospitals that encourage the organization of research interest groups; there are others that would view this type of activity as a waste of time.

It is essential for you to know how to find the research relating to your practice area. To do this, it is helpful to know the sources of previous work, what agencies collect such information, and efficient ways of finding the information you need. The basic sources of information include storage and retrieval systems, computerized data bases, indexes, and periodicals, books, and dissertations.

In order to use these sources, you must familiarize yourself with the library and its services. It is especially important that you know how the card catalogue is organized and where the needed periodicals can be found.

The *Cumulative Index in Nursing* is a valuable source for locating research articles from all nursing journals. The *Cumulative Index in Nursing* is divided into different sections—subject index, author index, and so forth. Most libraries have computerized access to the *MEDLINE* and *MEDLARS* retrieval systems. These systems enable you to conduct a literature search by means of a telephone call.

Several suggestions may help avoid disorganization while searching for the relevant literature. You should begin with the most recent studies in the field and work backwards through earlier works. With this approach you start with studies that have already incorporated the findings of previous research. These studies will also include references to earlier works and will direct you to sources you might otherwise overlook.

You can save much time by reading the abstract section of a report to determine if it is relevant to your practice setting. Additionally, you can save time by skimming a report before taking notes. Notes can be made directly on 5- by 8-inch file cards because they are easier to organize than sheets of paper. Bibliographic references should be written out completely for each work. If you know the library call number, this also facilitates finding the work again if it becomes necessary. No more than one reference should be placed on each card so that sorting and organization will be easier. Later these single cards can be sorted alphabetically. Direct quotes by authors should be indicated by quotation marks as compared to your paraphrasing of the information. You should also be careful to separate your evaluative comments from those of the authors.

Now that we have examined how attitudes and socialization into the research role either hinders or facilitates research efforts, let us relate the research process to the problem-solving method discussed in Chapter 2.

## Relationship between Research and Problem Solving

Sometimes you learn about one content area, and then go on to learn new but related subject matter without synthesizing or linking the two content areas. What links research to problem solving? The term *scientific inquiry* may not be frequently used by most nurses, but if you use the nursing process and are solving problems of individual, family, and community clients, you are making scientific inquiries. You may use different criteria than another person does to make an inquiry, but you are still using rules of the scientific method (and the process of scientific inquiry) to observe and explain the many activities we call "nursing."

If you will recall from Chapter 2, a figure for the problem-solving process was designed. We can depict very easily the link between research and problem solving by examining Figure 9–1. In comparing these two processes, we see the difference is that in the research process there is empirical testing of data as determined by the plan for analyzing data.

So far we have looked at the effect one's attitude may have on research and the relationship of the research process to problem solving. Now we will look at the relationship between the research process and the nursing process.

## Relationship between the Research Process and the Nursing Process

The steps of the research process correlate with the steps of the nursing process. We will examine each step to see these relationships.

*Assessing.* The identification of the problem and review of the literature of the research process coincide with the assessing step of the nursing process. For example, if you are caring for an oncology client who is experiencing a great deal of pain, you have identified a client problem as well as a problem that is worthy of researching. A review of literature can be the basis for selecting a conceptual framework for both processes. In the research process, the conceptual framework guides the research and is the basis

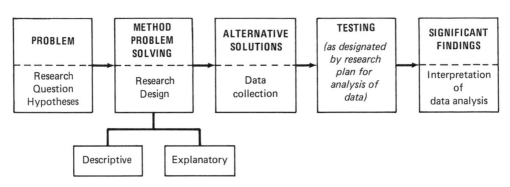

**Figure 9–1.** Relationship between the research process and the problem-solving process.

for deriving specific research questions or hypotheses. In the nursing process, the conceptual framework guides the assessment of the individual, family, or community client. Theories involve general principles whose application to specific nursing problems is still hypothetical until confirmed through research. Only through research can the generalizations contained within theories be translated into definite recommendations for nursing practice. An example would be: research has supported the assertion that bonding (a theory concerning mother–newborn attachment) is more positive in birthing rooms. This approach to researching nursing problems results in a productive means of expanding knowledge in a particular area.

*Diagnosing.* The diagnosing step of the nursing process correlates with the development and testing of the hypothesis. An example of how a hypothesis is tested may help you understand this process. Let us say you were interested in testing the hypothesis that verbal encouragement results in increased motivation on the part of clients. If this hypothesis is correct, it should be logical to assume that nurses' words of encouragement would be followed by improvement in diabetic clients' rate of compliance in testing urine for glucose. This assumes that increased motivation is indicated by improved compliance in testing urine. At this point, an example may be helpful.

- **Step One:** This deduced implication can be stated as: Nurses' verbal encouragement to diabetic clients results in improved compliance by performing urine testing. It is the relationship between the two variables—nurses' verbal encouragement and compliance in urine testing—that must be tested.
- **Step Two:** This type of hypothesis can be tested by means of an experiment. The researcher could randomly select two groups of diabetics to use in the study. For the diabetics assigned to Group A, the nurses would give verbally encouraging remarks concerning their urine-testing performance. (The remarks should not have anything to do with content or correcting mistakes, but such words as "Excellent," "You're doing great.") The diabetics assigned to Group B would receive no verbal comments at all during urine-testing performance.

  The nurses would keep a record of whether the clients in both groups in the experiment did not test their urine at the prescribed times. Then the independent variable (treatment) of verbally encouraging remarks would be introduced as described above to Group A. The nurses would keep a record of both groups comparable to the pretreatment record. The change from the first record to the second record would be ascertained for each client as well as the average gain for the group. It would then be possible through analysis of the data to determine whether average gains on the second record were related to the experimental treatment (nurses' verbally encouraging remarks concerning urine-testing performance).
- **Step Three:** If, as a group, the clients who received comments—Group A—achieved significantly higher gains than the group of clients that did not receive comments—Group B—then the results would support the hypothesis that nurses' verbal encouragement to diabetic clients results in improved compliance in testing urine.

We have acknowledged the significant contributions that nursing diagnosis offers to the practice of nursing. The adoption of approved diagnostic labels requires—mandates—that nurses using nursing diagnosis in their practices develop a critical, systematic inquiry for evaluating and testing them.

The beginning development of the classification system involved recalling and then inductively identifying diagnostic categories. Expert clinicians either generated diagnoses related to a particular body system (for example, the neurologic system) or to their professional experiences. This group-empiricism approach led to identifying defining characteristics and related sustaining factors. In the beginning this approach was important so that the diagnostic labels would reflect the phenomena on which nurses focused. The limitation to this approach is the limited scope of diagnoses accepted. The emphasis on frequently occurring diagnoses took precedence over those that require specialized skill to identify. This restriction reduces the development of a comprehensive taxonomy.

Research is needed to decrease a potential bias that may result from recollecting former client problems and their defining characteristics. There is a need to collect data systematically on clients during the time alterations in their health status occur—not retrospectively. This is to ensure greater accuracy in observing the presence or absence of every cue. Replications of the same type of study would allow for generalization of findings.

If you will recall the discussion about memory in Chapter 2, you can understand the necessity of a tightly planned research study to prevent the nurse from being susceptible to bias. When inductive methods such as group empiricism are used to determine diagnoses and defining characteristics, samples of clients may be recalled selectively by the clinicians—rather than recalling the total population. There is the danger of recalling separate data or patterns of data that have occurred more recently or that were unusual and impressive.[10]

To reflect support for researching the diagnoses, the National Conference Group amended the definition of nursing diagnosis to read, "a health problem amenable to nursing intervention which has been sufficiently refined for clinical testing."[11] You will therefore have to view the accepted list of nursing diagnoses as tentative hypotheses until they are empirically validated. After testing, they may be viewed as the most significantly effective way to describe the health alterations that nurses diagnose and treat.

Research on nursing diagnoses is conducted by the following method:

1. Data are gathered by direct or indirect means by using the senses. Data are treated empirically to arrive at some evidence.
2. A focus is defined for scientific inquiry. (This step as well as the third, fourth, fifth, and sixth steps allows the researcher to achieve control and order. It is important that the research study be carefully planned and executed.)
3. Predictions are then generated about the outcomes.
4. Data are collected according to a carefully designed plan.
5. Data are analyzed.
6. Conclusions are drawn.
7. Inferences or generalizations that go beyond the client focus under study can be established if the researcher uses well-defined assessment tools. There would also need to be a large sample of clients that have been randomly selected.
8. In place of a theory being developed as in other disciplines, a diagnosis is developed. This diagnosis expresses relationships among cues, risk factors, and the diagnosis.

Unlike some research it is crucial that the nurse–researcher maintain an active role in designing and conducting the research on diagnoses. The ability to recognize cue patterns is critical. Many times specific observational methods may be necessary. It is totally possible for even busy clinicians to systematically collect much data in their day-to-day practice if they have well-developed observational tools.

*Planning.* The planning step of the research process is as important to successful implementation of a research project as the planning step of the nursing process is to successful nursing intervention. The difference between the two processes is that the planning step of the research process is subject to formal review and approved guidelines for protection of human subjects. It would be impractical to have the same conditions operating for the nursing process. However, if similar safeguards were possible, clients' safety would be ensured.

*Implementing.* The implementing phases correspond in both processes. The proposed plan is tested in actual practice. The specific activities are different in each of the processes.

*Evaluating.* Both processes have evaluating steps. In the research process this step comprises analysis of research data and disseminating the findings. Both processes make use of reliable and valid measures to test the significance of the treatment or intervention in making a difference in the observed behavior.

Decisions must be made daily about the probable effects of nursing therapies on client behavior. The scientific approach to nursing practice holds that decisions about how to do things in nursing should be based on empirical evidence rather than upon impressions, feelings, or tradition. For example, does the back massage actually reduce tension? At present, research is attempting to determine the validity of this assumption.

The measures the researcher takes to validate nursing observations are necessary in practice. These observational methods may contribute to better decisions concerning client care. The methods as well as the knowledge derived from research are important. An example would be a research study conducted to validate the diagnostic label: Alteration in nutrition less than body requirements. Results of such a study may benefit the nutritional support of clients, but so would the data collection tool—a reliable and valid nutritional assessment tool.

Now that we have examined the relationship among the research process and problem solving and nursing process, we will explore ways nurses can use research knowledge and skills in their practice settings.

## Application to the Practice Setting

Your role in nursing will influence the way in which you use research. The level of educational preparation has an effect on the research skills you can apply. We will consider several basic ways in which you can use research in your practice setting.

*Critiquing Research Articles.* It is possible for you to undertake planned periodic critical readings of research articles that pertain to your practice. Many schools of nursing teach students how to critique. The areas that you would address as you critique an article are: (1) What are the purposes of the research, the research question, the related review of literature, and the conceptual framework? (2) What design and methodology was used? (3) How were the data presented and analyzed? and (4) What were the conclusions and recommendations?

*Using New Knowledge in Planning Care.* A complete and thorough knowledge of statistical techniques is not necessary to use published research findings. It is, however, necessary that you have access to research articles. You can either receive a personal subscription or read journals in a library. Although nurses seem to feel that research is important for improving quality of care, few actually seem motivated to carry out this independent activity and use research findings in planning care.

*Encouraging Nursing Peers to Become Involved in Research Activities.* To provide for continuity of care, more than one person should be involved in research activities. Continuing education departments need to incorporate research findings into their programs. Some institutions have nursing research committees that critique current nursing research for the purpose of using the findings in their practice setting.

You should make every effort possible to update your knowledge by reading nursing research articles. In addition, you should strive to incorporate research findings in caring for individual, family, and community clients.

## SUMMARY

In this chapter, we examined the nurse's role in relation to research. The general research process was explored; the relationship of this scientific process to problem solving and the nursing process was established.

There is an increase in the number of clinical findings that nurses can use to implement therapeutic interventions for clients. Professional nurses are being challenged to practice from a scientific base that will assure that individual, family, and community clients will be the recipients of effective nursing actions. Nurses are encouraged to read critically research articles and to maintain a supportive attitude toward incorporating research findings into their practice.

## STUDY GUIDE

1. List three research questions that are relevant to your last clinical experience.
2. Discuss your present attitude toward research.
3. Identify the steps in the research process that are the most difficult for you to comprehend. Explore possible reasons for this difficulty.
4. Project opportunities in nursing that are open to nurses who wish to become involved in nursing research.
5. Identify how clients, for whom you recently cared, would benefit from clinical research.

## REFERENCES

1. Abdellah, F. G., & Levine, E. *Better Patient Care Through Nursing Research* (2nd ed.). New York: Macmillan, 1979.
2. Bergstrom, N., Flinton, J., & Hansen, B. Issues in the conduct of clinical nursing research. In J. A. Williamson (Ed.), *Current Perspectives in Nursing Education.* St. Louis: C. V. Mosby, 1978, pp. 101–110.

3. Curran, C., & Mattis, A. Construction of a reliable instrument to measure attitudes. *Nurse Educator,* November/December 1978, 6–8.
4. Department of Health, Education and Welfare. The institutional guide to DHEW policy on protection of human subjects. Washington, D.C.: DHEW Publication No. (NIH) 72–102.
5. Diers, D. *Research in Nursing Practice.* Philadelphia: Lippincott, 1979.
6. Ferguson, G. Statistical Analysis in Psychology and Education (4th ed.). St. Louis: McGraw-Hill, 1976.
7. Fox, D. J. *Fundamentals of Research in Nursing* (4th ed.). Norwalk, Conn.: Appleton-Century-Crofts, 1982.
8. Lysaught, J. *Abstract for Action.* New York: McGraw-Hill, 1970.
9. Notter, L. E. *Essentials of Nursing Research* (3rd ed.). New York: Springer-Verlag, 1982.
10. Tanner, C. Factors influencing the diagnostic process. In D. Carnaveli, P. Mitchell, N. Wood, & C. Tanner (Eds.). *Diagnostic Reasoning in Nursing.* Philadelphia: Lippincott, 1984.
11. Tanner, C., & Hughes A. Nursing diagnosis: Issues in clinical practice research. *Topics in Clinical Nursing,* 1984, *1,* 30–38.

# BIBLIOGRAPHY

American Nurses' Association. *Research In Nursing: Toward a Science of Health Care.* Kansas City, 1976.
American Nurses' Association. *Guidelines for the Investigative Function of Nurses.* Code No. D-54 2500. Kansas City, 1981.
American Nurses' Association. *Research Priorities of the 1980's.* Kansas City, 1981.
American Psychological Association. *Publication Manual of the American Psychological Association.* Washington, D.C., 1983.
Armiger, B. Ethics of nursing research: Profile, principals, perspective. *Nursing Research,* 1977, *26* (5), 330–336.
Armstrong, G. Parametric statistics and ordinal data: A pervasive misconception. *Nursing Research,* 1981, *30* (1), 60–62.
Binger, J. L., & Jensen, L. M. *Lippincott Guide to the Nursing Literature.* Philadelphia: Lippincott, 1980.
Campbell, S. *Flaws and Fallacies in Statistical Thinking.* Englewood Cliffs, N.J.: Prentice-Hall, 1974.
Clinton, J. Nursing diagnosis research, methodologies. Presentation at North American Nursing Diagnoses Association (April 6, 1984).
Cook, T. D., & Campbell, D. T. *Quasi-Experimentation: Design and Analysis Issues for Field Settings.* Chicago: Rand McNally, 1979.
Creighton, H. Legal concerns of a reliable instrument to measure attitudes. *Nursing Research,* 1977, *26* (5), 337–341.
Diers, D., & Molde, S. Some conceptual and methodological issues in nurse practitioner research. *Research in N8ursing and Health,* 1979, *2,* 73—84.
Downs, F., & Newman, M. *A Source of Nursing Rewsearch* (3rd ed.). Philadelphia: F. A. Davis, 1983.
Fleming, J., & Hayter, J. Reading research reports critically. *Nursing Outlook,* 1974, *22,* 172—176.
Gordon, M. Historical perspective: The national conference group for classification of nursing diagnosis. In M. J. Kim, & D. A. Moritz (Eds.), *Classification of Nursing Diagnosis: Proceedings to the Third and Fourth National Conferences.* New York: McGraw-Hill, 1982, p. 6.
Gordon, M. Predictive strategies in diagnostic tasks. *Nursing Research,* January/February 1981, *29* (1), pp. 39–45.
Gordon M., & Sweeney, M. Methodological problems and issues in identifying and standardizing nursing diagnoses. *Advances in Nursing Science,* October 1979, *2* (1), 145.

Henderson, V. The nursing process. *Journal of Advanced Nursing,* 1982, *7,* 103–109.

Jacobson, B. Know thy data. *Nursing Research,* 1981, *30* (4), 254–255.

Jacox, A., & Prescott, P. Determining a study's relevance for clinical practice. *American Journal of Nursing,* 1978, *78,* 1882–1889.

Keppel, G. *Design and Analysis: A Researcher's Handbook* (2nd ed.). Englewood Cliffs, N.J.: Prentice-Hall, 1982.

Knapp, R. *Basic Statistics for Nurses.* New York: J. Wiley, 1978.

Kopf, E. Florence Nightingale as statistician. *Research in Nursing and Health,* 1978, *1* (3), 93–102.

Kriz, F., & Knafl, K. *Statistics for Nurses.* Boston: Little, Brown, 1980.

Leininger, M. The research critique. *Nursing Research,* 1968, *17* (5), 444–449.

Orlich, D. S. *Designing Sensible Surveys.* New York: Redgrave Publishing, 1978.

Orr, J. A. Nursing and the process of scientific inquiry. *Journal of Advanced Nursing,* 1979, *4,* 603–610.

Polit, D., & Hungler, B. *Nursing Research: Principals and Methods* (2nd ed.). Philadelphia: Lippincott, 1983.

Rosenthal, R. How often are our numbers wrong? *American Psychologist,* November 1978, 105–107.

Seaman, C. H., & Verhonick, P. J. *Research Methods for Undergraduate Nursing Students* (2nd ed.). New York: Appleton-Century-Crofts, 1982.

Shamansky, S. L., & Yanni, C. R. In opposition to nursing: A minority opinion. *Image,* Spring 1983, *15,* 47–50.

Sherman, K., & Kirsch, A. Research questions and answers. *Nursing Research,* 1978, *27,* 69–70.

Stetter, C. B., & Marram, G. Evaluating research findings for applicability to nursing practice. *Nursing Outlook,* 1976, *24,* 559–563.

Sweeney, M. A., & Olivieri, P. *An Introduction to Nursing Research.* (Part V: Using the Computer). Philadelphia: Lippincott, 1981.

Waltz, C. F., & Bausell, R. B. *Nursing Research: Design, Statistics and Computer Analysis.* Philadelphia: F. A. Davis, 1981.

Ward, M. J., & Fetter, M. E. *Instruments for Use in Nursing Education Research.* Western Interstate Commission for Higher Education, P. O. Drawer P, Boulder, Colo., 1979.

Ward, M. J., & Lindeman, C. (Eds.). *Instruments for Measuring Nursing Practice and Other Health Care Variables* (Vol. 1 and 2). U.S. Department of Health, Education, and Welfare, Public Health Service, Health Resources Administration, Bureau of Health Manpower, Division of Nursing, Hyattsville, Md., 1978.

Weiner, E. E., & Weiner D. L. Understanding the use of basic statistics in nursing research. *American Journal of Nursing,* 1983, *83,* 770–774.

Zielstorff, R. (Ed.). *Computers in Nursing.* Wakefield, Mass. Nursing Resources, 1980.

# 10

# Teaching Process: An Essential Component of the Nursing Process

A major activity of the nurse is health teaching designed to develop the health potential of individual, family, and community clients and to encourage their knowledgeable participation in the management of their own health care. The teaching process is generally conceptualized in the literature as a separate and whole process that nurses execute in addition to their other activities. Although it is true that the teaching process is complete and independent, it takes on a different perspective when used by nurses. It is important for nurses to conceptualize teaching as an integral part of the nursing process. We will present the total teaching process as part of the implementing step of the nursing process. This chapter will focus on teaching interventions, but we also will address the assessing, diagnosing, planning, and evaluating steps that are required with other nursing interventions. The nurse's responsibility in teaching clients will be discussed, and the assessment of learning needs, development of diagnostic statements, selection of teaching methodology, and evaluation methods will be explored.

Study of this chapter will help you to:

1. Discuss the historical and philosophical background of client teaching.
2. Define teaching and learning as it relates to client education.
3. List the goals of client teaching.
4. Explain the nurse's role in client education.
5. Perform an assessment of client learning needs.
6. Develop nursing diagnostic statements relevant to teaching.
7. Formulate learning goals and objectives.
8. Develop a lesson plan for client teaching.
9. Use a learning contract to teach clients.
10. Explain direct and indirect means of evaluating learning.

## Historical Background
During the middle and late 19th century, the focus of teaching was on control of environmental stressors contributing to disease. This approach was appropriate because there were no antibiotics, sanitation treatment plants, or quality control at that time.

During World War II, rehabilitation emerged as a specialization when veterans were treated with prostheses. The aim of teaching was to maximize their potential in spite of permanent deficits. Today, the emphasis in health care has shifted from an illness orientation to a health orientation. Individual, family, and community clients are taught to maintain health. Changes in today's health care system make it necessary to prepare clients to manage their health at home. Examples of these changes are shorter hospitalization and the increase in the number of clients with chronic illnesses. National goals have been established in relation to the prevention of illness and the promotion of health. Health teaching in these two areas is increasingly important as we learn more about the influence of health habits and life-style on our lives.

As early as 1918, there is documentation of the preparation of nurses to teach.[2] The teaching function began in the thoughts of nursing leaders, spread into schools of nursing, and lastly appeared in nursing practice. Today, the American Nurses' Association (ANA) describes teaching as a function of all nurses[1] regardless of the setting in which they practice. In the primary level of care, teaching is implemented to prevent illness and promote health. There is also a need for teaching clients in the secondary and tertiary levels of care. During the secondary level of care, teaching is done in relation to early diagnosis and prompt treatment of health concerns. In the tertiary level of care, teaching is for the purpose of preventing complications and restoring optimal functioning.

The historical background of client teaching is useful in understanding changes in the focus of health teaching. Of equal importance is the philosophical background.

## Philosophical Background
The teaching process rests upon particular philosophical beliefs concerning basic human nature. The differences revolve around whether a person is an active creature of instincts, a basically passive organism, or a purposive person who interacts with the environment. The philosophy of **logical empiricism** views a person as an active creature of instincts or as basically passive. The philosophy of **psychological empiricism** views a person as purposive and interactive with the environment.

*Logical Empiricism.*[3] Logical empiricists think there are absolutes or fixed natural laws that are unchanging. For them, truth does not change. Teachers who believe in this philosophy are critical, realistic, and fact-minded in their thinking and practices. The sciences are regarded as their models to imitate. Teaching that flows from logical empiricism is based on pure scientific facts. Nothing is considered true unless it has been objectively studied and verified through scientific research. They think in terms of stimuli (causes) and responses (effects). Logical empiricists think of people as machines that learn by accumulating memories. In terms of learning, they believe the environment will control the behavior and learning of the learner. Teachers that possess this type of philosophy select subject matter that is factual, but at the same time useful. They believe this type of subject matter causes a predictable effect.

*Psychological Empiricism.*[3] This philosophy contrasts sharply with logical empiricism. Instead of believing in an absolute reality that corresponds to fixed natural laws, psychological empiricists believe reality is relative, changeable, and gained through the senses. They believe that it is possible to construct a body of knowledge that over time will promote continual development and improvement of self and society. Psychological empiricists regard knowledge as insights, and they expect change. Teachers who believe in this philosophy are more flexible with respect to data—they go beyond the data available. Learning is viewed as a product of inner urges instead of a conditioning. Teachers who adhere to this philosophy emphasize interaction. Development occurs only when the individual interacts with the environment. They feel certain that persons will not learn unless they see the need to learn.

*Humanistic Perspective.*[10] A **humanistic approach** to client teaching is effective in increasing motivation. This philosophy holds that learners should take responsibility for determining what is to be learned and become more self-directing and independent. The teacher is no longer in a superior status to the learner; they are of equal status. The choice of what is to be learned is considered the learner's right.

The humanistic approach to teaching includes the belief that learners have a self-actualizing tendency. The humanistic perspective views persons as capable of managing their own learning. The teacher builds upon this tendency and organizes what learners need to learn so that they are put in contact with meaningful events. When this happens, learners will "wish to learn, want to grow, seek to find out, hope to master, desire to create."[22]

There are five basic assumptions to the humanistic approach to teaching. First, persons learn what they need and want to know. Second, learning how to learn is as important as acquiring factual knowledge. Third, the learner's own evaluation is the only meaningful judgment of the learner's work. Fourth, feelings are as important as facts, and learning how to feel is as important as learning how to think. And finally, learning takes place only when the learner does not feel threatened.

Now that we have examined the historical, philosophical, and humanistic background of teaching, we will discuss the definition and principles of learning.

## Definition of Learning

**Learning** is defined as the process whereby learners change their behavior as a result of experience. Since learning involves change, it takes time. To measure learning, you compare the way in which the learner behaves at one time with the way the learner behaves at a later time under similar circumstances. If the behavior differs on the two occasions, we infer that learning occurred. Written and verbal communication can be examined to determine whether changes in behaviors have occurred. Observation of talking, writing, and moving allow study of psychological behaviors such as thinking, feeling, wanting, remembering, and problem solving. In learning, change in behavior refers to the ability to remember or comprehend various things, and the tendency to have certain attitudes and values as set forth in statements of learning objectives.

The final component of the definition of learning is "as a result of experience." The term *experience* limits the kinds of changes in behavior that are representative of learning. It is easier to understand these limitations by discussing causes of change in behavior that are not considered to reflect experience. For example, changes in behavior that result from fatigue, sensory adaptation, drugs, and mechanical forces are not considered to be changes caused by experience—therefore, they are not considered representative of learning. Another process that reduces change in behavior for reasons other than learning is maturation. These changes occur in the normal process of physiologic growth and development.

## Principles about Learning

Principles of learning are derived from theory. There are three major categories of learning theories—behavioristic, cognitive, and information processing.[3,14] **Behavioristic learning theory** views learning as the reaction between a stimulus and a response.

**Cognitive learning theory** defines learning as an interactional process in which the person gains or restructures new insights or cognitive structures. **Information processing theory** holds that learning results when stimuli are processed by the central nervous system similar to the way a computer processes data.

These three groups of theories have common areas of agreement. All are scientific approaches to the study of persons. All view persons as basically neutral—neither innately good or bad. Each group of theories flows from a particular philosophical background. The behavioristic theories are derived from logical empiricism and cognitive theories originate from psychological empiricism. Information-processing theories probably flow from logical empiricism because they have factual inputs and outputs.

Learning principles based on these three groups of theories provide specific directives for teaching. In spite of the lack of a unified theory and a precise science of learning, knowledge of the learning process can be consolidated into the descriptive principles about learning that are listed in Table 10–1.

## Definition of Teaching

There are many different ways to conceptualize and define teaching. For our purpose, **teaching** will be defined as the act of transmitting intentionally structured and sequenced information from a human or nonhuman source to a recipient for the purpose of producing a change in behavior. If you look at Figure 10–1, you will see that the source of information (the teacher) does not have to be a human being. Examples of nonhuman sources are computers, programmed instruction books, and educational games. The depiction of teaching does not imply that learning actually took place; it merely states that change in behavior (learning) is the purpose of the teaching act.

---

**TABLE 10–1. FIFTEEN POINTS OF AGREEMENT AMONG LEARNING THEORISTS**[3,11,13]

---

1. To be effective, a learning program must consider what learners know how to do, and what they don't know how to do.
2. In deciding what should be learned, the capacities are very important. The prerequisite skills that have not been mastered are an important guide to what needs to be learned.
3. Motivated persons learn more readily than those who are not motivated.
4. Excessive motivation is less effective than moderate motivation for learning some kinds of tasks, especially those involving difficult discriminations.
5. Learning under intrinsic motivation is preferable to learning under extrinsic motivation.
6. Learning under the control of reward is preferable to learning under the control of punishment. Correspondingly, learning motivated by success is preferable to learning motivated by failure.
7. Tolerance for faiure is best taught through providing a background of success that compensates for experienced failure.
8. Learners need practice in setting realistic goals for themselves. Realistic goal-setting leads to more satisfactory improvement than unrealistic goal-setting.
9. The personal history of learners may hamper or enhance their ability to learn from a given teacher.
10. Active participation by learners is preferable to passive reception when learning.
11. Meaningful material and tasks are learned more readily than nonsense materials and more readily than tasks not understood by learners.
12. There is no substitute for repetitive practice in the learning of skills.
13. Information about the nature of a good performance, knowledge of the learner's own mistakes, and knowledge of successful results, aid in learning.
14. Transfer to new tasks will be better if, in learning, persons can discover relationships for themselves, and if they have experience during learning of applying the principles within a variety of tasks.
15. Spaced or distributed reviews have an important role to play in retention. If the learner has the opportunity to learn over time, the material will be retained for future use.

---

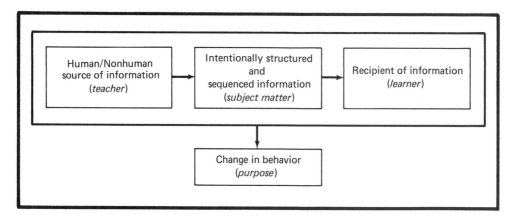

**Figure 10–1.** The teaching act.

Now that we have defined learning and teaching, we will examine the client–nurse learning–teaching process.

## Goals of Client Teaching

Teaching is more likely to be effective if goals are established. The first goal of client teaching is to assist clients to participate fully in planned teaching activities so they will be motivated to implement health maintenance measures. The second goal of client teaching is to guide clients in strengthening their role performance when they experience health alterations. The third goal of client teaching is to increase client awareness of available options.

In addition to the three broadly stated goals, more specific objectives are helpful in planning teaching activities for clients. Objectives of teaching can be categorized by the levels of health care. During the primary level of care (maintaining health and preventing disease) the nurse teaches such topics as preparation for childbirth, first aid, nutrition, and safety. During the secondary level of care (diagnosing and treating disease) the nurse teaches clients and families about disease, the need for treatment, and the medical care facility. During the tertiary level of care (rehabilitation or follow-through) the nurse teaches clients aspects of care at home such as medications, diet, and activity level.

## The Nurse's Role in Client Teaching

The teaching role of the nurse has gradually changed through the years. In the past, nurses were uncertain as to the degree of independence they had in initiating client teaching. In part, the lack of clarity about the nurse's teaching role resulted from confusion about the role of other health disciplines. For example, it was fairly routine for nurses to tell clients to ask their physicians to answer their questions. Since today the nurse's role in teaching is clearly described in the ANA Standards of Nursing Practice,[1] teaching is viewed as a function of all nurses and therefore an integral part of nursing.

Some hospitals that are committed to client teaching have developed a policy that allows nurses to teach clients who meet selective criteria unless the physician writes an order not to teach the client. The policy is drafted by nurses and sent to physicians for endorsement. Such policies acknowledge that client teaching is an independent function of the nurse.

Currently, there seems to be a trend for health agencies to use teaching as a marketing tool. Institutions are promoting their organization by offering teaching programs to the public. This practice is also used as a means of generating additional income. This trend raises an issue—should teaching programs be offered solely to maintain and promote health or can they be used as a means of increasing revenue and promoting the image of an institution? Teaching tools developed and used by one institution are being sold to others. This is not a negative action; there is merit in sharing effective teaching tools.

Now that we have examined the goals of client teaching and the nurse's role, let us analyze components of the teaching process. The first component is assessing learning needs.

## ASSESSMENT OF LEARNING NEEDS

You will recall that **assessment** is the act of gathering, verifying, and communicating data in a comprehensive and systematic manner for the purpose of accurately identifying needs. Assessment of learning needs does not have to be performed separately from other assessment activities—all data can be gathered at the same time. We will discuss assessment of physiological, psychological, and sociological needs of the learner.

### Assessment of the Learner
Some of the questions to keep in mind as you collect information are: (1) What does the client need to know? (2) What attitudes, values, and beliefs should you explore with the client? (3) What psychomotor skills does the client need to maintain health? (4) What environmental barriers are preventing the client from performing desired behaviors?

*Assessment of Physiological Needs.* Learning and maturation are closely associated. Persons cannot learn unless their physical development is adequate enough to comprehend information and to make necessary changes. Various motor and sensory capacities are required to learn. If physiological alterations are present, they may interfere with readiness to learn.

Normal aging is an example of the relationship between learning and maturation. Adults who are older than 65 years of age have the capacity to learn. While they retain their general intelligence and problem-solving and creative abilities, they have physiological changes which may disrupt learning. Some mature learners have memory loss for recent events and experience difficulty in ordering time sequences of recent events. They may also have difficulty in the immediate recall of new learning. Older adults may also have trouble choosing alternatives (decision making); they require more time. Sensory loss in some older adults may lead to misinterpretation of material being taught. In addition, they may have decreased interest and motivation for learning.

Based on knowledge of normal growth and development, you could anticipate these disruptions and plan teaching in a way that would support learning. An example of an effective method to use with older adults is to give them more direction.

Other physiological alterations disrupt learning. In conditions that result in increased levels of waste products (for example, acute renal failure), certain intellectual functions such as attention and concentration are impaired. Temporary conditions such as pain, anxiety, and medication cause shortened attention span. Each client's health history and physiological examination will provide you with data needed for identifying potential disruptions to learning.

***Assessment of Psychological Needs.*** Preparation for teaching requires a careful assessment of the learner's psychological needs. Three areas will be examined for their relevance to learning—assessment of the learner's developmental needs, intellectual level, and readiness to learn. In discussing readiness to learn, we will focus on motivation, experience, skills, attitudes, and abilities to learn.

The developmental level of the learner influences readiness to learn, and readiness to learn is dependent on maturation. Knowledge of the learner's state of development therefore enables you to develop a relevant and individualized teaching program.

A number of theoretical frameworks are available for assessing development. For example, outlined in Table 10–2 are the eight stages of man identified by Erikson.[9] The developmental tasks for each age group include the normal expectations in the areas of motor control, cognitive functions, and expression of feelings.

If you look at Table 10–2, you see that the first stage of development is trust versus mistrust. By providing for a child's needs for physical care and love, the child learns to place trust in people in the future. In the second stage, autonomy versus shame, children strive for autonomy, build cognitive and psychomotor skills, and gain independence and control. In the third stage, initiative versus guilt, children continue to take initiative and master skills. They have a need to gain independence without guilt. Although children at these early stages have limited skills, the knowledge you gain from the assessment data increases the likelihood of setting realistic and attainable expectations. Assessed data may be useful in devising methods for gaining the child's cooperation and acceptance.

In the fourth stage, industry versus inferiority, the child learns how things are made and how they work. The child needs to be encouraged and given a sense of accom-

**TABLE 10–2. ERIKSON'S EIGHT STAGES OF MAN**

| Stage | Age |
| --- | --- |
| Trust versus mistrust | Age 0–1 |
| Autonomy versus shame | Age 1–2 |
| Initiative versus guilt | Age 3–5 |
| Industry versus inferiority | Age 6–Puberty |
| Identity versus role confusion | During Adolescence |
| Intimacy versus isolation | Early Adulthood |
| Generativity versus stagnation | Adulthood |
| Ego-integrity versus despair | Maturity |

*(From Erikson, E. H. Childhood and Society. W. W. Norton, 1950, with permission.)*

plishment rather than feelings of failure. In the fifth stage, identity versus role confusion, identity emerges with the integration of roles. Role models and peer pressures are strong influences at this time. Learners in the fourth and fifth stages are capable of understanding causality and can participate more fully in a teaching program. Your assessment should be detailed enough to determine if the learner can make responsible decisions and perceive relationships between different ideas.

In the sixth stage, intimacy versus isolation, courtship and starting a family are important, and the roles of spouse or parent are developed. Learners in the sixth stage of development benefit from informal discussions that allow time for them to thoroughly spell out their questions and problems.

In the seventh stage, generativity versus stagnation, adults value productivity and contributing to society. In the eighth stage, ego-integrity versus despair, reflection on one's life accomplishments takes place, as well as dealing with death and dying. Persons in the seventh and eighth stages are adult learners. Adult learning refers to informal learning rather than formal schooling. Knowles[15] proposed four assumptions concerning adult learners that distinguish adults from children:

1. Adults are self-directed and see themselves as capable of making their own decisions and managing their own lives.
2. Adults have an accumulation of life experiences that act as a resource for learning.
3. Adults have a readiness to learn that is oriented to their developmental tasks and social roles.
4. Adults are problem-oriented learners who require immediate application of knowledge.

Adult learners respond well to support groups comprised of persons who are experiencing similar circumstances. Adults learn by reflecting on their problem, becoming aware of alternative solutions, and applying newly gained insights to their own situation.

In addition to assessing the learner's developmental needs, it is important to assess cognitive development. For learning to occur, learners must be capable of perceiving, thinking, and communicating their thoughts and feelings. A lack of intellectual capabilities interferes with emotional and social development.

An assessment of the learner's cognitive development enables you to formulate realistic and attainable objectives. It also helps you to determine the proper level of presentation.

A theoretical framework can be used to assess the learner's cognitive development. Piaget[18] is credited with describing the changes in cognitive functioning throughout development. Piaget's theory can help you to understand how one behavior must develop in order that another can follow, and how the abilities to categorize, generalize, and discriminate grow with an individual's experience. Intellectual development has four main phases: sensorimotor, preoperational (which is subdivided into preoperational and intuitive), concrete operational, and formal operational (Table 10–3).

Piaget's theory has a bearing on how you should teach because thinking changes according to chronological age. The following implications are derived from the study of cognitive development:

1. Intellectual Empathy. Children should not be viewed as young adults in their thought processes. Children think in ways that adults can no longer remember; they make errors that adults have difficulty predicting. Therefore, you need to

**TABLE 10–3. PIAGET'S STAGES OF COGNITIVE DEVELOPMENT**

Stage I (Birth to 2 years): Sensorimotor Stage

During this stage, learning is based primarily on immediate experience through the five senses. The child has perceptions and movements as his only tools for learning. Lacking language, the child does not yet have the ability to represent or symbolize thinking and, thus, has no way to categorize experiences. One of the first sensorimotor abilities to develop is that of visual pursuit (i.e., the ability to perceive and hold a visual object with the eyes). Later, the child develops the capacity of object permanence (i.e., the ability to understand that an object can still exist, even though it cannot be seen). Lacking vision during this period prevents the growth of mental structures.

Stage II (2 to 7 years): Pre-operational or Intuitive Stage

During this stage the child is no longer bound to the immediate sensory environment, and it builds upon abilities (such as object permanence) from the sensorimotor state. The ability to store mental images and symbols (e.g., words and language as a structure for words) increases dramatically. The mode of learning is a freely-experimenting, intuitive one that is, quite generally, unconcerned with reality. Communication occurs in collective monologues, in which children talk to themselves more than they do each other. Use of language during this stage is, therefore, both egocentric and spontaneous. Although use of language is the major learning focus at this stage, many other environmental discoveries are made by the child, who uses a generally free-wheeling, intuitive approach to the environment.

Stage III (7 to 12 years): Concrete Operational Stage

During this stage there is a dramatic shift in the child's learning strategy from intuition to concrete thought. Reality-bound thinking takes over, and the child must test out problems in order to understand them. The difference between dreams and facts can be clearly distinguished, but that between an hypothesis and a fact cannot. The child becomes overly logical and concrete, so that once its mind is made up new facts will not change it. Facts and order become absolutes during this stage.

Stage IV (12 years and older): Formal Operational Stage

At this stage the child enters adolescence, and the potential for developing full, formal patterns of thinking emerges. The adolescent is capable of attaining logical-rational (or abstract) strategies. Symbolic meanings, metaphors, and similes can now be understood. Implications can be drawn, and generalizations can be made.

*(From Piaget, J. The Origins of Intelligence in Children. New York: International University Press 1952, p. 142.)*

make a special effort to put yourself in the child's place so that you can view problems in the way the child sees them. This type of "intellectual empathy" is not easy but can be achieved by interviewing and observing children.

2. Concrete Objects. Preschool and early school children learn from working with concrete objects, materials, and events. Words are less effective than things in promoting understanding at these ages. If children are given the chance to manipulate, act, touch, see, and feel things, they acquire an understanding of concepts and relationships in ways that are more beneficial than more abstract forms of learning.

3. Sequenced Instruction. Piaget's theory of sequence of development suggests that instruction be sequenced across time and begin with a "messing around" stage (that is, a touching period with pieces of equipment that are to be discussed). The second part of the sequence involves developing perceptual clarity. This can be accomplished using audiovisuals extensively and pointing out important objects or events. The final instructional stage in this sequence is the verbal stage. In this stage, discussions are encouraged. A knowledge of this sequence is especially beneficial if you experience difficulty teaching a particular learner. In most of the stages described by Piaget, language is the instrument of thinking.

4. Amount of Fit of New Experience. The new experience should fit in with what the learner already knows. The information should be novel enough not to bore the learner, but not so new that it bewilders the learner.

5. Self-Paced Instruction. Learners need to be allowed to proceed through the sequence of instruction at their own pace. They should regulate or direct their own learning instead of it being forced in ways for which the learner is unprepared. This means that individualized instruction is preferred over teaching methods that carry an entire group of learners along at the same rate. Some learners need more assistance, different kinds of help, and more time. In this case, your role is to arrange opportunities and materials that the learner can use to acquire knowledge.
6. Value of Interaction. Interaction with others has cognitive as well as affective values. Through social interaction, learners' own views give way to more valid ideas, and they receive information about how other people see things.
7. Error Analysis. Piaget's theory suggests that you gain more information about learning needs when learners make errors than when they are correct. Therefore, if you analyze and interpret the errors that learners make, rather than inform them of the errors, they would learn more.

Piaget's theory also has implications for teaching adult learners who have not had certain experiences: you need to develop the teaching plan to include taking the learners through each of Piaget's stages of development by means of specific activities.

For learning to be effective, it is essential that readiness be assessed. Assessment of readiness is comprised of two aspects—emotional readiness (motivation) and experiential readiness (experiences, skills, attitudes, abilities).

**Motivational readiness** or emotional development is necessary for learners to be capable of developing awareness and acceptance of themselves. It also enables learners to interact with others and their environment and to be responsible for their own behavior. Learning requires motivation.

The term **motivation** describes what energizes learners and what directs their activity. Energy and direction are central to the concept of motivation. Environmental and personal facts affect a learner's behavior and therefore learning. (See Fig. 10–2 and Fig. 10–3). The environmental factors are external to the learner, but they influence

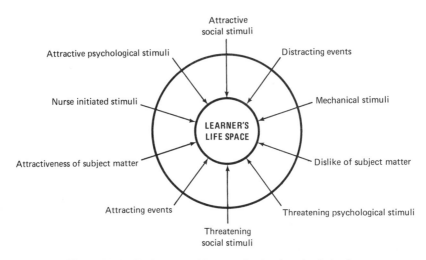

**Figure 10–2.** Environmental factors affecting learning behavior.

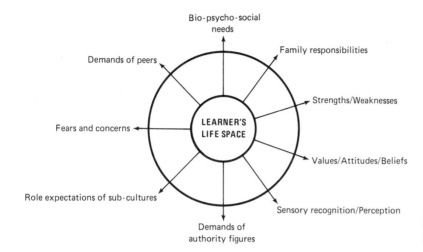

**Figure 10–3.** Personal factors affecting learning behavior.

the energy or direction of learning behavior, or both. Personal factors are internal to the learner, and they too influence learning behavior. For example, when learners desire to achieve particular goals that are important to them (a personal factor), they are compelled to carry out purposeful activities that are goal-oriented. Another example is when the chance for a life of fuller quality causes a person to follow a strict diet and exercise regime (environmental factor). Learners become highly motivated when personal and environmental factors work together and foster behavior that leads to the same goals. Motivation, which is one of the goals of teaching, serves as a means for achieving learning objectives. It is one of the purposes of teaching and if present results in effective learning.

Motivation is linked to other factors that influence the energy and direction of behavior. These influencing factors are interest, need, value, attitude, aspiration, and incentive.

1. Motivation and interest. Learners who are interested in a particular area tend to pay attention to it. Their attention level is high, and their satisfaction is great. **Interest** refers to selecting and attending to stimuli. Things will not be noticed or attended to unless the learner is interested in the area.
2. Motivation and need. Learners who have needs lack something that a given activity can provide. Thus, a learner's need for achievement can be met, with a corresponding increase in satisfaction, by success in attaining some goal requiring effort. A learner's need for affiliation is satisfied by friendly relationships with other persons.
3. Motivation and values. A **value** can be defined as an orientation toward an entire class of goals that are considered important in one's life. The value is labeled with the name of that class of goals. A set of categories of values was developed by Spranger:[24] (1) the theoretical value, or truth for its own sake; (2) the economic value, or wealth for its own sake; (3) the esthetic value, or beauty for its own sake; (4) the political value, or power for its own sake; (5) the social value, or the welfare of other people; (6) the religious value, or a mystic unity with the supernatural world.

Each culture holds to a differing value system; therefore, this aspect should be explored with the learners. In the United States, some values include democracy, economic productivity, fairness, and material wealth and comfort. Being a "well-rounded" person in the sense that one is not overly devoted to any one life goal also seems to be a value held by many Americans. Whatever a learner's values are, they have a motivating function. They energize and direct the learner's activity toward certain goals.

4. Motivation and Attitude. The learner's **attitude** toward something consists of feelings for or against what that thing is conceived to be. An attitude, therefore, involves emotions (feelings), directionality (for or against), an objective (the something), and cognitive elements (what the learner conceives the object to be). If learners like to be sociable, it means that they get pleasure out of being involved in activities that represent sociability. They seek out activities toward which positive attitudes are held. Attitudes, like motives, arouse and direct purposeful activity.

5. Motivation and Aspiration. A learner's **aspiration** is hope or longing for a certain type of achievement. With a certain level of aspiration, a learner will try; without it, little effort will be made.

6. Motivation and Incentive. An **incentive** is something the learner perceives as having the capability of satisfying an aroused motive. It draws the learner to action aimed at acquiring the incentive. The learner motivated by curiosity has knowledge as an incentive. If achievement is the motive, then success and honor will serve as incentives. The fact that incentives arouse activity suggests that behavior modification techniques use this aspect of motivation to the fullest.

The concept of motivation helps one understand and explain certain intriguing facts about behavior and learning. All learners have common needs that must be satisfied. Learners are more motivated to learn when they can identify their own needs and contribute to a planned educational program that is individually designed.

**Experiential readiness** of learners must also be assessed before learning needs can be identified. Certain experiences, skills, attitudes, and abilities may need to be present before learners can be taught new information. For example, before a woman is taught breast-feeding technique, it is necessary to determine if certain prerequisites exist:

1. Attitude. Does she desire to breast-feed or was she talked into it?
2. Experience. Has she had other children who were breast-fed? Has she observed others breast-feed?
3. Ability. Does she know how to relax?
4. Skills. Can she understand simple instructions? Can she pay attention to a series of commands?

Skills may refer to cognitive, psychomotor, or affective skills. The learner must have these necessary prerequisites before an objective of breast-feeding is realistic.

***Assessment of Sociological Needs.*** Learners, who are social beings, must have their sociological needs met before learning can be effective. Knowledge of the learner's attitudes, values, and beliefs will enable you to understand the learner's behavior. For example, you may unintentionally formulate objectives that are unacceptable to the learner's social value system. Learners who are strongly committed to certain social values will not perform behaviors they consider wrong.

Other areas that are important to assess are communication and interaction patterns. Generally, the social class of learners influences the abstractness and complexity of the language they use and understand. Also, assessment of communication and interaction patterns will enable you to be aware of your own use of verbal and nonverbal communication and to determine their influence on changing behavior.

The sociological needs vary among different age groups. For example, in children it would be important to concentrate on play patterns. In middle-aged adults, you need to assess their work patterns. And in mature older adults, leisure patterns may be most helpful in assessing sociological needs. These areas give important clues to what learners' attitudes and values are.

A family assessment, which was discussed in Chapter 4, is helpful in gathering information about the learner's social roles, patterns of interacting with others, and reaction patterns to change. Your use of the information will vary depending on the age and role of the learner. For example, you can learn about a child's sociological needs by studying the family because they prescribe patterns of expected behavior for the child. For a young adult, you can determine the amount and nature of internal and external pressures that may interfere with learning new behaviors. For the older adult, you can assess if they have frequent contact with others or if they are socially isolated.

We have discussed some needs that should be assessed before teaching preparation begins. The most valuable tool is the nursing health history and physical assessment. You can examine the information for clues about the learner's knowledge and beliefs, socioeconomic status, amount of education, and development tasks. Information about learners and their family will enable you to anticipate receptivity to learning. This information also will help you structure an environment that supports learning.

## Assessment of Learning Environment
Environment means surroundings. When we speak of **learning environment,** we are referring to factors that are external to the learner that influence learning. The environment in which teaching is implemented should provide for physical and psychological comfort.[6,14] Learners need to feel accepted, valued, and encouraged to contribute their thoughts, ideas, and past experiences.

Earlier, we discussed some early environmental influences that affect learning and which must be assessed. These were the physiologic, psychological, and sociological needs of the learner. Now we will concentrate on the immediate environment of a learning situation which influences attention, motivation, and perception. Some of the influences cannot be manipulated (for example, age, sensory functioning), so we will examine those that can.

*Instruction Modes.* The method of teaching and the materials used to stimulate learning are part of the environment and can be changed to maximize learning. (We will discuss teaching methods later in this chapter.) Assessment of learner's cognitive styles and preferences enables you to establish an individualized learning environment by selecting appropriate means.

*Human Interaction.* The teacher is responsible for establishing a conceptual environment as well as a physical one. This cognitive component of environment deals with the learners' feelings, attitudes, emotions, and psychosocial needs. Human relations affect learning and teaching. You must assess the emotional climate, which needs to be positive and supportive of learning. The amount and quality of interaction will indicate whether the environmental climate is positive or negative. To promote acquisition and retention of learning, you must control as many external stimuli as possible.

***Physical Conditions.*** You need to assess the physical space where learning will be taking place. Generally, a cool, well-lighted, adequately ventilated area does not distract the learners' attention. Other aspects to assess are noise level, presence of odors, and general appearance of the physical setting. You will need to know the learners' preferences in some instances, such as temperature of the room.

There are variations in what constitutes an effective learning environment. For example, the environment for children requires more concrete objects. Adult learners enjoy an informal and friendly environment where they are called by name and valued as individuals. Knowledge of normal growth and developmental needs of the various age groups will enable you to establish a suitable learning environment.

So far we have discussed assessing the learner and the learning environment. Now we will turn our attention to assessing learning needs. It is at this point that the teaching process will be applied to the implementing step in the nursing process.

### Assessment of Learning Needs

After you have completed your assessment of clients–learners and their environment, an assessment of their learning needs must be made. Clients may be aware of what they need to know as well as what they want to know. An example is when persons want to start an investment program. They realize that they need more knowledge about the subject, so they attend a local seminar on the topic.

If clients lack the necessary awareness, motivation, or knowledge to identify their own need to know, you must help them identify their learning needs. This is accomplished by observing and making inferences from the data collected from the nursing health history and physical assessment. Testing may also be appropriate.

You may find it beneficial to ask: What does the client need to know based on the assessment data? Why does the client wish to learn this information or skill? Who and what would provide the best instruction? Where would the client feel most comfortable while learning? When is the best time for learning this information? How will the client learn the most? After these learning needs are identified, they are formally stated.

## DIAGNOSIS OF LEARNING NEEDS

After data are collected, a diagnosis is made of learning needs. We will discuss analysis of data, derivation of conclusions, assignment of diagnostic label to conclusions, identification of sustaining factors, and formulation of diagnostic statement (refer to Chapter 5 for a thorough discussion of diagnosing).

### Analysis of Data

You need to separate and organize the subjective and objective information that was collected from the client. Outlined in Table 10–4 are samples of subjective and objective data that are organized according to the three domains: cognitive, psychomotor, and affective. The **cognitive domain** concerns the intellectual abilities and the development of thought processes. The **affective domain** concerns emotional development and is re-

**TABLE 10–4. SUBJECTIVE AND OBJECTIVE DATA CATEGORIZED ACCORDING TO DOMAINS**

| Domain | Subjective Data | Objective Data |
|---|---|---|
| Cognitive domain | Verbalizes a deficiency in knowledge | Level of education<br>Ability to read<br>Ability to understand written and verbal languages<br>Age<br>Ability to write<br>Sex |
| Psychomotor domain | Verbalizes a deficiency in skill<br>Does not perform correctly a desired skill | Ability to write<br>Ability to hear<br>Ability to see<br>Ability to taste<br>Ability to feel |
| Affective domain | Verbalizes a lack of motivation<br>Verbalizes ineffective coping patterns<br>Expresses unhealthy health practices and/or beliefs | Traditions<br>Life-style<br>Health care beliefs<br>Health care practices<br>Ethnic origin<br>Motivation<br>Coping patterns<br>Adherence/non-adherence |

lated to interests, attitudes, values, and goals. The **psychomotor domain** concerns motor activities and skills. A set of learning objectives in all three domains serves as a guide to you and the client in setting up a teaching program. If you examine Table 10–4, you will notice that both positive and deficit responses are included. This enables you to build on the learner's abilities. The same procedures are used regardless if an individual, family, or community client is the learner.

After the data are organized, you need to determine if there are inconsistencies and omissions within the data. If so, gather additional information. Next you need to examine the subjective and objective data for patterns. Compare these patterns of data with established norms, standards, and theories. When you compare your assessment data to standards, you need to consider the learner's perception of what is expected as well as what the literature states.

## Derivation of Conclusions

Once you have analyzed data, you are ready to derive conclusions about the learner's abilities and needs. You use reasoning to arrive at your conclusions. (Refer to the discussion of synthesis and inductive and deductive reasoning in Chapter 2.)

The last aspect of diagnosing is determination of the learner's need. For example, you may conclude from the subjective data listed in Table 10–4 that there is a deficit of knowledge in all three domains. Agreement upon learning needs, factors affecting behavioral change, and setting priorities for identified needs and problems are necessary before a diagnostic label is assigned.

## Assignment of Diagnostic Label to Conclusions

You may use a standard diagnostic label such as knowledge deficit or you may develop your own that more specifically describes the learner's need. Outlined in Tables 10–5, 10–6, and 10–7 are nursing diagnostic labels for the three domains—cognitive, psycho-

**TABLE 10–5. NURSING DIAGNOSTIC LABELS ADAPTED FROM BLOOM'S COGNITIVE DOMAIN**

| Level I | Inability to remember facts |
|---|---|
| Level II | Inability to state information in own words |
| Level III | Inability to apply learned information to new situations/real life situations |
| Level IV | Inability to determine the most important aspects of presented material |
| Level V | Inability to synthesize material |
| Level VI | Inability to make judgments concerning the accuracy of presented information |

*(Adapted from Bloom, 1956.[5])*

motor, and affective. Each domain is divided according to level of complexity. if the learning response is not an actual one, it should be labeled as potential. This indicator will identify that the learner risks developing a knowledge deficit unless measures are instituted. Actual diagnostic labels must be substantiated by assessment data obtained from the client. If you do not have adequate data to validate a label, or if you are uncertain when it is a threat to the learner, you may identify this label as probable.

## Identification of Sustaining Factors
The second part of the nursing diagnosis is the sustaining factor. Sustaining factors can also be categorized according to the domains (Table 10–8). To arrive at a sustaining factor, you must reevaluate the assessment data. You use the same cognitive processes to arrive at sustaining factors as you used to derive conclusions—synthesis, inductive reasoning, and deductive reasoning.

## Formulation of Diagnostic Statement
After the sustaining factor is determined, a diagnostic statement can be formulated. The diagnostic statement consists of the client's identified learning need related to a probable cause or sustaining factor. (The general rules concerning the format for stating nursing diagnoses can be found in Chapter 5.)

After you have diagnosed the learner's needs, you are ready to plan the activities that will bring about learning.

**TABLE 10–6. NURSING DIAGNOSTIC LABELS ADAPTED FROM DAVE'S PSYCHOMOTOR DOMAIN**

1. Inability to imitate an observed skill

2. Inability to follow directions (verbal or written) in performing a selected skill

3. Inability to perform a skill independently with high degree of accuracy

4. Inability to perform a skill competently and accurately within a given time limit

5. Inability to perform a skill spontaneously without stress

*(Adapted from Dave, 1970.[8])*

**TABLE 10–7. NURSING DIAGNOSTIC LABELS ADAPTED FROM KRATHWOHL'S AFFECTIVE DOMAIN**

1. Lack of awareness of existing situation

2. Nonacceptance of the necessity of performing a task

3. Lack of motivation to perform a behavior

4. Failure to develop and rank a value system consistently with desired behavior

5. Inability to incorporate value system into life-style

*(Adapted from Krathwohl, 1964.[16])*


# PLANNING OF LEARNING ACTIVITIES

Learning is more likely to occur if you carefully plan the activities before implementing them. A **plan** is a method for accomplishing something. In this circumstance, the accomplishment is learning. This step gives you the opportunity to intentionally establish goals and objectives, plan content, and select learning materials.

## Formulation of Learning Goals
Establishing goals is essential to the success of teaching. During the assessment phase, data were obtained concerning where the client was in terms of knowledge, skills, and attitudes. Goal-setting is the activity that allows the client to accomplish what he or she wishes. **Goals** are broad statements of what is to be accomplished and flow from the nursing diagnoses. (For a more thorough discussion of goals see Chapter 6.)

## Formulation of Learning Objectives
**Learning objectives** are statements containing observable behaviors that describe the change that should be evident in the learner. They provide the basis for organizing the learning content, selecting learning methods and materials, preparing evaluation meth-

**TABLE 10–8. CATEGORIZATION OF SUSTAINING FACTORS ACCORDING TO DOMAINS**

| Domain | Sustaining Factor | |
|---|---|---|
| Cognitive domain | Language differences | |
| | Decreased short-term memory | |
| | Increased learning time | Secondary to aging |
| | Increased recall time | |
| | Decreased mentation secondary to prescribed medication | |
| Psychomotor domain | Decreased motor skills | |
| | Decreased coordination | |
| | Decreased manual dexterity | |
| | Sensory deficits | |
| Affective domain | Lack of motivation | |
| | Conflict with value system | |
| | Conflict with customs | |
| | Ineffective coping | |

**TABLE 10–9. CLASSIFICATION OF OBJECTIVES IN THE COGNITIVE DOMAIN**

| Level | Emphasis | Objective | Verbs to Use |
|---|---|---|---|
| I. Knowledge | Recognition and recall—ability to remember facts in a form close to the way they were first presented | Show that you know | List, tell, define, identify, label, locate, recognize |
| II. Comprehension | Grasp the meaning and intent of information—the ability to tell or translate in your own words | Show that you understand | Explain, illustrate, describe, summarize, interpret, expand, convert, measure |
| III. Application | Use of information—ability to apply learning to new situations and real life circumstances | Show that you can use what is learned | Demonstrate, apply, use, find solutions, collect information, perform, solve, choose appropriate procedures |
| IV. Analysis | Reasoning—ability to break down information into component parts and to detect relationships of one part to another and to the whole | Show that you perceive and can pick out the most important points in material presented | Analyze, debate, generalize, conclude, determine, distinguish |
| V. Synthesis | Originality and creativity—ability to assemble separate parts to form a new whole | Show that you can combine concepts to create an original or new idea | Create, design, plan, produce, compile, develop |
| VI. Evaluation | Criteria or standards for evaluation and judgment—ability to make judgments based on criteria or standards | Show that you can judge and evaluate ideas, information, procedures, and solutions | Compare, decide, evaluate, conclude, contrast, develop criteria, appraise |

ods, and directing self-learning. Objectives tell you and the learner what needs to be done to attain the goal. Outcome criteria may also be used in addition to goals and objectives. **Outcome criteria** are defined as standards used to determine the responses to or results of teaching interventions. (For a detailed discussion of these three aspects of planning see Chapter 6.)

Learning objectives vary in detail depending on the area of learning they encompass. It is recommended that each learning objective cover a limited area of content or skills to be learned.

In the context of a total teaching program, learning objectives may be arranged in several different ways. (1) Objectives can be organized by content areas. For example, certain content has a logical order to it, and the objectives would be correlated with the content area. (2) Objectives can be grouped into units. Each unit is free-standing, but can be a part of a larger content area. The objectives in this instance would be for the unit and thus are more general than those correlated to content areas. (3) Objectives can be sequenced into learning levels. For example, the first objective would emphasize recall while the last objective would emphasize creativity.

Objectives are organized into three domains. These three domains—cognitive, affective, and psychomotor—comprise a classification system for learning objectives. Behaviors that are complex fall at the upper end of the taxonomy and are synthesis and evaluation. Simple behaviors fall at the lower end and are knowledge. The most complete taxonomy that has been developed in the classification of objectives is the cognitive domain[5] (Table 10–9).

## Lesson Planning

In informal or spontaneous teaching, lesson planning does not occur but thought must always be given to the content to be taught. For formal group presentations you may want to map out the learning objectives, content to be covered, and learning activities. Nurses are often asked to speak at community affairs on health topics. In these situations there are usually time limitations, which necessitate more formal planning. Lesson planning has many benefits: (1) defines objectives to be accomplished, (2) insures preparation, (3) provides for a specific method of teaching, (4) provides for planned questioning, (5) provides for summarization, (6) provides for active learning and motivation, and (7) provides for individual differences. A sample of a lesson plan can be seen in Figure 10–4. Sample teaching plans are included in Appendix J. They were developed by Saint Elizabeth Medical Center, Granite City, Illinois.

## Selection of Learning Materials

You need to choose learning materials that ensure transfer of learning to the actual situation and help meet the learning objectives. The more senses learners use, the more likely they will learn the content. Dale's cone of experiences (Fig. 10–5) illustrates how you can determine what materials to use in teaching.[7]

The most concrete learning experiences are those using physical objects that the learner sees as relevant and has the opportunity to manipulate as they are explained. For example, you could have the diabetic client hold the syringe and examine it closely. If you merely showed the client a photograph of the object, which lacks dimensionality, the learning experience would be less concrete. If you verbalized what you wanted to teach the client without any visual aids, this would be a highly abstract learning experience and less likely to transfer to a real situation.

| LEARNING OBJECTIVES | CONTENT OUTLINE | LEARNING ACTIVITIES |
|---|---|---|
| | | |

**Figure 10–4.** Lesson-plan format.

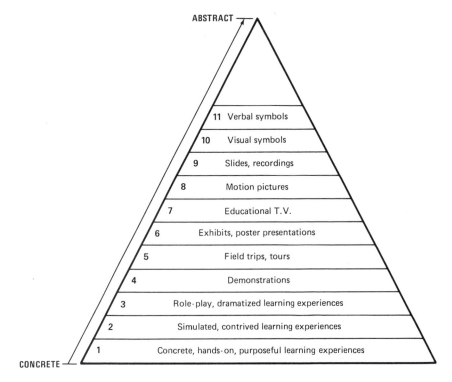

**Figure 10–5.** Levels of learning experiences. *(From Dale, 1976.[7])*

Motion pictures are a suitable learning aid when motion is essential for teaching a particular procedure. When you plan to use a film, you should order it early enough to preview it. A short discussion prior to showing the film will facilitate learning. In addition, a short discussion afterwards will increase learning further.

When you use written materials as teaching tools, there are a number of factors to consider. You should assess the size of print and factors that affect readability, and match the vocabulary and sentence structure to the learner's ability. Also of great importance is whether the information is accurate or whether it expresses only your point of view. To be useful, the written materials should meet one of the learning objectives. You need to decide if the material meets the objectives before you use it as a learning aid. Meaningful material is learned more readily and retained longer.[12] Assessment is necessary to determine what would be meaningful to the learner. For example, some pamphlets are designed for health providers and for clients. It is especially important that you read the pamphlet to see if it is appropriate.

After planning is completed, the teaching program is implemented. You need to remember that the plan is a guide and may need to be adjusted if it is not meeting your objectives.

## IMPLEMENTATION OF TEACHING PLAN

An important decision you must make is the selection of a method for teaching the client. We will discuss various methods that can be used with individual, family (small group), and community clients (large group).

### Selection of Appropriate Method
In most learning situations, you want clients to transfer new information to their life situation. There are two ways of teaching for transfer. The first way is to teach directly what you want the learner to understand by means of the lecture method. The second way of teaching for transfer has to do with generalized training. An example of this type of transfer is to teach broadly applicable concepts, principles, and procedures such as problem-solving skills. Most teaching involves only the first method but there is no reason why both methods cannot be combined.

The following is a guide for transfer of new information to clients:

1. Real life similarity. Make the learning situation as similar to the real world as possible. If it is impossible to simulate reality, describe a new situation so that clients are not bewildered when they encounter it.
2. Practice opportunities. Provide many practice opportunities of the original procedure before the transfer task is attempted. This guide should be adhered to strictly in teaching potentially dangerous procedures.
3. Related practice. Provide practice on a related set of problems. If you are requiring interpretation of signs and symptoms, provide examples of many different types of signs and symptoms to make the client aware that in the midst of changing conditions some constants remain.
4. Early learning. Emphasize the early learning of basic information. If related to a chronic disease, it may be teaching briefly the pathophysiology so that the importance of carrying out a particular treatment is emphasized. Once the client masters certain early information, transfer of knowledge to related tasks is easier.
5. Examples. Whenever a principle or generalization is stated, provide a variety of examples.
6. Applications. Ask clients to make some of the applications. Invite them to determine how learning the signs and symptoms of diabetic shock has potential use. Ask them whether the particular procedure reminds them of anything they are familiar with.

Positive transfer takes place most often when you try different explanations of events, use many different examples, provide practice, teach rules with wide applicability, provide many examples of a principle in action, and provide realistic settings for teaching.

Regardless of the method you select to teach, there are some general principles that will guide your selection of learning activities:

1. Learning activities should provide an opportunity to practice the kind of behavior implied by the objectives (interest, skill, etc.).

**TABLE 10–10. NURSING STRATEGIES FOR FACILITATING SELF-DIRECTED LEARNING**

| Nursing Activities | Self-directed Learning Activities |
|---|---|
| Organize a process, such as contracting, to structure time and effort. Set expectations and limits. Help to explore alternative activities. | Client self-assessment: diagnosis of skills necessary for successful performance and identification of the instruction needed to correct shortcomings. shortcomings. |
| Teach new skills required such as goal-setting, time management, and resource identification. | Begins writing contract and practicing skills. |
| Establish one-to-one conferences to discuss the client's learning style and learning tasks. | Begins to study the group interaction process. |
| Clarify new roles. | Small groups form for discussion of emerging difficulties. |
| Discuss purpose and direction, provide a general program structure. Help but do not rescue. | Launch small-group projects to allow for modeling leadership in activities. |
| Renegotiate learning contracts, setting more realistic goals and deadlines. | Combine activities for personal development with activities for development of intellectual and procedural skills. |
| Reinforce any sign of success; help to identify with exemplars and to build a self-fulfilling prophecy of success. Model respect for learning and encourage respect among the clients. | Overcomes apathy by completing a task successfully. (Nurse helps client to finish any task by any means.) |
| Secure written commitment in learning contract. | Launches challenge experiences. |
| Conduct conferences to establish pattern of self-evaluation, to identify internal rewards, and to deal with the future. | Discusses behavioral changes achieved and successes accomplished. |
| Increase freedom and responsibility of client. Implement self-evaluation and reporting. | Demonstrates accomplishments to the nurse. This is followed by self-evaluation sessions. |

2. Learning activities provide the client with satisfaction from carrying out the kind of behavior implied by the objectives.
3. The reactions desired in the activity are within the range of possibility for the client.
4. Several activities can be used to attain the same learning objectives.
5. The same learning activities will usually bring about several outcomes.

An assessment of the client and the learning needs will enable you to select the most appropriate method of presenting information. We will examine methods that are appropriate for individuals, small groups, and large groups.

## Teaching Individuals

Three methods of learning that are appropriate for individuals are self-directed learning, programmed instruction, and computer-assisted instruction.

***Self-directed Learning.*** Perhaps one of the teaching methods that best reflects humanistic principles is self-directed learning. Self-directed learning is vastly different from teacher-directed learning. The client decides what should be learned, how it should be studied, and how the accuracy and value of the accomplishment should be judged.

Your role is to instruct the client in designing and managing the learning process and in your giving assistance to the client. This places the responsibility for learning strictly on the client.

You need to assess whether the client values self-direction. If there is no desire to become self-directed, the client will lack the motivation to take the initiative and to persevere in the face of difficulty. But even with desire and initiative, the client needs the skills of organization, planning, and interacting with others. The question is, How can you help clients develop the attitudes, characteristics, and skills they need to become self-directed learners? Table 10–10 outlines specific strategies to assist the client in becoming a self-directed learner.

Learning contracts seem to be a very promising method of motivation. This method depends heavily upon a one-to-one relationship. Knowledge of general counseling principles therefore is helpful to you. Contracting systems, used with clearly stated objectives and incorporating personal contact between you and the client, seem to improve the motivation to learn. The learning contract is one of several methods that allows clients to actively participate in defining their own needs and goals. This format for learning is particularly successful for adult clients. A drawback to using a learning contract is the possibility that one or both persons may not fulfill their responsibility. In addition to motivational readiness, the client must possess experiential readiness for learning to be effective. In Figure 10–6, a sample learning contract is suggested for your use.

The following eight steps will help you plan a self-directed teaching program for your client.

*Step 1: Diagnose Learning Needs.* A **learning need** is the gap between where the client is and where he or she wants to be in regard to a particular set of competencies. A **competency** can be thought of as the ability to do something at some level of proficiency and is usually composed of a combination of knowledge, understanding, skill, attitude, and values.

After the client decides what set of competencies to achieve, the next task is to as-

| This is a learning contract for: Name: _____ Goal: _____ | | | |
|---|---|---|---|
| LEARNING OBJECTIVES | LEARNING RESOURCES AND STRATEGIES | EVIDENCE OF ACCOMPLISHMENT OF OBJECTIVES | MEANS FOR VALIDATING EVIDENCE |
|  |  |  |  |
|  |  |  |  |

**Figure 10–6.** A sample learning contract.

sess the gap between where the client is now and where the client should be in regard to each competency. This can be done alone or with help.

*Step 2: Specify Learning Objectives.* Each learning need diagnosed in Step 1 should be translated into a learning objective. The objectives should describe what the client will learn, not what the client will do.

*Step 3: Specify Learning Resources and Strategies.* When clients have finished listing their objectives, they describe how they propose to go about accomplishing each objective. They should identify the resources (material and human) they plan to use and the strategies (techniques, tools) they will employ in making use of them.

   An example of a learning objective might be, "Improve my ability to give an insulin injection efficiently so that I can accomplish it accurately and safely 100 percent of the time." The client could list the following in the "Learning Resources and Strategies" column:

1. Find and read books and articles in the library on how to give insulin injections.
2. Interview three diabetics on how they give their injections, then observe them for one day each, noting techniques they use.
3. Select the best techniques from each, plan an injection, and have the nurse and other diabetics observe me for a day, giving me feedback.

*Step 4: Specify Evidence of Accomplishment.* After completing the second column, the client completes the third column, "Evidence of Accomplishment of Objectives," and describes what evidence is to be collected to indicate the degree to which each objective has been achieved. Examples of evidence for different types of objectives can be found in Table 10–11.

*Step 5: Specify How the Evidence Will Be Validated.* After clients have specified what evidence is to be gathered for each objective in column 3, they complete column 4,

**TABLE 10–11. RELATIONSHIP BETWEEN OBJECTIVES AND EVIDENCE OF ACCOMPLISHMENT**

| Types of Objectives | Examples of Evidence |
| --- | --- |
| Knowledge | Report of knowledge acquired, as in oral presentations, audio-visual presentations, annotated bibliographies |
| Understanding | Illustrations of utilization of knowledge |
| Skills | Performance exercises, video-taped performances, etc., with ratings by observers |
| Attitudes | Attitudinal rating scales; performances in real situations, role playing, simulation games, critical incident cases, etc., with feedback from participants and observers |
| Values | Value rating scales; performance in value clarification groups, critical incident cases, simulation exercises, etc., with feedback from participants and observers |

"Means for Validating Evidence." For each objective, they should specify the means by which the evidence will be judged. The means will vary according to the type of objective. For example, appropriate criteria for knowledge objectives might include comprehensiveness, depth, precision, clarity. For skill objectives more appropriate criteria may be speed, flexibility, precision, imaginativeness. After they have specified the criteria, the means that they will use to have the evidence judged according to these criteria should be indicated.

*Step 6: Review the Contract with Consultants.* After clients have completed the contract, it will be helpful to review it with two or three other expert resource people to get their reactions and suggestions.

*Step 7: Carry Out the Contract.* The client now simply does what the contract calls for. As the client works on it, notions about what the client wants to learn and how to learn it may change. The client should not hesitate to revise the contract.

*Step 8: Evaluate Learning.* When clients have completed their contract they will want to get some assurance that they have learned what they set out to learn. The simplest way to do this is to ask the consultants used in Step 6 to examine the evidence and validation data and give their judgment about their adequacy.

***Programmed Instruction.*** Another method of self-learning is programmed instruction. Programmed instruction is a method that arranges learning material in a series of frames or sequential steps.[6] The learner is presented with familiar information initially and then is guided to more complex material. There are different formats for programmed instruction—books, films, filmstrips, computer printouts.

This method of instruction is an active way of learning. Generally, reinforcement in the way of feedback is built into the materials. This method may be boring to some learners but is gaining in popularity because of its effectiveness and low expense.

***Computer-Assisted Instruction (CAI).*** This self-learning method is a form of programmed instruction and shares many of the advantages.[6,23] It is, however, relatively expensive. Well-designed CAI individualizes learning activities for each learner. It is therefore possible to accommodate different learning rates and intellectual levels.

## Teaching Small Groups

Most teaching occurs on an informal basis. Whether you teach an individual or a small group, knowledge of the question-and-answer method[4,10,12] is beneficial. The most common uses of the question-and-answer method are to:

1. Set the stage for group discussion, role-playing, or other teaching–learning activities.
2. Identify learning needs and problems, interests, work habits, and levels of development.
3. Review previous instruction.
4. Pretest to explore client background.
5. Secure and maintain client interest.
6. Draw upon client experiences.

7. Develop and reinforce concepts and generalizations.
8. Involve nonresponsive clients in group activity.

You need to master the following techniques of questioning to effectively use the question-and-answer method.[10,12,18,20] (Review communication skills in Chapters 4 and 7.)

1. Begin each question with a word or phrase that calls for thought.
2. State questions in simple, straightforward language.
3. Ask questions which challenge the client to apply knowledge rather than repeat facts.
4. Limit questions to those within the client's experience and knowledge.
5. Organize the sequence of planned questions around a core and key them to the objectives of the lesson.
6. Develop an attitude of client responsibility for answering questions from other group members.
7. Maintain an attitude during questioning which is natural, friendly, and conversational.
8. Allow questions to point up the important aspects of the lesson.
9. When practical, try to discuss client's questions when they are asked, rather than at some later time.
10. Do not hesitate to say "I do not know" in response to a client's questions.
11. Avoid a pattern of calling on clients in turn.
12. Allow clients time to answer without interruption.
13. Draw out answers to questions by saying, "Do you agree?" "What do you think?"
14. Encourage clients to give answers to the group, not to you.
15. Direct all of your responses to questions toward the entire group and not to individual clients who asked the questions.

These guidelines take practice but are very useful. Next, we will examine methods of teaching large groups.

## Teaching Large Groups

Although many methods are impractical to use with large groups, the lecture can be an effective method for large community groups as well as for people who do not learn effectively through reading.

Many clients do not learn effectively through reading, but the lecture can introduce them to the subject matter. You can repeat material in different words when necessary, whereas books can provide only one wording of an explanation.

Clients can be reinforced by the warmth, humor, logic, enthusiasm, and attention as well as knowledge and comprehension they obtain from the lecture method. Clients in a classroom may obtain a sense of security through being assured that their own attendance and attention are appropriate. The effectiveness of teaching methods is often measured by how much people learn in the form of knowledge and comprehension of subject matter. But the lecture situation may also provide social reinforcement, esthetic pleasure, and emotional reassurance. The lecture method[10,12] is appropriate when (1) the basic purpose is to disseminate information, (2) the material is not available elsewhere, (3) the material must be organized and presented in a particular way for a specific group, (4) it is necessary to arouse interest in the subject, (5) the material need be remembered for only a short time, and (6) it is necessary to provide an introduction to an area or directions for learning tasks to be pursued through some other teaching method.

The lecture is inappropriate when (1) objectives other than acquisition of information are sought, (2) long-term retention is desired, (3) the material is complex, detailed, or abstract, (4) client participation is essential to the achievement of the objectives (5) higher cognitive objectives such as analysis, synthesis, or integration are being sought, or (6) the clients are average or below average in intelligence or educational experience.[10]

There are many different ways to organize a lecture. We will examine two ways that are appropriate to large group teaching.

***Sequential Relationships.*** This way of organizing the lecture refers to chronological, cause-and-effect, building-to-a-climax, and topical sequences. Here you use a given basis for arranging a series of ideas in a certain order. Once this basis is understood, the sequence is easier to remember (Fig. 10–7).

***Problem-centered Lecture.*** This organizational format begins with a set of facts that create a question or problem. You then present information about an argument for each of several possible solutions. Such problem-centered lectures can be highly motivating and tension arousing. Dramatic puzzlement can be heightened through rhetorical questions, skillfully timed introduction of new pieces of evidence, and careful explanations of the way in which the hypothesized solutions follow from the evidence.

We have discussed how teaching can be effectively implemented for an individual, small group, or large group. After teaching has been implemented, the learner's achievement of the objectives is evaluated.

## EVALUATION OF THE TEACHING–LEARNING PROCESS

Evaluation is an integral part of the teaching–learning process. It is not something tacked on at the end of a teaching unit; it is not limited to the measurement of the amount of factual material retained; it is not limited to paper-and-pencil examinations. Evaluation is a continuous, comprehensive process which utilizes a variety of procedures and which is inescapably related to the objectives of the teaching program.

**Evaluation** can be defined as the process by which the nurse and the client determine to what extent the learning objectives were accomplished. The purpose of evaluation is to project how a client will behave in the future. We have already discussed developing learning objectives for the purpose of evaluation. The sequence of steps shown in Figure 10–8 summarizes a general procedure for relating evaluation techniques to objectives.

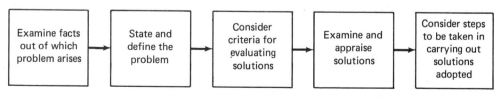

**Figure 10–7.** Sequential relationships lecture method.

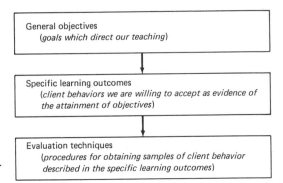

**Figure 10–8.** Relationship of evaluation to learning objectives

These procedural steps clarify the importance of relating the evaluation techniques directly to the specific learning outcomes being evaluated. This is the only way you can have any certainty that you are evaluating client progress toward the objectives selected as teaching objectives.

There are numerous ways to evaluate whether a client has learned a particular subject area. We will consider two methods—direct and indirect measures.

## Direct Measures

Observation of whether the client is accomplishing an objective is an example of a direct means of evaluation. Psychomotor skills and affective behaviors are more easily observed than cognitive skills. Rating scales or checklists are other direct means of evaluating learning objectives. To record client behaviors that express attitudes, anecdotal records are helpful. Over a period of time, you can judge whether a change in behavior has occurred.

## Indirect Measures

Since you cannot always be present when the actual behavior occurs, you may use indirect measures to evaluate the attainment of an objective. These indirect measures of evaluation are written, verbal, or performance reaction to a simulated situation. Video tapes can also be used.

Regardless of the method of evaluation used to measure the change in client behavior, the following steps[4,17,19,20] are essential in the evaluation process:

1. Examine objectives to be assessed in terms of content and implied behavior.
2. Identify situations that are likely to provide opportunities for the demonstration of the behaviors to be assessed.
3. Examine available evaluation instruments or experiences to determine the extent to which they may satisfy the purpose of evaluation desired.
4. Determine the aspects of behavior to be evaluated and the terms in which each aspect will be summarized.
5. Establish means for collecting, interpreting, and using data and results.

Evaluation is not an ending point, but rather another starting point in a continuous process that is aimed at providing optimal care to clients.

## SUMMARY

The teaching process is an essential component of the nursing process. A thorough assessment of learners, their environment, and learning needs are the basis for planning teaching interventions. A number of methods are available for appropriate use with individuals, small groups, and large groups. The content, method of presentation, learning materials, and evaluation methods are based on the type of objectives formulated. While the teaching process is complete in itself, it is part of the implementing step of the nursing process.

## STUDY GUIDE

1. Write on one page your beliefs about client education. Incorporate into your answer the type of interaction desired between the nurse and the client. Explain the type of environment that you consider most conducive to teaching–learning.
2. Imagine you were working on the pediatric unit and had the responsibility of teaching two clients aged 4 and 12. If all other things were equal, how would your assessment differ?
3. Write one objective representing each of the three domains for a client you cared for this week.
4. Identify two learning principles you use on a consistent basis. Can you isolate factors that prevent you from fulfilling your role as client educator?
5. Evaluate your role as a client educator. Are your teaching activities directed toward prevention, restoration, or promotion?

## REFERENCES

1. American Nurses' Association. *Standards of Nursing Practice.* Kansas City: American Nurses' Association, 1973.
2. Bell, D. F. Assessing educational needs: Advantages and disadvantages. *Nurse Educator,* 1978, *3,* 15–21.
3. Bigge, M. L. *Learning Theories for Teachers* (4th ed.). New York: Harper & Row, 1981.
4. Bille, D. A., (Ed.). *Practical Approaches to Patient Teaching.* Boston: Little, Brown, 1981.
5. Bloom, B. S., Englehart, M.D., Furst, E. J., et al. (Eds.). *Taxonomy of Educational Objectives: Handbook I, Cognitive Domain.* New York: D. McKay, 1956.
6. Clark, C. C. *Classroom Skills for Nurse Educator.* New York: Springer-Verlag, 1978.
7. Dale, P.S. *Language Development* (2nd ed.). New York: Holt, Rinehart & Winston, 1976.
8. Dave, R. H. Psychomotor levels. In *Developing and Writing Behavioral Objectives.* Tucson, Ariz.: Educational Innovators Press, 1970.
9. Erikson, E. H. *Childhood and Society.* New York: W. W. Norton & Co., Inc., 1950.
10. Gage, N. L., & Berliner, D. C. *Educational Psychology* (2nd ed.). Chicago: Rand McNally, 1979.
11. Gagne, R. M., & Leslie, J. B. *Principles in Instructional Design* (2nd ed.). New York: Holt, Rinehart, & Winston, 1979.
12. Glaser, R. Learning. *Encyclopedia of Educational Research.* New York: Macmillan, 1969.
13. Hilgard, E. R., & Gordon, H. B. *Theories of Learning* (4th ed.). Englewood Cliffs, N.J.: Prentice-Hall, 1975.
14. Huckabay, L. M. *Conditions of Learning and Instruction in Nursing.* St. Louis: C. V. Mosby, 1980.

15. Knowles, M. S. *The Modern Practice of Adult Education*. (Rev. ed.). Chicago: Association Press, 1980.
16. Krathwohl, D. R., Bloom, B. S., & Masia, B. B. *Taxonomy of Educational Objectives: The Classification of Educational Goals: Handbook II: Affective Domain*. New York: D. McKay, 1964.
17. Narrow, B. *Patient Teaching in Nursing Practice*. New York: Wiley, 1979.
18. Piaget, J. *The origins of intelligence in children*. (M. Cook, trans.) New York: International Universities Press, 1952, p. 142.
19. Rankin, S., & Duffy, K. L. *Patient Education: Issues, Problems and Guidelines*. Philadelphia: Lippincott, 1983.
20. Redman, B. *The Process of Patient Teaching in Nursing* (4th ed.). St. Louis: C. V. Mosby, 1980.
21. Reilly, D. E. *Behavioral Objectives: Evaluation in Nursing*. New York: Appleton-Century-Crofts, 1980.
22. Rogers, C. Significant learning: In therapy and education. *Educational Leadership*, 1959, *16*, 232–242.
23. Southern Council on Collegiate Education for Nursing. *Computer Technology and Nursing Education*. Atlanta, Ga.: SCCEN, 1984.
24. Spranger, E. *Types of Men*. New York: Stechert, 1928, p. 370.

## BIBLIOGRAPHY

Cross, K. P. *Adults as Learners*. San Francisco: Jossey-Bass, 1981.
delBueno, D. J. Competency-based education. *Nurse Educator*, 1978, *3*, 10–14.
deMeneses, M. Split brain theory: Implications for nurse educators. *Nursing Outlook*, 1980, *28*, 441–443.
Gronlund, N. E. *Individualizing Classroom Instruction*. New York: Macmillan, 1974.
Herje, P. A. Hows and whys of patient contracting. *Nurse Educator*, 1980, *5*, 30–34.
Hyman, R. T. *Ways of Teaching* (2nd ed.). Philadelphia: Lippincott, 1974.
Johnson, N. Teaching dental health to children. *Pediatric Nursing*, March/April 1978, 20–23.
Jones, P., & Oertel, W. Developing patient teaching objectives and techniques: A self-instructional-program. *Nurse Educator*, September & October 1977, *2*, 3–18.
Kaufman, J. S., & Woody, J. W. For patients with COPD: Better living through teaching. *Nursing '80*, 1980, *10*, 57–61.
Leighton, A. O. Ten steps to better patient teaching. *RN*, 1976, *39*, 76–79.
Linde, B.J., & Jany, N. M. Effect of a teaching program on knowledge and compliance of cardiac patients. *Nursing Research*, 1979, *28*, 282–286.
Luciano, K., & Shumsky, C. Pediatric Procedures—The explanation should always come first. *Nursing '75*, 1975, *5*, 49–52.
Mager, R. F. *Measuring Instructional Intent*. Belmond, Calif.: Lear Siegler, 1973.
Maslow, A. *Motivation and Personality*. New York: Harper & Row, 1954, p. 379.
McLagan, P. A. *Helping Others Learn*. Reading, Mass.: Addison-Wesley, 1978.
Milhollan, F., & Forisha, B. E. *From Skinner to Rogers*. Lincoln, Neb.: Professional Educators Publications, 1972.
Morris, L., Hitchcock, L., Kucera, J., & Vernon, K. Student-made, student-played games. *American Journal of Nursing*, 1980, *80*(10), 1816.
Mosston, M. *Teaching: From Command to Discovery*. Belmont, Calif.: Wadsworth, 1972.
National League of Nursing Education. *Standard Curriculum for Schools of Nursing*. Baltimore: Waverly Press, 1918, p. 6.
Pidgeon, V. Characteristics of children's thinking and implications for health teaching. *American Journal of Maternal-Child Nursing*, Spring 1977, *2*, 1–8.
Shafer, S. Teaching via the play-discussion group. *American Journal of Nursing*, 1977, *77*, 1960–1961.

Smith, C. E. Planning, implementing and evaluating learning experiences for adults. *Nurse Educator*, 1978, *3*, 31–36.

Sovie, M. D. Investigate before you educate. *Nurse Educator*, 1981, *6*, 17–22.

Squyre, W. D. *Patient Education: An Inquiry into the State of the Art.* New York: Springer-Verlag, 1980.

Tarnow, K. G. Working with adult learners. *Nurse Educator*, 1979, *4*, 34–40.

Thompson, D. Teaching the client about anticoagulants. *American Journal of Nursing*, 1982, *82*, 278.

Toth, J. C. Effect of structured preparation for transfer on patient anxiety on leaving coronary care unit. *Nursing Research*, 1980, *29*, 28–34.

Tough, A. M. *The Adult's Learning Projects.* Toronto: Ontario Institute for Studies in Education, 1971.

Treloar, D. M. Ready, Set—Go: Something is missing from pediatric pre-op preparation. *American Journal of Material—Child Nursing*, 1978, *3*, 50–51.

Zander, K. A., et al. (Eds.). *Practical Manual for Patient-Teaching.* St. Louis: C. V. Mosby, 1978.

# 11

# Decision-making Process: A Method for Selecting Alternatives within the Nursing Process

Although decision making is used in each step of the nursing process, the focus of presentation in this chapter will be on the planning and diagnosing steps of the nursing process. As professional nurses become increasingly independent in their practices, they make more complex decisions—decisions for which they are responsible and accountable. The decision-making process is useful in determining the relevance of assessment data, in facilitating the organization and analyses of data, in selecting appropriate interventions, and in evaluating the effectiveness of these interventions. Also, nurses are involved in managing the care of clients—individuals, families, and communities. Effective managers must of necessity be decision makers. The decision-making process is an integral part of management. Effective nurses distinguish themselves by their ability to reach logical decisions. Although nurses may be scholarly and have a caring attitude toward clients, they are ineffective as managers without the ability to reach timely decisions.

In this chapter, we will examine the characteristics of effective decision makers and different models of decision making. The relationship of decision making to problem solving and the nursing process will be explored.

Study of this chapter will help you to:

1. Define the decision-making process.
2. Explain the phases and conditions of the decision-making process.
3. Identify the characteristics of an effective decision maker.
4. Discuss the steps of the decision-making process.
5. Differentiate between individual and group decision making.
6. Describe the following decision-making models: Kepner-Tregoe, Bower, Easton, Vroom-Yetton, and Bailey and Claus.
7. Relate the decision-making process to the following processes: problem solving and nursing process.

## DECISION MAKING

A distinction needs to be made between decision making and problem solving. Many authors use these terms interchangeably. In Chapter 2 we said that problem solving involved a given situation, a desired situation, and the method of moving from one to the other. Inherent in problem-solving activities are decisions.

**Decision making** can be defined as a deliberate and systematic analysis used to select a particular course of action. Decision making usually involves a conscious choice on the part of the person. By making a choice, you come to a conclusion and select a particular course of action from two or more alternatives that are available. In some instances, that choice is not conscious. You may select a particular behavior pattern on the basis of habit or "rule of thumb." In this chapter, we will restrict our discussion of decision making to conscious choices in which a person perceives the alternatives and consciously makes a choice.

There is a tendency to focus on the final moment wherein the decision maker selects a course of action. For example, a decision is announced that a new branch of a local bank will be built in a particular part of the city. A decision has been made. This focus upon the final choice obscures the fact that decision making is in reality a process in which the choice of a particular solution represents only the final step. Investigation, analysis, deliberation, evaluation, and thought are involved[5,8,13] in the various steps in the decision-making process as well as the final choice of alternatives.

Decisions are more complex than they appear on the surface. For example, opening a new branch of a bank involves extensive analysis by the sales department, production, and several officials before the final choice of a site is made. Numerous subsequent decisions will be required in implementing the plan to construct the new branch.

Decision making is a much slower process than most people imagine. This slowness can be attributed to the analysis required in making an effective decision. **Analysis** is the act of isolating various elements that are associated with the primary concern, as well as the factoring of these variables as a basis for arriving at some type of judgment. To isolate various elements, one must consider carefully all the data that are collected about the primary concern. Inherent in the decision-making process are making judgments and choosing one among many options. These judgments and choices are based on an accurate knowledge base.

### Phases of Decision Making

There are three broad phases of the decision-making process: deliberation, evaluation, and thought.[5,8,13] During the deliberation phase, the decision maker uses inductive and deductive reasoning to organize and interpret isolated pieces of information. For example, if bank officials want to determine the most desirable site for the new branch, they may conduct surveys of area residents. They would then organize and interpret the responses to see if there was a need for a new branch. If there is, what would be the most desirable location? As many alternatives as possible would be generated. During the evaluation phase, statements about the focus area that were formulated in the deliberation phase are scrutinized, and hypotheses are developed. This means that decision making involves more than rational analysis of isolated facts. Judgment or intuition can be used in the process of assessing the importance of the information.

In the last phase, thought or discrimination, a careful selection of the best solution is made on the basis of an evaluation of alternatives.

## Conditions of Decision Making

Three conditions under which decisions are made have been described:[8,11] (1) When you know the outcome of each alternative course of action, decisions are made with certainty. An example would be the launching of a space shuttle. Actions are based on research and are fairly predictable. Several research studies conducted at different times and using different space shuttles would determine that if certain conditions exist particular events will happen. (2) If the chance of an outcome can be estimated, but you do not know the outcome with certainty, the decision is made under risk. For example, when you use established principles of communication, perception, and interpersonal relationships in your interactions with friends, you cannot be certain precisely how others will respond because of the unpredictability of human behavior. (3) When the outcomes are unknown and factors are uncontrolled, the decision is made with uncertainty. In major catastrophic situations, for example during an earthquake, you really cannot project the outcome of your decisions or control the effects that occur.

## Characteristics of Effective Decision Makers

Certain characteristics help to reduce the risk and uncertainty of making decisions. These characteristics include the ability to use selective perception, awareness, creativity, risk-taking, and to make value judgments that are based on facts.

**Selective perception** is the mental process that you use to select, categorize, and interpret data. For you to perceive data, you must be (1) alert and attentive, (2) able to detect a stimulus, (3) capable of receiving the stimulus into your sensory storage, and (4) able to interpret the processed data in your brain. Many times, perception is selective because the information may be in conflict with your personal values, attitudes, and beliefs. If, however, you validate your observations and inferences with others, you can increase the accuracy of your perceptions. (See Chapter 4 for additional information on selective perception.)

**Selective awareness** is a knowledge or perception that results from experiences, feelings, and exposure to ideas. As you accumulate knowledge, your awareness is enhanced, and your ability to make decisions improves.

**Creative thinking** is the ability to form an opinion that is novel and imaginative. This characteristic is required to devise solutions to problems. In regard to decision making, creative thinking assists you in making inferences from data and in seeing new patterns and relationships. Creativity develops when you are in close touch with your feelings and perceptions. By being in touch with yourself, you are open to new perceptions of what is occurring around you.

**Risk-taking** or trial-and-error behavior in thought often accompanies enhanced creativity. By accurately perceiving data, you are more inclined to be certain about the decisions you make and unafraid of taking a risk. When you allow yourself to take risks, you open yourself up to potential loss as well as potential growth. In other words, risk-taking can be painful as well as growth producing.

**Making value judgments** often is the basis on which the decision-making process is based. Values can be defined as the standards and principles that stem from one's beliefs about one's self and others. Although decisions are deliberate actions based on objective norms, standards, or criteria, they are still dependent on value judgments. Several authors agree that the beliefs and standards (values) that decision makers consider to have intrinsic worth are the basis of their judgments or decisions.[6,9,12,14] For example, if you were asked to list the things (places, persons, items) that you considered worthy of your effort, time, and money, you would have a list of "valuables" that you cherished. They are probably, consciously or unconsciously, the driving force behind the decisions you make. Any time you hear yourself say, "They should do . . . " or, "I really think it would be best if . . . ," you are expressing a value you cherish and feel should serve as the basis for decisions and actions.

*Values Are Learned.* Social learning theory states that we learn by what we see (observation) and by what we do (experience). This is the reason your choice of employment (a decision) is extremely important. When you observe particular behaviors in the work setting, you learn that this behavior is possible. If you have a strong, positive reaction to the behavior, you are likely to incorporate this behavior into your own life-style. When you decide to perform a behavior—after observing and experiencing it a couple random times—you receive either negative or positive feedback. This negative or positive feedback from yourself and others determines if you repeat the behavior. We have not mentioned the social system in which learning values occur. Individual, family, and community values have already had an influence on your decision making. Professional values are also learned and can influence the decisions you make. You learn these professional values by observations and experiences. The school you choose for learning and the place you choose for employment are extremely influential in shaping the professional value system that forms the basis for decision making. It is a consoling thought that values, even once learned, are subject to change through continuing growth and new learning.

Who you are and what you are influence the decisions you make. Several personal characteristics of effective decision makers have already been discussed. Some of these characteristics are professional integrity, humanistic concern and involvement, effectiveness in communication, effectiveness in problem solving, competence, sense of responsibility and accountability, and autonomy.

Up to this point, we have discussed decision making in general terms and have examined the characteristics of effective decision makers. Now we will take a look at the decision-making process itself.

## THE DECISION-MAKING PROCESS

The three phases of the decision-making process—deliberation, evaluation, and thought—[5,10,13] reflect the cognitive skills that are required to implement the decision-making process. These cognitive functions are activated through problem solving.

### Steps in Decision Making
First, we will discuss the five steps of the decision-making process that occur during the deliberation phase.

*Identify the Problem.* The stimulus for the decision-making process is an issue that surfaces and necessitates a decision. You become aware that something is wrong (reactive) or that adjustments need to be made for optimal functioning (proactive). On a daily basis, you are confronted with issues that are threatening and in need of preventive measures. You may lack adequate information needed to ensure effective functioning. Once the focal issue is identified, information about the problem needs to be collected.

***Collect Information.*** Wasting much time developing solutions to the wrong problems is of concern to many persons. Data collection is extremely important because it helps you see all facets of the problem. An exploration is made of the conditions calling for action. Questions may be posed such as: What characterizes the condition requiring a decision to be made? What are the attributes of the problem?

***Establish Objectives.*** After information has been collected about the nature of the problem, terminal and enabling objectives are established. These objectives direct the course of action and are stated in terms of effectiveness. To determine objectives, you need to ask these three questions: What do you want to accomplish by the decisions you make? Do you want to maintain anything by the decisions you make? What consequences do you wish to avoid by the decisions you make?

***List Alternatives.*** Whether you list the alternatives or merely think them through mentally, it is possible to brainstorm and come up with a number of alternatives. Every attempt should be made to generate as many alternatives as possible to avoid making a poor decision. It requires creativity to think of new solutions that capitalize on the positive aspects of several alternatives.

***Choose Decision Rules.*** Before completing the deliberation phase, a method for making decisions is selected. For example, you could use a 10-high scale for rating alternatives and projecting the numerical value that constitutes the basis for decision. When you use a scientific approach to decision making it is possible to consider several alternatives rather than jumping immediately to a conclusion concerning only one choice. Fortunately (or unfortunately), there are no set rules that are appropriate for making all decisions. You can, however, select a means of further analyzing the situation so that you can determine the best alternative for that given situation. In addition to a rating scale like the one mentioned in the previous example, you could develop criteria on which to base your decision. For instance, you could project (1) if the alternative involves minimal, moderate, or a great deal of personal risk taking; (2) if the alternative is minimally, moderately, or highly desirable in comparison to other alternatives; or (3) if the alternative has the potential of being minimally, moderately, or highly successful. In using this type of rule, it is necessary to weight criteria according to the significance to a particular situation. The weighting would vary from situation to situation although the criteria would remain the same.

The next four steps of the decision-making process comprise the evaluation phase.

***Analyze Optional Courses of Action.*** The analysis of alternatives as well as the consequences of the alternatives is done in relation to the objectives you established earlier. This analysis also reflects your personal values because the objectives are based on value judgments. This means that the criteria you consider important will differ from those of others. The method of analysis can be a trial-and-error approach, an intuitive approach, or a systematic and scientific approach. By using a decision rule such as the one described in an earlier step, you are more systematic in your approach and less likely to experience frustration, failure, and loss of time. Your knowledge and skills will increase your ability to analyze alternatives. To assist you in analyzing possible consequences, try to brainstorm the answers to the following questions.

1. What do you think could go wrong? List all the possible problems you can project as a result of this course of action.
2. What is the probability that each of these problems will occur? What impact will they have if they do occur?
3. What proactive measures can be taken to manage each potential obstacle?

**Rank Optional Courses of Action.** In this step you rank the possible alternatives according to how successful you think a particular course of action will be in achieving the objectives most efficiently and expediently. As you review the objectives, you will be able to separate those that are essential and most important in fulfilling the purpose from those that are desirable but not absolutely necessary. For example, if you have 10 objectives and are using the 10-high rating scale for the decision rule, the objectives ranked 1 through 5 would receive a high numerical value of 6 through 10. These objectives would constitute the essential and most important category. The greater your deliberation and analysis, the more effective your ranking will be and thus the more effective the decision. To select the most relevant course of action, you again could use the 10-high rule to rank the options and make a tentative choice that you feel best meets your objectives and fulfills your purpose.

**Select a Tentative Course of Action.** In this step you want to choose the course of action that will optimally meet the objectives. Before a decision is made and the actual course of action is implemented, however, it is important to test the tentative course of action. You need to determine how well each alternative meets each criterion. In using the 10-high decision rule, this would be determined by multiplying the rating of each objective by the rating of each alternative course of action. Then you would total the scores for each alternative and compare the results. The choice occurs when you select one alternative with its consequences over the others, based on this systematic method. Prior testing is important because your knowledge of consequences may be somewhat fragmented. Consequences reside in the future and it is impossible to anticipate them accurately.

**Determine Alliances.** It is helpful to determine people in support of your tentative decision. What do others think about the proposed course of action? Decision making is a group process and seldom is restricted solely to the decision maker. It is important to consider the people that will be affected by the tentative decision. Will they be satisfied as a result of the proposed action? The success and effectiveness of the decision also may rely heavily on those who will be asked to provide necessary financial and material support. It is important to include the people who will be affected by or involved in implementing the decision. On the other hand, a wise move may be to find out who opposes the tentative course of action. You can use their feedback to further analyze the usefulness of the tentative decision, or you may have the opportunity to persuade those in opposition to support your efforts.

The final phase of the decision-making process—thought—encompasses the last three steps necessary to arrive at a decision.

**Determine a Course of Action.** Based upon systematic deliberation and evaluation you have completed the planning step. At this point you are now ready to decide what is the choice of action. You deliberately choose one of the alternatives you generated earlier as the one you think will best achieve desired outcomes. The tentative course of action becomes a reality as the means to achieve the designated end.

***Implement the Decision.*** During implementation, the decision is carried out. It is important to continue to search for cues to analyze the changes resulting from the decision during this step. It is helpful to continue gathering additional information and reassess your choice of alternatives. All inputs are important to determine the reliability and validity of the chosen course of action. Do the people involved seem satisfied? You should continue to make judgments concerning the effects of implementing the particular decision.

***Evaluate the Effectiveness of the Decision.*** In this final step of the decision-making process, it is important to determine if all of your efforts worked. Did the decision cost too much to implement? Was the decision successful in achieving the stated objectives? Evaluation is the valid measurement of the effectiveness of the decision to achieve predetermined objectives. The approach used to implement the decision also is evaluated. Perhaps collaboration was not done often enough and unpredicted consequences resulted that could have been prevented. Essentially, what occurs in this final step is a reappraisal of the entire decision-making process. You may discover that you lacked additional information needed to come up with better alternatives.

The three phases of decision making have several commonalities and represent an interrelated cycle of events. All three phases suggest a cycle (1) search for alternatives that requires deliberate action and ordering, (2) analysis and evaluation of alternatives and their consequences to formulate an answer to circumstances needing action, (3) selection of the best alternative for a particular situation, and (4) exploration for new information to alter the original situation requiring a decision.

Now that we have discussed the steps of the decision-making process, we will examine the differences between individual and group decision making.

## Individual versus Group Decision Making

We have focused on individual decision making up to this point. It is equally important that you understand the dynamics of group decision making. A **group** is defined as two or more people who can be identified as having a common purpose and who act as one unit. Group members are interdependent in achieving a particular goal. Although types of groups may vary, their functions and problems are similar. Some groups are formally structured and meet over an extended period of time. Other groups may meet only for the length of time it takes to complete an assigned task.

You are more effective in group decision making if you possess a knowledge of group dynamics. A knowledge of group process also facilitates cohesion. When you understand how a group functions and what your role is, you are more likely to make constructive contributions. Also, there is less tendency to feel manipulated by social pressures.

***Characteristics of a Group.*** All groups have some similar characteristics. Three characteristics distinguish an effective group from an ineffective one—cohesiveness, cooperation, and commitment.

**Cohesiveness** is the quality of sticking together. This characteristic describes the magnetic drawing power the group has on its members. Members find the group appealing and as a result they are motivated to work together. Belonging to the group meets personal needs of the members. An example of group cohesiveness is shown when a disaster occurs and people band together because they have shared similar experiences.

**Cooperation** is the joint action of one person with another. This characteristic refers to the participation and interaction patterns of members as they work together. The quality of interaction can be described in terms of the amount of conversation, the directional flow of communicated messages, and the balance between listeners and speakers.

**Commitment** is a pledge or vow to a particular cause or course of action. In a group the commitment is in reference to the goal that group members desire to achieve. Members are also committed to each other as they work together to meet each other's needs. Members develop a sense of purpose when they are committed. Commitment implies that strong intrinsic motivation is present to propel members toward each other and toward the established goal.

Groups experience similar problems regardless of the type or composition. We will examine the expressions and causes of three of the most common group problems: lack of agreement, lack of interest, and ineffective decision making.

**Lack of agreement** is expressed in the following ways:

1. Members become impatient with one another and attack ideas before they are completely expressed.
2. Members take sides, refuse to compromise, and cannot arrive at a consensus about plans and suggestions.
3. Members are very intense and emotional when they make contributions or react to the comments of others.
4. Members feel the group cannot function because of lack of knowledge and experience to accomplish a task or because of the size of the group.
5. Members hear only parts of other members' contributions.

There are several possible reasons for lack of agreement within groups.

1. The group was given an overwhelming task which frustrates the members, and causes them to feel inadequate to meet the demands requested of them. This problem frequently happens when the group is a committee of a larger organization. The task seems insurmountable because there are not enough members or because the charge is unclear.
2. The primary concern of some members is to attain status within the group. Although the group is working on some task, members use the task as a means of competing for power. Members establish cliques or attempt to suppress certain people. When this occurs, certain members oppose one another on issues without reasonable cause.
3. Members feel involved and work hard on a problem. Members frequently exhibit impatience, irritation, or disagreement because they feel strongly about the issue being discussed. They fight for a certain plan because it is important to them—this fight may take the form of irritation with others because they refuse to go along with a suggestion which (to the member) is the best one. As long as there is a clearly understood goal and continuing movement toward resolving a problem, this kind of fighting contributes to effective decision making.

**Lack of interest** is another frequent problem experienced by groups. Members may display a range of behaviors. For example, members may act completely indifferently to the task and show evidence of marked boredom. Lack of interest may take the form of a decrease in genuine enthusiasm for the task, a failure to exert much energy, a lack of persistence, and contentment with poor work. Lack of interest is expressed in the following ways:

1. Members yawn frequently, slouch in their seats, and are restless.
2. There is minimum participation as well as frequent lulls in the conversation.
3. Members arrive late, are frequently absent, and do not make necessary preparations for meetings.
4. The group makes decisions too quickly.
5. Members are reluctant to assume responsibility and fail to follow through on decision making.

Common reasons for lack of interest are:

1. The assigned task does not seem important to the members, or it is less important than other problems on which they would prefer to work.
2. The group has inadequate procedures for making a decision.
3. Members feel they do not have power to influence final decisions.

**Ineffective decision making** is the final group problem we will discuss. Ineffective decision making is expressed in the following ways:

1. Members have difficulty in deciding anything. When they do decide, their decisions are made too rapidly and at the last minute.
2. The group is not clear as to what the decision is. Members disagree about where the consensus is and leave decision making to the leader.
3. Members refuse responsibility and allow the discussion to wander.

Common reasons for ineffective decision making are:

1. The decision was too difficult or the leader called for a decision prematurely.
2. The decision area presents a threat to the group.
3. The group lacks confidence and cohesiveness.

Since the focus of this chapter is on decision making, we will examine this final group problem more closely. It is important to realize that group decision making is beneficial for two reasons. First, the knowledge, experience, and talents of all group members are mobilized to accomplish the task. The pooling of resources results in higher quality decisions than if any one member made the decision alone. Second, group decision making benefits the members by giving them a sense of accomplishment. This sense of ownership promotes commitment to the decision.

To increase the effectiveness of group decision making, you must first diagnose the problem (ineffective decision making). After the problem is diagnosed, data about the group are collected: What is the group's basic problem for which information is needed? Of the pertinent information, what is most important? What is the minimum of essential material the group needs?

Observation is probably the simplest method to use for data collection on a group. A simple check list can be used to summarize your observations. Categories of observations could be (1) the leader's actions, (2) the members' contributions, (3) the overall emotional climate of the group, and (4) a summary and analysis of the group's activities including goals, methods, accomplishments, and quality of work.

Goals should be evaluated to determine if they are realistic and specific enough to give direction to the group. Goals need to be relevant to the members so they will be motivated to participate. It is important that group goals are adapted to emerging needs of the group. To prevent diversion, the goals should be kept at hand so each member has a clear understanding of them.

The methods used to assist the group in making decisions should be flexible, but not so flexible that the group loses sight of its task. It is important that individual needs are satisfied and group productivity achieved. Once the group makes the decision, reviewing the entire process is important so revisions can be made.

We have examined individual and group decision making, and now we are ready to look at some decision-making models that can be used by individuals and groups.

## Decision-making Models

Numerous decision-making models have been developed to guide people in making effective decisions. Outlined in Table 11–1 are five models that were developed by different authors to explain the decision-making process. Although the decision-making models vary as to the number and description of the steps, six elements are similar in all five. Each model provides for the (1) need to make a decision, the objective or goal of a decision, or the identified problem calling for a decision; (2) generation of alternatives; (3) analysis of alternatives; (4) selection of a choice or decision; (5) implementation of the decision; and (6) evaluation of the effectiveness of the decision.

Of these six elements, three stages emerge that represent the analytical processes involved in the formation of a decision—the identifying, generating, and testing stages. *The identifying stage* comprises problem recognition, goals and objectives, identification, and diagnosis. The cognitive processes operating in this stage are recognition, identification, and analysis. These processes operate to establish meaningful patterns of relationships among isolated data that are collected prior to the identifying stage. There are several approaches you can take to analyze the problem once it has been recognized and identified. You can seek to identify or isolate the factor(s) involved in the problem. These factors may need to be considered in defining the problem. You may compare the problem under study with the experiences of others. What have others done in similar situations? You may use an implicit or explicit rule or standard to analyze the problem. What should be, ought to be, or must be the standard? Lastly, you may analyze the problem by considering the probable type of consequences which will follow a particular course of action.

*The generating stage* comprises the search for alternative solutions and the listing of alternatives. The cognitive processes operating in this stage are inquiry, synthesis, and ideation. Ideation triggers the generation of alternatives. Ideas are generated by matching the known problem with data derived from the identifying stage.

*The testing stage* encompasses evaluating all possible alternatives that were generated during the second stage, considering the consequences of each alternative, and selecting a tentative course of action. The cognitive processes operating during this final stage are testing, evaluating, and selecting. The Decision Analysis plan, developed by Kepner, Tregoe, Inc., a New Jersey-based consulting firm, can help you make choices.[7]

**TABLE 11–1. COMPARISON OF DECISION-MAKING MODELS**

| Kepner & Tregoe[a] (1965) | Bower[b] (1972, 1977) | Easton[c] (1973) | Vroom & Yetton[d] (1973) | Bailey & Claus[e] (1975) |
|---|---|---|---|---|
| 1. Establish objectives<br>2. Classify objectives as to importance | 1. Determine what blocks goal attainment | 1. Recognize need for change<br>2. Diagnose the problem<br>3. Identify affected interest groups; define decision objectives; assign numerical weights to objectives | 1. Consider problem attributes<br>2a. Determine type of problem | 1. Overall needs and goals<br>2. Define problem<br>3. Determine constraints and capabilities<br>4. Specify approach<br>5. Establish objectives |
| 3. Develop alternative actions<br>4. Evaluate alternatives against objectives | 2. Generate possible solutions<br>3. Determine consequences of each solution<br>4. Estimate likelihood of consequences occurring<br>5. Determine desirability and risk of each consequence | 4. Identify all feasible alternatives<br>5. Predict and evaluate outcomes for alternatives | 2b. Determine feasible set of alternatives | 6. List solutions<br><br>7. Analyze options |
| 5. Tentative decision is alternative that best meets the objectives<br>6. Explore tentative decision for future possible adverse consequences<br>7. Take action to prevent adverse consequences, and make sure decision is carried out | 6. Choose best solution | 6. Select a rule for choosing<br>7. Compute and make choice<br><br>8. Implement | 3. Apply decision rules<br>4. Choose best alternative<br><br>5. Implement decision | 8. Choose; apply decision rules<br><br>9. Control and implement decision<br><br>10. Evaluate effectiveness of action |

*(From Bernhard & Walsh, 1981, p. 115, with permission.[2])*
[a] See reference 7.
[b] See reference 3.
[c] See reference 4.
[d] See reference 16.
[e] See reference 1.

You must first state your goal, then divide your objectives into "musts" and "wants." Musts are criteria that each choice has to meet; wants are those that would be nice but are not essential. Instead of comparing one alternative with another, you compare each possibility with your original list of "musts" and "wants." This method allows you to limit your choices and keep your goals in mind. After a tentative course of action is selected, it is implemented and evaluated. (Fig. 11–1.)

The decision-making process has been presented as a three stage cognitive process that is part of the planning and diagnosing steps of the nursing process. Although the assessing, implementing, and evaluating steps are part of the decision-making process, the emphasis was placed on the planning and diagnosing steps. Next, we will discuss how the decision-making process relates to the problem-solving process and the nursing process.

## APPLICATION OF THE DECISION-MAKING PROCESS

Knowledge of the phases, conditions, and steps of the decision-making process will enhance your understanding of the interrelatedness of decision making and problem solving and the nursing process.

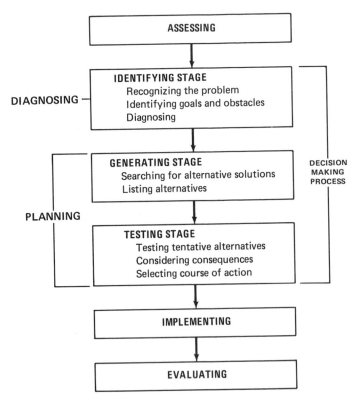

**Figure 11–1.** Analysis of the decision-making process.

## Relationship to the Problem-solving Process

Both decision making and problem solving use the rational and intuitive modes.[15] The **intuitive mode** has greater flexibility and is based on intuition, values, and feelings. The **rational mode** is based on a set of logical relationships among problems, solutions, actions, and so forth. The relationships are used as a means of clarifying, structuring, and ordering ideas. It is not necessary to apply them in a systematic fashion. It is possible to alternate between idea generation (intuitive mode) and idea structuring (rational mode). For example, you could start brainstorming and loosely explore all possible ideas about a particular situation. This action permits you to freely use the intuitive mode. After you clarify relationships between ideas, you can switch to the rational mode to structure and refine your ideas. The intuitive and rational modes are complementary.

In Chapter 2, problem solving was presented as a method of proceeding from a given situation to a different situation. In other words, problem solving is the method of achieving a solution to a problem. Decision making is also a method. It enables you to make choices between alternative courses of action. Both processes can be used to solve problems. Two types of problems are restructuring and straightforward. The restructuring type of problem could be solved by both processes if the rational mode were used.

Now that we have established relationships between decision making and problem solving, we will examine the relationship between decision making and the nursing process.

## Relationship to the Nursing Process

Decisions are made throughout the nursing process. Earlier we said that the focus of presentation was on the planning and diagnosing steps. Now all of the steps of the nursing process will be discussed in relationship to the decision-making process (Fig. 11–1).

*Assessing.* The decision-making process is used to decide what variables will be assessed. Decisions are also made as to when an assessment needs to be performed and what tools should be used. The assessing phase of the nursing process and the deliberation phase of the decision-making process involve searching. Both processes examine conditions requiring some type of action. The processes also are instrumental in identifying alternatives and their consequences.

*Diagnosing.* In the nursing process, a nursing diagnosis is made from data. The diagnosing step is similar to the evaluation or judgment step of the decision-making process. Decisions are necessary to determine what information is relevant and if the problem is a potential or actual threat. Judgments are required throughout the diagnosing step. Judgments are used to determine inconsistencies and gaps in the data. A decision must be made as to whether intervention is needed. During this phase, you must decide whether the client's response is healthy or unhealthy. Also, it is necessary to decide where the focus of decision making rests—with the nurse, the client, or both.

*Planning.* In the planning phase of the nursing process, goals are linked with the means to achieve them. This phase relates to the thought or choice phase of the decision process. Both processes involve group dynamics and are more effective when mutual planning occurs. Decision making is used to establish priorities and to determine what framework to use. Decisions concerning the prognosis of each nursing diagnosis and appropriate alternative courses of action are selected by applying the decision-making process.

*Implementing.* During the implementing step, the choice made in the previous planning stage becomes a deliberate action and is used to achieve a goal. The methods used to implement care require decisions, and continual analysis and decisions are made to determine the effects of the implementations. Decisions also are made concerning who will implement nursing actions and when implementation will occur. If families are to be involved, decisions are needed to determine how much involvement to allow.

*Evaluating.* In the evaluating step of the nursing process, the deliberate action that was implemented is measured for effectiveness. The decision-making process is used to make judgments, select the proper tool, determine realistic objectives, and decide what revisions are necessary.

## SUMMARY

The decision-making process is emphasized in the planning and diagnosing steps of the nursing process. Decision making is a deliberate and systematic method of choosing an alternative. The three phases of the decision-making process—deliberation, evaluation, and thought—relate very closely to the problem-solving process and the nursing process. The phases of the decision-making process are divided into steps that are cyclic and interrelated.

Decisions are made by groups as well as individuals. The nurse, therefore, needs to be knowledgeable about the role and functions of group members. Effective groups have three identifiable attributes—cohesiveness, cooperation, and commitment. Ineffective groups experience three common problems—lack of agreement, lack of interest, and ineffective decision making. Groups can become more effective if measures are taken to avoid these three problems.

## STUDY GUIDE

1. Attend a small group meeting. Perform an assessment using the information given in this chapter. Diagnose the group's problem and determine measures that will make the group function more effectively.
2. Discuss ways you can use the decision-making process to improve client care.
3. Identify three characteristics you possess that help you make effective decisions. Identify three characteristics that hinder you from making effective decisions.
4. Read one current nursing journal about decision making. List the steps the author used to make an effective decision.

## REFERENCES

1. Bailey, J. T., & Claus, K. E. *Decision-Making in Nursing.* St. Louis: C. V. Mosby, 1975.
2. Bernhard, L. A., & Walsh, M. *Leadership: The Key to the Professionalization of Nursing.* New York: McGraw-Hill, 1981.

3. Bower, F. L. *The Process of Planning Nursing Care: A Theoretical Model.* St. Louis: C. V. Mosby, 1972.
4. Easton, A. *Complex Managerial Decisions Involving Multiple Objectives.* New York: Wiley, 1973.
5. Griffith, J. W., & Christensen, P. J. *Nursing Process: Application of Theories, Frameworks, and Models.* St. Louis: C. V. Mosby, 1982.
6. Hawley, R. C., & Hawley, I. L. *Human Values in the Classroom: A Handbook for Teachers.* New York: Hart Publishing Co., 1975, pp. 210–211.
7. Kepner, C. H., & Tregoe, B. B. *The Rational Manager.* New York: McGraw-Hill, 1965.
8. Longenecker, J. G. *Principles of Management and Organizational Behavior.* Columbus, Ohio: Chas. E. Merrill, 1964.
9. Matson, H. N. Values: How and from where? *Nursing Digest,* September 1974, *46,* 36–38.
10. McFarland, G., Leonard, H., & Morris, M. *Nursing Leadership and Management.* New York: Wiley Medical, 1984.
11. Mitchell, P. H., & Loustau, A. *Concepts Basic to Nursing.* New York: McGraw-Hill, 1981.
12. Rubinstein, M. F. *Patterns of Problem Solving.* Englewood Cliffs, N.J.: Prentice-Hall, 1975, pp. 474–476.
13. Schaefer, J. The interrelationship of decision making and the nursing process. *American Journal of Nursing,* October 1974, *74* (10), 1852–1855.
14. Smith, D. W. The effect of values on clinical teaching. In J. A. Williamson (Ed.), *Current Perspectives in Nursing Education.* St. Louis: C. V. Mosby, 1976, p. 93.
15. Stone, S., Firsich, S., Gordon, S., et al. *Management for Nurses* (3rd ed.). St. Louis: C. V. Mosby, 1984.
16. Vroom, V. A new look at managerial decision making. *Organizational Dynamics,* 1973, *1,* 66–80.

# BIBLIOGRAPHY

Barnard, C. The environment of decision. *Journal of Nursing Administration,* 1982, *12* (3), 25–29.

Bernhard, L. A., & Walsh, M. *Leadership: The Key to the Professionalization of Nursing.* New York: McGraw-Hill, 1981.

Claus, K., & Bailey, J. Facilitating change: A problem solving decision making tool. *Nursing Leadership,* 1979, *2,* 30–39.

del Bueno, D. J. Doing the right thing: Nurse's ability to make clinical decisions. *Nurse Educator,* Autumn 1983, *8* (3), 7–11.

del Bueno, D. J. Values enrich nurses' role, complicate decision making. *Hospital Progress,* May 1983, *64* (5), 22–25.

Ehrat, K. S. A model for politically astute planning and decision making. *Journal of Nursing Administration,* September 1983, *13* (9), 29–35.

Francoeur, R. T. Teaching decision-making skills in biomedical ethics for the allied health student. *Journal of Allied Health,* August 1983, *12* (3), 202–209.

LaMonica, E., & Finch, F. Managerial decision making. *Journal of Nursing Administration,* 1977, *7,* 20–22.

Lane, I., Mathews, P., Chancy, C., et al. Making the goals of acceptance and quality explicit: Effects on group decision. *Small Group Behavior,* 1982, *13* (4), 542–554.

McKay, P. S. Interdependent decision making: Redefining professional autonomy. *Nurse Administration Quarterly,* Summer 1983, *7* (4), 21–30.

Pryor, T. A., et. al. The HELP system. *Journal of Medical Systems,* April 1983, *7* (2), 87–102.

Sampson, E., & Marthas, M. *Group Process for the Health Professions* (2nd ed.) New York: Wiley, 1981.

Schweiger, J. *The Nurse as Manager.* New York: Wiley, 1980.

Tappan, R. M. *Nursing Leadership: Concepts and Practice.* Philadelphia: F. A. Davis, 1983.

Taylor, A. G. The decision-making process and the nursing administrator. *Nursing Clinics of North America*, September 1983, *18* (3), 439–470.

# 12

# The Change Process: A Method for Promoting Planned Change within Nursing Practice

Professional nurses are involved in the process of change every time they assist their clients toward a higher level of health. In this chapter, the process of planned change will be discussed in relationship to its use with individual, family, and community clients. Specific theories will be explored to illustrate the use of theory in planning change, and the role and functions of the nurse as change agent will be examined. Lastly, we will look at the relationship of planned change to the nursing process—especially during the planning and implementing steps.

Study of this chapter will help you to:

1. Define planned change as it relates to the role of the professional nurse.
2. Describe the different levels, cycles, and phases of planned change.
3. Discuss different theories of change that may be used in the care of individual, family, and community clients.
4. Identify the characteristics and functions of the professional nurse who assumes the role of a change agent.
5. Assess the need for planned change in the practice setting.
6. Diagnose conditions that require planned change.
7. Plan the outcomes of planned change.
8. Implement planned change strategies while caring for individual, family, and community clients.
9. Evaluate the effectiveness of the change model.
10. Recommend revisions and methods for stabilizing planned change.

## THE CONCEPT OF PLANNED CHANGE

We will be focusing on **planned change**, which is a deliberate action that has as its goal the modification of the present structure and process of a social system. This planned modification requires people within the social system to relearn how to perform their roles.[7] The more complex the change, the less likely that others will accept it. If, therefore, the change fits the particular situation psychologically, culturally, and socially others are more likely to accept it.

In contrast, **unplanned change** refers to changes or modifications that take place without being wanted. The outcomes of the modifications are not intentional and are unpredictable. Unplanned change is upsetting to most people because it cannot be anticipated.

To enact planned change, it is important for you to understand the consequences and characteristics of planned change. This knowledge will enable you to prepare for possible resistance to change, to avoid or surpass barriers to change—whether these barriers are the attitudes of others or fiscal constraints—and to accomplish your goal of achieving planned change.

## Consequences of Planned Change

It is possible to forecast the consequences of planned change. These consequences may be viewed as the positive and negative outcomes one might expect, the positive and negative effects upon people involved in the change, and the significance such a planned change would have upon all concerned. An example would be: a university wishes to change from a quarter system to a semester system (the planned change). The developers of the proposal may list the money the university would save in copying syllabi less frequently, in decreasing registration expenses, and so forth (consequences). The modifications and changes have the potential of being beneficial or detrimental. Many changes are reversible, or they may be discontinued if not effective. Their consequences, therefore may be considered temporary.

## Characteristics of Planned Change

It may be helpful to think of the term *characteristics* as individual or distinctive attributes of planned change. Eight characteristics of planned change will be discussed.

*Advantages.* Planned change provides certain advantages. There are no reasons to change existing actions or circumstances if there are not at least some advantages. To determine if the planned change is needed, you may ask yourself these questions: Will this change provide a benefit that is not covered by existing ideas? Does the planned change provide the needed improvement? Have others also identified both the planned change and the needed improvement?

*Social Relationships.* Planned change has an impact on social relationships. Effective interaction skills are essential to encourage dissemination of the change. To determine mine the impact of the planned change, you may ask yourself the following questions: Will it be necessary to establish new interaction patterns? Will it be important to form new relationships? Will new roles be created as a result of the planned change?

*Divisibility.* Planned change is more effective when divisibility is present. Before a wide-scale change is implemented, it is wise to test it out on a smaller scale. This is important even though the change has been well planned in advance of implementation. For example, you will see planned change occurring in a large department store in one section at a time rather than in all sections simultaneously. It is important to ask yourself these questions: Is it possible to try the planned change on a trial basis? Can the planned change be tested on a limited scale?

*Reversibility.* Planned change is more effective when it is reversible. This characteristic is important because you may not be able to forecast all the consequences of the planned change. In the event you discover the planned change is not going to be a beneficial one once implementation occurs, you would want to be able to terminate the action and return to the original state. The following questions are useful in determining reversibility: Can the planned change be discontinued? Will there be permanent consequences as a result of the planned change?

*Implementation.* Planned change is more successful when the implementation is not complex. Often a planned change fails because only the designer of the plan understands it well. The persons directly involved in implementing the planned change have not been adequately prepared for the implementation. To avoid this dilemma, it would help to ask yourself: Will the planned change be too complex to implement? Will it be difficult to communicate the planned change to others because of its complexity?

*Target Population.* Planned change is more effective when it is compatible with the target population. Often your planned changes will involve working with individuals and groups. Their involvement in implementing the plan will ensure that the planned change continues. Persons within a group adhere to varying attitudes, values, and beliefs that merely conflict with the change you plan to implement. To determine if your change "fits" the target population, you need to ask: Is the planned change consistent with the target group's values? Will the change be sympathetic to the group's beliefs?

*Communication.* Planned change is more effective when communication needs are considered. Again, communication is of utmost importance in implementing planned change. The more difficulty you have in communicating, the less likely that the change will succeed. The characteristic is closely linked with the complexity of the change. It is more difficult to communicate highly complex ideas. The following questions will assist you in determining the communicability of the planned change: Can the change be conveyed by word of mouth? Does the planned change require a working knowledge of new terminology?

*Time Factors.* Planned change is effective when the time factor is considered. On paper the planned change may appear to be highly useful. If an effective planned change is not implemented at the correct time or at the correct pace, however, it will not be as effective. You should therefore ask yourself: Is this the best time to implement this planned change? After implementation occurs, this question is important to consider: Is the planned change occurring too rapidly?

Now that we have discussed the possible consequences and some of the characteristics of planned change let us explore the process of change.

## THE PROCESS OF PLANNED CHANGE

The word **process** refers to the dynamic movement of bringing about a change. The movement is in a specific direction, which is determined by the source, the goals, and way in which the change is implemented. In order to implement change effectively, you need to consider the levels, cycles, phases, and strategies of change.

## Levels of Planned Change

Four levels of change have been described by Hersey and Blanchard.[1] These levels are changes in knowledge, changes in attitude, changes in behavior, and changes in performance.

*Changes in knowledge* result from acquiring new information and intellectual skills. Every effort should be made to gain new knowledge as it becomes available. What you read has the potential of changing your knowledge. As you gain new information, from multiple sources, the intellectual skills of synthesizing and analyzing become more efficient.

*Changes in attitude* refer to altering one's value system and are more difficult to accomplish. You must plan for a change in attitude before an individual or a group will be receptive to what you have to say.

*Changes in behavior* are more difficult to bring about. Modifying behavior involves unlearning one behavior in order that another one can be learned. It can be very threatening to people when they are asked to change a behavior. Supportive measures are important if you desire consistent behavior after a change is implemented. Changes in the performance of groups or organizations are the most difficult to accomplish because the behaviors are more ingrained.

## Cycles of Planned Change

Cycles of change must also be considered before a change is implemented. Hersey and Blanchard[1] described two change cycles: directive change and participative change.

A **directive change cycle** is one that is imposed on a target population by an external force. In a directive change cycle, the target population is not involved in any part of the decision to change the behavior. There are times when the directive cycle may be the most effective one to use. This cycle is most effective when used with persons who are seen as dependent, less motivated, less knowledgeable, and less willing to assume responsibility.

People using the directive cycle are significantly more powerful than those with whom they are working. Although this cycle can be implemented in a shorter period of time, the change is maintained only for the length of time that it is enforced. This type of cycle tends to provoke hostility and resistance within the target population.

In most instances, a participative change cycle may be more effective in attempts to modify behavior than the directive change cycle. A **participative change cycle** begins when new information is made available to the target population. The next step is when a decision is made to (1) accept the new information, (2) determine what behaviors are to be changed, and (3) decide the best way to bring about these behavior changes. In contrast to the directive cycle, the participative cycle is more effective with people who are motivated, independent, knowledgeable, and responsible.

People using the participative cycle are more effective if their levels of expertise and knowledge are perceived by others as equal to or greater than those with whom they are working. It takes more time to accomplish change using the participative cycle, but there is a greater commitment to the change, and it tends to last longer.

## Phases of Planned Change

The phases of planned change propel movement toward the identified goal. Lewin[3] and Schein[6] identified three phases in the change process: unfreezing, changing, and refreezing. Knowledge of these phases will help you to decide how the levels and cycles inter-act at different times during the change process.

The *unfreezing phase* is aimed at motivating a person to accept the proposed change. This desired readiness implies that one sees a need to change one's behavior and is ready to change. During this phase, information must be provided that will en-able one to see the projected change as more positive than previously believed. People need to become aware of behavior that is incongruent with the goal of the change, and assumptions that directed their previous behavior may have to be altered. This phase is cognitive in nature because the person is exposed to the idea that change needs to occur. The person asks this question: What is wrong? This question is a form of diagnos-ing the problem. Once the problem is identified, the person must determine the best solution among many alternatives. According to Lewin's theory, three possible mecha-nisms give the initial impetus to create change—lacking confirmation, inducing guilt–anxiety, or creating psychological safety. In other words, the person becomes aware of the need to change because: (1) the person's expectations have not been met (lack of confirmation), (2) the person is uncomfortable about some particular action or inaction (guilt–anxiety), or (3) a previous barrier to the change has been removed (psychological safety).

The *changing phase* is comprised of two methods of changing: identification and in-ternalization.[1] After one is motivated to change, one is open to receiving information that will help change behavior. Identification takes place when one learns the desired behavior changes from a resource person. Internalization takes place when the environ-ment is changed in ways that require use of the new behaviors to function effectively.

In this second phase of change—the actual changing—the person develops new re-sponses based on collected information. The person seeks this information to clarify and identify the problem. According to Lewin, looking at the problem from a new perspec-tive (cognitive redefinition) occurs through identification. During identification, an es-pecially knowledgeable, respected, or powerful resource person influences the individ-ual's decision as to possible modes for solving the problem. During this second phase of planned change, the change is mapped out in detail and then initiated. (Strategies as well as other details about this particular phase are discussed later.)

The *refreezing phase* results when the new behavior is incorporated into one's life-style. New behavior must be reinforced to maintain the change and to prevent it from becoming extinct. In groups, refreezing must take place within each member as well as within the group as a whole. Maintaining change in a group will not take place until the new behavior becomes part of the norms and standards for that particular group.

During this final phase of change, people involved in the change integrate the idea into their own value system—the change becomes integrated and stabilized. The change is so much a part of themselves that it is perpetuated.

Lewin also spoke of forces that either facilitated or impeded the process of planned change. The forces that facilitated change were referred to as driving forces; the forces that impeded change were referred to as restraining forces. When driving forces are identified in a planned change, they can be consciously used to an advantage. In con-trast, it is just as important to note the restraining forces so that they can be either avoided altogether or modified so they will not interfere with the planned change.

## Strategies of Planned Change

Plans of actions that bring about unfreezing, changing, and refreezing are referred to as **strategies of planned change**. The master plan or strategy you develop will be comprised of various tactics. These **tactics** are activities aimed at implementing the different parts of the overall plan.

Both strategies and tactics are dependent on the goal of the planned change. Some general guidelines may assist you to develop effective strategies and tactics.

1. Strategies should incorporate the general principles from the levels and cycles. For example, strategies need to be developed for people to acquire knowledge, take on new attitudes and values, and incorporate new behaviors into their lifestyle. These strategies flow from the level of change. If you are using the participative cycle, it would be important to develop strategies that would imply that the individual has an active role in making decisions and planning the change.
2. The cost of implementing the change should be considered in developing strategies. For temporary changes, it would be impractical to plan expensive changes.
3. The time element should be taken into account. The strategies should reflect whether the change will be a gradual, slow one over a long period of time or a rapid change over a short period of time.
4. The scope and magnitude of the planned change should be considered before strategies are formulated. Will this change take place in one state or will the entire nation be affected?
5. The resources necessary to implement the planned change need to be projected. Will the planned change require additional personnel? Will more space be required? What about supplies, materials, and equipment?

To begin the unfreezing phase of planned change, several strategies may be useful. It is important for a target population that is about to become involved in the planned change to modify their attitudes and acquire knowledge. A beneficial strategy may be to hold up an ideal model of another target population that has successfully undergone the planned change. Another effective strategy may be to ask for volunteers to participate in the planned change on a trial basis. Regardless of the strategy that is used during the unfreezing phase, it should be kept in mind that the intent of this phase is to create a disequilibration. Extreme strategies that promote defensiveness and resistance, however, will be destructive because they could impede the planned change.

During the changing phase of planned change, there may be problems in providing positive reinforcement for new behaviors. Strategies that are directed toward identifying meaningful rewards are necessary. Also, strategies aimed at creating an environment that is supportive, nonthreatening, and educative are germane to this phase.

We stated that refreezing involved stabilizing the change and incorporating the new behaviors into the value system of the target population. Some strategies that may be effective during this phase are positive feedback and constructive remarks.

Strategies also need to be devised to maintain a balance between the driving and restraining forces. Change occurs when the driving forces are increased while at the same time the restraining forces are decreased. For example, a strategy that may increase the strength of the driving forces could be the provision of support and guidance; a strategy that may decrease the strength and number of restraining forces could be frequent meetings that allow for open discussion.

Now that we have discussed the process of change, we will examine the role of the change agent in bringing about effective change.

# THE ROLE OF THE CHANGE AGENT IN NURSING

Today, nurses must make many difficult decisions about the health care extended to clients, families, and communities. An awareness of this responsibility will compel you to implement change to better serve clients. One who assists members of a social system to modify their own behavior or that of the system is called a **change agent**. It is possible for you to function as a change agent regardless if you are in a staff nurse position or an official leadership position. When you work with members of the health team to change attitudes, circumstances, and behavior you act as a change agent.

## Functions of the Change Agent

When nurses take on the role of change agent, they perform many functions. These functions involve problem solving and decision making, as well as interpersonal competency. Change agents are not given a job description with a listing of what they are to do. Some key words, however, that can be associated with the functions of the change agent are: influence, support, initiate, and participate. Nurses can *influence* or persuade others to change their behavior. They accomplish this action through use of interpersonal relationships. To be effective, change agents should be socially adept, interested in others, and competent in their interactions with others. Change very seldom occurs in a vacuum or merely on a piece of paper. It involves working with other individuals who have feelings. If nurses as change agents are aware of their attitudes and behaviors, how they approach other persons, and how they feel about change, they are more likely to succeed in promoting planned change.

Since change is frightening to many, nurses need to *support* those affected by the change. This action helps to stabilize the new behavior. An important role of the change agent is to gather together potential allies that are in favor of the proposed change. There will most certainly be some resistance to a change. The change agent needs to be sensitive to the needs of the target population for support and be available and willing to provide that support.

Nurses who function as change agents must *initiate* actions rather than passively wait for the change in behavior to occur by itself. Inaction and frustration are inevitable aspects of the change process. The change agent needs to be flexible, persistent, and yet realistic about what can be accomplished. While the nurse as change agent initiates action, it is important that others involved in the change feel that they are contributing.

From the action verbs used to describe the functions of change agents, it is apparent that they are not delegating their functions to others. Change agents actively participate in the process. Nurses who are active in the change process participate by using their knowledge and skills to set the thermostat for the tone of the proposed change.

Effective change agents realize that change does not just happen by itself. They also are convinced that it is possible to change attitudes, values, and behaviors. Successful change agents practice change on a consistent basis and are aware that change is a skill that can be learned. The more developed the skill, the fewer unknown consequences one encounters.

## Risk Taking and Effective Change

Nurses often feel they know how to bring about change. But lasting change in attitudes, values, and behaviors is more than switching or exchanging one act for another. Lasting change requires personal risk taking, and not all persons are risk takers. The word **risk** implies that one cannot be guaranteed that the change will be successful. Many people are afraid of doing anything unless they are relatively assured of success. Sometimes nurses talk themselves out of potentially effective interventions because they are afraid to risk failure—perhaps it is more accurate to say to risk "lack of success" rather than "failure."

You need to work through your personal feelings about how you might feel if you were to fail while attempting to implement a change. Would you acknowledge the fact that lack of success does not mean you are a failure, but that the planned change needs different strategies and tactics? Change can make you vulnerable because you may not meet your goals. The potential for meeting goals can be more certain and less risky if you systematically follow the steps of the change process.

How can you learn the skill of taking risks and making effective changes? These suggestions are offered:

*1. Reflect on Your Feelings about Change.* Some people think a person is weak if the person changes. If this is the way you feel, you need to work toward modifying your perceptions before you can be receptive to learning about the change process. Comments such as, "He's wishy-washy" and, "She's always changing her mind," imply that change is an undesirable characteristic. Comments like, "He's steadfast," or, "You always know where she stands," are often reflective of sterling qualities of character rather than resistance to change.

*2. Determine What Prevents You from Practicing Change.* You may be eager to assume the role of change agent, but you do not know where to begin. Assess in what areas of change you need guidance. Do you need to develop skill in assessing relevant areas in need of change? Are you comfortable and knowledgeable about goal-setting? It may be necessary to gain information about these skills before you study the basic steps of the change process.

*3. Develop the Practice of Being Proactive Rather Than Reactive.* There are times when we tolerate unwanted and nonproductive situations. Then we find ourselves reacting emotionally, irrationally, and desperately. It is far more beneficial to be proactive by having a clear goal. If you know what you want, how much you want it, and how much effort you are willing to exert, you will be actively engaged in initiating proactive measures to reach your goal.

To a great extent, your philosophy about man influences whether you will be reactive or proactive. If you believe that you are not capable of making a difference, that you are "acted upon" by others, or that you need to "roll with the punches" to make it through life, you may find it difficult to initiate change. You are reacting to the actions of others. If you believe that you "make your own destiny," that you can change the course of events through a concerted effort, you are prepared to actively initiate measures that will meet your goal.

*4. Analyze Your Reactions to Potential and Actual Risks.* Not only must you become aware of how you feel about change, but you must also develop an awareness of how you react to perceived risks. No change is made without some risk. You have probably heard comments like, "I break out in a cold sweat just thinking about what I would do if I lost my job." Just thinking about a particular change may bring on overwhelming fear and anxiety. There is an optimal amount of change each of us can endure. Even if a change is desirable and positive, it may not be the optimum time to take on an extra burden. Even positive changes are stressful.

Also, you need to determine if you need the support of others when you initiate change. If you need support, or if the particular change calls for added support that will not be available, it may not be the right time for a change.

5. *Assess Your Attitude Toward Asking for Assistance from Others.* When planning change, it is essential to gather as much information as you can. You need to ensure that your knowledge and skills are adequate to bring about the proposed change most effectively. It is important for you to realize that you may not have all the information you need, and that you need to take advantage of those with more expertise. Some nurses have the attitude that they are expected to know the answers to everything, and that seeking the advice of others is an admission of inadequacy. For nurses to perpetuate such an attitude is merely a reflection that their needs are more important than those of clients. If you are genuinely concerned about making planned changes to attain the optimum welfare of clients, you will prepare yourself.

Preparation also encompasses the emotional extremes that often accompany change. Other nurses, who have practiced longer than you, can offer their support and thus decrease the stressfulness of the change. The more prepared you are for the change, the more realistic your expected outcomes will be, and the more reasonable your risks.

6. *Calculate Your Potential for Impulsiveness and Making Rash Judgments.* An aspect of a change plan is to allow time for incubation to occur between the planning stage and the implementation. The change agent must attentively wait for an idea to become systematically plotted out in its entirety before it becomes reality. There are times when you may feel uncomfortable about waiting a day or so before the tentative plan for change is judged to be appropriate. This delayed action will be especially difficult if you usually make hasty decisions and impulsively jump into things that you later regret. The ability to wait for the plan to incubate will label you—the change agent—as decisive and confident.

7. *Push Yourself into Action.* There are many people who have all of the important prerequisite characteristics for practicing change . . . except one. They plot out an intelligent change plan and know what they want to do. They are aware of all the consequences. But they never implemented the plan.

As we implied earlier, as the implementation step draws near, it provokes anxiety. In addition, hesitancy to act may be attributed to the fear that the changes are irreversible. The person promoting the change may have difficulty accepting the idea of irreversibility. Remember it is true that you cannot reverse some of the changes you carry out. But many changes are not irrevocable; they are merely less effective. Once change agents complete implementation of the change process, they feel very good about themselves. They begin to see that they can take charge and improve a situation.

8. *Profit from Your Experience.* If you want to increase your skill at initiating change, you need to learn from your experiences. By reflecting on and evaluating your past actions, you can determine if the strategies and tactics were beneficial, if you had adequate support, and if you should continue to use the present plan. As you continue to

initiate planned change, you will find it much easier each time. Evaluating and reflecting are also means of rewarding yourself for reaching your goal. You are intentionally being made aware of your success.

We have completed our discussion of the risks that nurses must take when functioning as change agents. Now let us take a look at some of the barriers nurses must overcome to become effective.

## Barriers to Becoming an Effective Change Agent

The major barrier to becoming an effective change agent is a restricting fear. Fear may cause you to make impulsive moves without considering all the consequences. Fear may be preventing you from implementing planned change. To overcome this barrier, practice initiating change. In time, your fear will lessen, and you will start feeling comfortable about participating in change. (See Table 12–1 for fears that are barriers to change.)

Barriers other than fear also prevent you from participating in change. Some persons who are resistant to change deny their true feelings about the proposed change. The denial acts as a barrier. The desire to continue with the present circumstances may act as a barrier. People feel secure and comfortable with predictable routines that they can anticipate. Lack of self-worth also may prevent people from planning and implementing change.

We have completed our examination of the role of the nurse as a change agent. We will now see how the process of planned change can be applied to nursing practice.

## APPLICATION OF PLANNED CHANGE

Usually as nurses become more confident in their professional role, they wish to make planned change. Nurses who are knowledgeable, motivated, independent, and responsible will want to become involved in planning and implementing change.

## Relationship to the Nursing Process

Although the change process corresponds very closely with the entire nursing process, planned change is related most closely to the planning and implementing steps of the process (Table 12–2).

### Assessing

*1. Determining the Need for a Change Program.* Even though the nurse (change agent) may see a need for change, the individual, family, or community client must also feel

**TABLE 12–1. FEARS THAT ARE BARRIERS TO CHANGE**

1. Fear that others will think poorly of you if you fail.
2. Fear of what others will expect of you if you succeed.
3. Fear that you can't do something, even if you try.
4. Fear of the unknown.
5. Fear of inconvenience resulting from change.
6. Fear that the reward will not be worth the cost of the change.
7. Fear of appearing foolish to others.
8. Fear of opposition from others.
9. Fear that others will not like you if you succeed.

**TABLE 12–2. COMPARISON OF CHANGE PROCESS AND NURSING PROCESS**

| Nursing Process | Change Process |
|---|---|
| Assessing | Determining the need for a change program |
| | Establishing contact with target population |
| Diagnosing | Diagnosing the problem |
| Planning | Formulating goals for change program |
| | Selecting alternative courses of action |
| Implementing | Implementing change program |
| | Maintaining change program |
| Evaluating | Evaluating effectiveness of change program |
| | Disengagement of change agent |

that a problem exists. Throughout the change process, the client needs to be actively involved and see the outcome as relevant. Also, an accurate assessment needs to be made of the target population and the target setting. Some aspects in need of assessment may include organizational structure, policies and procedures, cultural limitations, personalities, and so forth. Restraining forces such as finances may need to be considered.

2. *Establishing Contact with the Target Population (individual, family, or community client).* Because you must work with and through the client to bring about the change, it is important to establish a trusting relationship. Your credibility must be established and apparent to the client. Interpersonal skills as well as other skills discussed in earlier chapters will facilitate acceptance of the change. As many sources as possible should be consulted for input into the assessment of the target population.

## Diagnosing

3. *Diagnosing the Problem.* The problem should be seen from the perspective of the individual, family, or community client—not merely from the perception of the nurse. Proper diagnosis of the problem is very important. All who are involved in the process of planned change should participate in identifying the problem. All concerned need to be committed to the proposed change. Their commitment results from their personal participation.

## Planning

4. *Formulating Goals for the Change Program.* After the problem is diagnosed, goals are mutually formulated by the client and nurse. Some form of outcome criteria will need to be set so it will be possible to determine if the goals were met. This planning stage needs to be as specific as possible with timetables established. Determining deadlines is helpful in assisting the target population to move toward the goal.

5. *Selecting Alternative Courses of Action.* The nurse acts as a facilitator by presenting to the client a number of alternative approaches for reaching the goal. It is the client who should make the decisions. By allowing the client to decide, the change is more likely to become stabilized and remain after the nurse terminates the change relationship. This implies that the nurse will have to help others to make decisions. Brainstorming is a helpful technique in determining alternatives. Identifying and using relevant resources is also important.

## Implementing

*6. Implementing the Change Program.* When the plan of action is carried out, it is important that the client feels positive about the entire experience. This will ensure continuance of the change program after the change agent ends the relationship. Creating motivation is important during this stage because the behaviors will be new and tentative at this time.

The use of a specific theory will specify the approach to use in the planning and implementing steps. Use of a theoretical framework is helpful in progressing toward an identified goal.

*7. Maintaining the Change Program.* If the nurse gives reinforcement to the client during this step, the program is more likely to become permanent. Reinforcement is the responsibility of the change agent. Communication is also important in perpetuating the change. A mechanism should be developed to provide frequent feedback to those involved in the change. Feedback helps to sustain others' interest in the change even after the change agent terminates the relationship.

## Evaluating

*8. Evaluating the Effectiveness of the Change Program.* The goals and outcome criteria set down during an earlier step are used to determine the effectiveness of the change program. Evaluation can be scheduled at specified intervals during the implementation phase of the change as well as at the end of the planned change. Revisions can be made after each evaluation period to make the change more effective.

*9. Disengagement of Change Agent.* After the change has been evaluated as effective and measures have been taken for its continuance, the change agent terminates the relationship with the client. Disengagement of the change agent needs to be considered from the beginning of the planned change so that the client is prepared and capable of continuing the new behaviors. Gradual withdrawal is most effective for the continuance of a change. As the change agent withdraws, designated persons within the setting should assume the functions of the change agent.

Now that we have seen the relationship of planned change to the nursing process, we will examine how various theories can be helpful in working with individual, family, or community clients.

## Change Theory for Individual Clients

A model described by Lippitt, Watson, and Westley[4] is a useful frame of reference to use when planning for change in the attitudes and behaviors of individual clients. Change is described by Lippitt and associates as a purposeful decision to bring about improvement in a social system. Improvement (the goal) in a social system (the individual) is accomplished with the help of professional guidance (the change agent). For example, let us assume the nurse (change agent) wants to control a client's increased arterial pressure (hypertension) by having the client adhere to a therapeutic regime (goal). You could work toward the goal by following the seven phases in the change process identified by Lippitt and associates.

*1. Development of a Need for Change.* During this phase, the change agent designs specific interventions (tactics) to increase the client's awareness[5] of an actual (or potential) increase in blood pressure that needs to be controlled. Also, you may want to explore what the client perceives as the attitudes and behaviors that the client needs to change in order to adhere to the therapeutic regime and thereby control the hypertension.

*2. Establishment of a Change Relationship.* At the completion of the first phase, the client has developed a basic awareness of the need for a change in attitudes and behaviors. In the second phase, the change agent demonstrates an understanding of the client's needs, identifies resistance, demonstrates expertise in the area of need, and negotiates the conditions, expectations, and responsibilities of working toward a change relationship.[5]

To increase understanding of client needs, you could complete a health history (a tactic). By using a nondirective interview (a tactic), you would be able to identify areas of resistance to change. Your expertise can be demonstrated by your knowledge of management of increased arterial pressure (intellectual skill), by your ability to perform correctly procedures such as taking blood pressure readings and administering antihypertensive medications (psychomotor skills), and by the professional and therapeutic manner in which you convey a helping and caring attitude (interpersonal skills). By mutually setting expected outcomes with the client, and negotiating how the client can cooperate with you, there is more likeliness that the change will be effected.

*3. Diagnose the Problem.* The basic process of this phase is collaboration between the client and the change agent in generating and analyzing information in order to diagnose the problem.[5] You could review with the client the information related to increased arterial pressure that you collected from the health history. Together, the client and nurse can analyze this problem-related information.

Many times, the medical diagnosis is the first thing known to clients. They may not have been told what their blood pressure was, or whether it was slightly elevated or seriously elevated, but they were told the medical diagnosis. The practice of reviewing the assessment data and relating these to the known medical diagnosis establishes important links for the client and ensures greater adherence.

*4. Action Planning.* During this phase, specific plans are made, evaluation criteria are formulated, and progressive change objectives are selected. Together with the client, the change agent should identify the strategies that will move clients from where they presently are to the new attitudes and behaviors they wish to attain. The strategies are based on the type of goals to be reached.[5] In the example, the goal was to control increased arterial pressure by adherence of the client to a therapeutic regime.

*5. Action Implementation.* The change agent is the main force behind change in this phase. Change will not occur without involvement of both the nurse and client.[5]

A time chart for implementing the plan may be established that both you and the client perceive as reasonable. This will accomplish several things. It will enable the client to see that there is an end in sight, at which time the client will be expected to follow the program independently. Clients are usually more cooperative if they know what is expected and when it is expected. The time chart also will assist you in organizing and initiating the planned strategies and tactics.

After the change strategies and tactics have been implemented, the results are evaluated for effectiveness. By comparing the results with the expectations set by both client and yourself, it can be determined if revisions are needed in the change program.

Many times, the decision is made to discontinue the plan by impulsively and emotionally thinking that it did not work. A more objective evaluation is necessary to accurately judge the effectiveness of the plan.

*6. Maintenance of Change.* At this point, after the change plan has been in place and adjustments made, measures should be taken to ensure that the new behaviors will continue.[5] In the example, adherence to a therapeutic regime for maintaining the client's blood pressure may be accomplished by reinforcing the change plan periodically with scheduled conferences with the client, asking that a diary be kept for reviewing problems with adherence, or establishing periodic telephone visits to maintain the probability of adherence.

*7. Termination.* The final phase of planned change using this model is termination. It is important to plan for the time when you (the change agent) withdraw from the change relationship, and the client continues to manage the new behaviors independently of professional guidance. The termination time should be known by the client from the very beginning of the plan. A note of thanks for the client's cooperation could be left before the end of the change program to signal the beginning of the termination phase.

Now that we have examined a change theory for individual clients, let us look at one for the family.

## Change Theory for Family Clients

Earlier we discussed the phases of planned change from Lewin's perspective. Now we will discuss Lewin's change model as a theory for implementing change for families.[3]

In this model, effective change is dependent upon change in the attitudes and values (norms) of a group. The example which will illustrate this model is the family's perception of the sexual functioning of a 45-year-old father who is paralyzed from the waist down.

We have already stated that change involves a certain amount of anxiety and often causes resistance. This view continues to be important as we consider this model. A feeling of need also must be present prior to the time a family engages in change.

Lewin's model involves the following three steps:

*1. Unfreezing.* This first phase is aimed at motivating others and is very important. If unfreezing does not occur, change will not occur. A possible problem in this stage is that the family may not be motivated to change—they may not be aware of the need to change. You (the change agent) need to motivate the members of the family in progressing in the direction of the desired change. In this example, the desired change would be the realistic perception of the father's sexual functioning. The family's knowledge about sexual functioning will need to be assessed. You can use the subjective comments they make as well as your own objective observations to identify the cues that problems may exist in the way the family perceives the father's sexual functioning. The family may have to undergo a change in knowledge in addition to a change in attitude before they can become motivated to modify their behavior. These changes (in knowledge and attitudes) may be threatening in the case of sexual functioning.

Remember that the manner in which the change agent introduces the change is important in this phase. The more positively the change is viewed, the more likely the change will be accepted.

*2. Changing.* This phase is aimed at learning the desired behavior change from a role model (identification), and altering the environment to reinforce the change behaviors (internalization). Movement toward the change is based on information from multiple sources. This information supports the change and a unified plan of action.[2]

During identification, goals, objectives, and outcome criteria are defined, measures are planned for fulfilling the objectives, and implementation of the plan occurs. The presence of a role model (the change agent) is important to facilitate effective change within a reasonable time frame. During internalization, planned rewards provide incentives for the family to change and help to combat resistance to change. Again, subjective information from family members and your own observations gained through frequent interactions with the client can provide the cues to identify problems in carrying out a program to change the family's perception.

*3. Refreezing.* Acceptance of the planned change, which involves maintaining and stabilizing the change, concludes the cycle. Even though this phase implies that the change has occurred and is stable, you need to plan ways to assure the permanency of the change.

One way of stabilizing change is through reinforcement. Examples of reinforcement are giving the family positive feedback and providing necessary guidance. Consistent and continuing reinforcement needs to be offered initially and then intermittently as the planned change becomes stabilized.

To maintain the change, ongoing evaluation is necessary. Goals and objectives developed in phase two will determine the specific direction planned change takes. Outcome criteria identified in that phase will enable you to measure the family's progress toward meeting the goals and objectives.

We have examined change theories for the individual and family. Now, let us look at a theory that can be used to promote planned change within the community.

## Change Theory for Community Clients

The general systems theory[7] may be used to analyze and understand how components of the community work toward planned change. As discussed in Chapter 3, a system is a set of interacting and interdependent parts. The community is an example of an open social systems model.

In Figure 12–1, two subsystems are depicted: one that safeguards physical safety and one that safeguards environmental safety. In turn, each of these two subsystems is composed of component parts or subsystems. This example illustrates that each system is a subsystem of another larger system.

Let us examine what happens when one system is affected and thus others are affected. When there is a breakdown in the efforts to safeguard a community from pollutants, there may be an effect on food, water, and milk. These effects may also spread to other systems. The physical safety of the community could also be affected. The feedback that results from inside and outside the system can help to change the behaviors that caused the problems. If changes are not made, even greater and lasting consequences will result.

When a geographical community is assessed, both the content and the process are addressed. Earlier in Chapter 3, we defined content as the sum of the discrete parts that are organized to accomplish a particular goal. Process was defined as the functions or series of sequential events by which the discrete parts work together. Through assessment, subjective and objective data are collected on the content of the community. Sub-

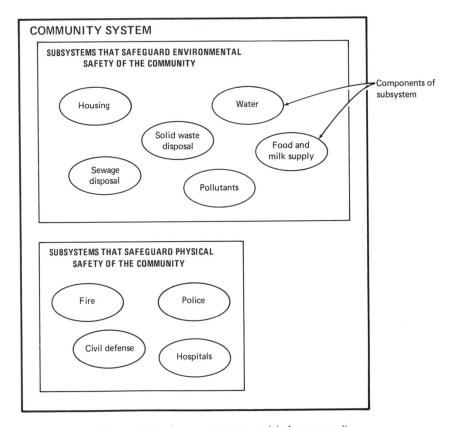

**Figure 12–1.** An open-systems model of a community.

jective data are obtained by speaking with the residents of the community. Objective data can be obtained from the census report and other official reports. It is important that you assess process, or how the geographical community functions, so the interactions among the subsystems may be known.

Each system obtains its *inputs* from the environment. The *outputs* (energy and waste products) go to other subsystems and out into the environment. The subsystems are interrelated and interdependent. If one subsystem is affected, others will be affected. The process that converts inputs into outputs is called *throughputs*. At any point within the system, *feedback* can occur. If feedback is heeded, the system can change itself and become more effective. (This process of change is called *cybernation*.) The feedback mechanism within an open-systems model is depicted in Figure 12–2.

Let us look at two ways we can use systems theory to bring about change in the community.

1. *Situation Where Problem Exists.* The change agent would need to understand what the problem of the community is. After the community problem is identified, the purpose of the change is established. A community assessment (sub-

**Figure 12–2.** Feedback mechanism within an open-systems model.

jective and objective) is made of the inputs, process, outputs, and the initial consequences. It is possible to initiate reactive changes at this point before lasting consequences result.

2. *Situation Where Problem Does Not Exist.* If the community change is to be proactive, the change agent can identify the goal of the desired community change and structure the inputs, process, and outputs in a way that would accomplish the purpose of the proposed change. Feedback would be used to maintain and stabilize the change and thereby make it permanent. Measures would be initiated to maintain the change.

We have completed our discussion of how change theory can be used with individual, family, and community clients. Now let us see how the process of planned change relates to the other processes used in nursing and those presented in this book.

## Relationships among Planned Change and Other Processes Used in Nursing

Today, planned change is part of the nurse's role. It is vitally important for the nurse to develop the ability to identify and effect change so that the needs of individual, family, and community clients are met. Implementing change is an integral part of the nursing process as well as the other processes nurses use. If you examine Table 12–3, you will see how closely the steps of planned change relate to the other processes that have been discussed in this book.

**TABLE 12–3. RELATIONSHIP AMONG PLANNED CHANGE AND OTHER PROCESSES USED IN NURSING**

| | Change Process | Decision-making Process |
|---|---|---|
| Assessing | Determining the need for change program | Identifying the problem |
| | Establishing contact with target population | Collecting information about the attributes of the problem |
| Diagnosing | Diagnosing the problem | (In decision making, the problem is diagnosed at the onset of the process) |

*(Continued)*

**TABLE 12–3. Continued**

| | Change Process | Decision-making Process |
|---|---|---|
| Planning | Formulating goals for change program<br>Selecting alternative courses of action | Establishing terminal and enabling<br>objectives in ranked order<br>Listing alternative courses of action<br>proposed to meet the objectives<br>Choosing decision rules<br>Analyzing optional courses of action that<br>relate to the objectives<br>Ranking optional courses of action<br>Selecting a tentative course of action that<br>best meets the objectives<br>Determining alliances and points of view<br>Determining a course of action |
| Implementing | Implementing change program<br>Maintaining change program | Implementing the decision |
| Evaluating | Evaluating effectiveness of change program<br>Disengagement of agent | Evaluating the effectiveness of the decision |

| | Teaching Process | Research Process |
|---|---|---|
| Assessing | Assessing readiness to learn<br>Assessing developmental level<br>Assessing cognitive development<br>Assessing learning needs | Identifying the problem<br>Stating the problem |
| Diagnosing | Diagnosing learning needs<br>Analyzing data<br>Deriving conclusions<br>Assigning diagnostic labels<br>Identifying sustaining factors<br>Formulating diagnostic statements | Stating the hypotheses |
| Planning | Planning learning activities<br>Formulating learning goals<br>Formulating learning objectives<br>Lesson planning | Developing a proposal<br>Selecting the design<br>Selecting the instruments<br>Selecting the sample |
| Implementing | Implementing teaching plan<br>Selecting learning method<br>Selecting audiovisual aids | Collecting the data<br>Organizing the data<br>Describing the data |
| Evaluating | Evaluating the teaching–learning process<br>Identifying behaviors to be assessed<br>Selecting instruments and methods for<br>measuring achievement of objectives<br>Establishing means of collecting,<br>interpreting, and using data and results | Analyzing the data<br>Preparing the report |

| | Problem Solving | Theory Development |
|---|---|---|
| Assessing | Understanding the problem<br>Collecting data | Forming a basic assumption about a<br>phenomenon<br>Conceptualizing<br>Observing a phenomenon<br>Grouping observations |
| Diagnosing | Formulating the hypothesis | Developing a theoretical statement<br>(hypothesis) |
| Planning | Preparing a plan for testing the hypothesis | Planning for the testing of the theoretical<br>statement |
| Implementing | Testing the hypothesis | Testing the theoretical statement |
| Evaluating | Interpreting and evaluating the results | Evaluating the theoretical statement |

## SUMMARY

Nurses are in an important position in the health care system to bring about planned change. Planned change can result in both positive and negative changes. Change is most effective when it is directed toward an improvement, when it can be initiated on a smaller scale first, and when it is simple enough to communicate to others. The attainment of a change is facilitated by a change agent who allows the target population to participate in each step of the process. An effective change agent initiates the change process, attempts risks, and interacts well with others. Change theory is applicable to individual, family, and community clients.

The systematic and logical steps in the nursing process as well as the other processes discussed in this book should enable nurses to fulfill their role in assisting individual, family, and community clients to attain health and well-being.

## STUDY GUIDE

1. Assess your ability to take risks comfortably. Compare your findings with someone you consider a risk taker.
2. List two planned changes you made this past week. Discuss the outcome.
3. Write a list of the barriers that prevent you from making changes.
4. Arrange for one of your classmates to observe you for 2 days in a clinical setting. Ask your classmate to keep a log of the instances when you planned a change or implemented a change.
5. Develop a list of five barriers you would like to overcome to enable you to make changes more comfortably.

## REFERENCES

1. Hersey, P., & Blanchard, K. Planning and implementing change. In *Management of Organizational Behavior* (4th ed.). Englewood Cliffs, N.J.: Prentice-Hall, 1982.
2. Lancaster, J., & Lancaster, W. *Concepts for Advanced Nursing Practice: The Nurse as a Change Agent*. St. Louis: C. V. Mosby, 1982.
3. Lewin, K. Frontiers in group dynamics: Concept method and reality in social sciences: Social equilibria and social change. *Human Relations*, 1976, *1*(1), 5–41.
4. Lippitt, R., Watson, J., & Westley, B. *The Dynamics of Planned Change*. New York: Harcourt, Brace, & World, 1958.
5. Lippitt, R., Hooyman, G., Sashkin, M., & Kaplan, J. *Resource Book for Planned Change*. Michigan: Human Resources Development Associates of Ann Arbor, 1978.
6. Schein, E. H. The mechanisms of change. In W. G. Bennis, E. H. Schein, F. I. Steek, & D. E. Berlow, (Eds.), *Interpersonal Dynamics*. Homewood, Ill.: Dorsey Press, 1964, 362.
7. von Bertalanffy, L. *General Systems Theory*. New York: George Braziller, 1968.

## BIBLIOGRAPHY

Bailey, B. J. Using change theory to help the diabetic. *Diabetes Educator*, (Fall 1983), *9* (3), 37–39, 56.
Bennis, W., Benne, K., Chin, R., & Carey, K. *The Planning of Change* (3rd ed.). New York: Holt, Rinehart & Winston, 1976.

Carner, D. C. Managing change . . . Carner's codes. *Hospital Forum*, (November–December, 1982), *26* (6), 59–62.

Douglas, H. E. III. Changing the guard: A methodology for leadership in transition. *Journal of Allied Health*, (May 1983), *12* (2), 141–150.

Dowling, W., & Sayles, L. *How Managers Motivate: The Imperatives of Supervision*. New York: McGraw-Hill, 1978.

Falk, D. S. The challenge of change. *Hospitals*, (April 1983), *57* (7), 92, 94, 96.

Goeddel, L. E. Quality-of-work-life efforts help hospitals manage change. *Hospital Managers*, (January–February 1984), *14* (1), 6–8.

Green, C. P. Teaching strategies for the process of planned change. *Journal of Continuing Education*, (November–December 1983), *14* (6), 16–23.

Huffman, M. L. The process of change . . . nurse managers. *Critical Care Nurse*, (September–October 1983), *3* (5), 44–46.

Klein, D. Some notes on the dynamics of resistance to change: The defenders role. In W. Bennis, K. Benne, R. Chin, & K. Carey, (Eds.), *The Planning of Change* (3rd ed.). New York: Holt, Rinehart & Winston, 1976, 117–124.

Lancaster, J. An ecological orientation toward change: Consideration for leadership in nursing. *Nursing Leadership*, 1980, *3* (4), 12–15.

Loomis, M., & Dodenhoff, J. Working with informal patient groups. *American Journal of Nursing*, (September 1970), 1939–1943.

Mackety, C. J. Strategy for change in the OR. *Todays OR Nurse*, (January 1984), *6* (1), 28–31.

Morgan, G. G. Practical techniques for change . . . service for children. *Journal of Child Contemporary Sociology*, (Summer 1983), *15* (4), 91–104.

Owen, G. M. The stress of change. *Nursing Times*, (February 23–March 1, 1983), *79* (8), (4) 44–46.

Shaw, M. E. *Group Dynamics: The Psychology of Small Group Behaviors* (2nd ed.). New York: McGraw-Hill, 1976.

Ward, M. J., et al. Resistance to change: Recognize, respond, overcome. *Nurse Manager*, (January 1984), *15* (1), 30–33.

Young, M. S., et al. Nursing diagnosis: Common problems in implementation. *Topics of Clinical Nursing*, (January 1984), *5* (4), 68–77.

Zaltman, G., & Duncan, R. *Strategies for Planned Change*. New York: Wiley, 1977.

# Medical Historian Form

## ST. LUKE'S HOSPITALS' MEDICAL HISTORIAN PROTOCOL

Name _____ Birthdate _____ Age _____ Date _____

Past Medical History (Use back of page if necessary)

1. List all hospitalizations, childhood to present, for illnesses, operations, tests or injuries. Include outpatient surgery:

| Year | Reason for Admission |
|------|---------------------|
| _____ | _____ |
| _____ | _____ |
| _____ | _____ |
| _____ | _____ |

2. List past injuries and fractures:

| Year | Injury |
|------|--------|
| _____ | _____ |
| _____ | _____ |

3. List allergies or adverse reactions to drugs, anesthesia, chemicals, pollens, adhesive tape, etc.:

| Substance | Reaction |
|-----------|----------|
| _____ | _____ |
| _____ | _____ |

4. What medications have you taken in the last six weeks? Include vitamins, laxatives, aspirin, birth control pills, etc.:

| Drug | Frequency of Use | Dates |
|------|-----------------|-------|
| _____ | _____ | _____ |
| _____ | _____ | _____ |
| _____ | _____ | _____ |
| _____ | _____ | _____ |

Have you ever been a smoker? _____ How much? _____ Dates _____

How much alcohol do you drink? _____ For how long? _____

Do you have a history of drug use? _____

**Review of Systems:**

1. Have you had any serious eye, ear, nose or throat problems? _____ Frequent colds or sore throats? _____ Sinus congestion? _____ Trouble swallowing? _____ Voice change? _____ Significant loss of vision? _____ Cataracts? _____ Glaucoma? _____ Wear contact lenses? _____ Significant loss of hearing? _____

2. Circle and give the year if you have had: Mononucleosis _____, Scarlet fever _____, Malaria _____, Shingles _____, Strep throat _____, Pneumonia _____, TB _____

3. Have you had any heart, lung or circulatory problems? _____ When? _____
   Describe _____
       Have you had: Chest pain? _____ When? _____ Location _____
       Describe the pain (dull, sharp, burning, heavy, etc.) _____ Does the pain move
       around? _____ Where? _____ How long does it last? _____
       How often? _____ Does cough or deep breath make the pain worse? _____
       Intensity of the pain: Mild _____ Moderate _____ Severe _____ Have you had: Heart attack? _____
       Irregular heartbeat? _____ Heart murmur? _____ Rheumatic fever? _____ A recent EKG? _____
       Result _____
       Have you had: Shortness of breath? _____ At rest? _____ With exertion? _____ Awaken you at night?
       _____ Wheezing? _____ Asthma? _____ Emphysema? _____ Pleurisy? _____ Chronic bronchitis?
       _____ Persistent cough? _____ Cough up something? _____ Cough up blood? _____ An abnormal
       chest x-ray? _____
       Have you had: High blood pressure? _____ Swollen Ankles? _____ Leg cramps? _____
       When? _____ Blood Clots? _____ Sores that failed to heal on feet or legs? _____
       Phlebitis? _____ Varicose Veins? _____ Recent fatigue or weakness? _____ Ever fainted or blacked
       out? _____

4. Have you had recent severe or continuing digestive or bowel problems? Change in your bowel habit? _____
   Describe _____
   Bright red blood in stool? _____ Abdominal pain, swelling? _____ Black stools? _____ Belching, rectal gas?
   _____ Nausea? _____ Vomiting? _____ Heartburn? _____ Food intolerance? _____ Lactose
   intolerance? _____ Loss of appetite? _____ Recent weight change? _____ Hemorrhoids? _____
   Diverticulosis? _____ Colitis? _____ Ulcer? _____ Gallbladder trouble? _____ Hernia? _____ Liver
   trouble? _____ Jaundice? _____ Hepatitis? _____ Had recent GI series? _____ Result _____

5. How many meals do you eat daily? _____ Do you eat meat, fruits, vegetables daily? _____ Do you eat large amounts of (circle) salt, sugar, soft drinks, coffee, tea? Do you eat a special diet? _____ Describe _____
   _____

6. Have you had recent severe or continuing kidney or bladder problems? _____ Pain or burning with urination?
   _____ Blood in your urine? _____ Difficulty with urination? _____ Difficulty controlling urine? _____
   Frequency of urination? _____ Urgency? _____ How many times do you get up at night to urinate?
   _____ Had recurring urinary tract infections? _____ Kidney stones? _____
   Syphilis, gonorrhea or herpes simplex? _____ When? _____ Treated? _____
   *Men Only:* Have you had any problems involving the genitals? _____ Sores on genitals? _____
   Discharge from penis? _____ Prostate problems? _____ Testicle problems? _____ Impotence? _____ Other _____

7. *Women Only:* Date of last menstrual period _____ Date of last pap test _____ Result _____
   At what age did menstruation begin? _____ Frequency of menstruation _____
   Duration _____ Is menstrual flow: Light _____ Moderate _____ Heavy _____ Do you usually have
   pain or cramps with your period? _____ Have you bled between periods? _____
   When? _____ Have frequent vaginal infections? _____ Had painful intercourse? _____ Had lumps or
   discharge from breasts? _____ Used IUD? _____ Dates used _____ Used birth control
   pills? _____ Dates used _____ Any side effects? _____ No. pregnancies _____ No. live births _____ No. miscarriages _____ No. abortions _____
   No. stillbirths _____ No. Caesarean sections _____ Complications during pregnancies? (High blood pressure,
   anemia, toxemia, etc.) _____
   Are you having menopausal symptoms? _____ Describe _____
   Have you taken hormone shots, pills, creams? _____ Dates used _____

8. Have you had recent, severe or continuing bone or joint problems? _____ Arthritis? _____ Bursitis? _____
   Gout? _____ Swollen or painful joints? _____ Which joints? _____ When? _____
   Back trouble? _____ Describe _____
   Treatment _____
   Bone disease or infection? _____ Describe _____
   Treatment _____

9. Have you had blood problems? _____ Describe _____
   Poor clotting? _____ Sickle cell trait? _____ Adverse reaction to a blood transfusion? _____
   Anemia? _____

10. Have you had severe skin problems? (Rashes, itching, eczema, psoriasis, acne, etc.) _____ Treatment _____
    Have you had serious problems with: Hair? _____ Nails? _____

11. Have you had tumors? _____ Cysts? _____ Where? _____
    When? _____ Benign/malignant; Treatment _____
    Had X ray treatments or chemotherapy? _____ Had moles removed? _____ When? _____
    Where? _____ Do you have moles that are changing in appearance, size, shape or color?
    _____ Where? _____

12. Have you had thyroid or goiter problems? _____ When? _____ Describe _____
    Have you had diabetes? (Sugar in blood or urine) _____ Hypoglycemia? (low blood sugar) _____ Had a
    recent fasting blood sugar test? _____ Result _____
    Have you been told you have hormone imbalance? _____ Do you tend to be warm? _____ Cold? _____
    Excessively hungry? _____ Excessively thirsty? _____ Sluggish? _____ Jumpy? _____ Have night sweats?
    _____ Recent fever? _____ Change in energy? _____

13. Have you had any neurological problems? _____ Do you have frequent or severe headaches? _____ How
    often? _____ Balance trouble? _____ Muscle weakness? _____ Speech difficulty? _____ Dizzy
    spells? _____ Loss of consciousness? _____ Convulsions? _____ Significant memory loss? _____
    Paralysis? _____ Double or blurred vision? _____ Neuritis? _____ Numbness/tingling in arms or legs?
    _____ Sciatica? _____ Tremor? _____ Stroke? _____ Circle: Right/Left handed

14. Have you been treated for mental illness or nervous disorder? _____ When? _____
    Hospitalized? _____ How treated? _____
    Have electric shock treatments? _____ Are you in treatment now? _____

## CURRENT LIFE SITUATION
Marital status: S _____ M _____ D _____ Sep _____ W _____ Occupation _____
Work full or part-time? _____ Who lives in your household? _____
Do you spend time in leisure activities? _____ How? _____
Are there stressful situations in your life at this time? _____ Describe _____

## FAMILY MEDICAL HISTORY
Have your parents, grandparents, brothers, sisters, aunts, uncles or your children had the following?

| Disease | Who | Paternal/ Maternal | If Deceased Give Cause and Age at Death |
|---|---|---|---|
| Cancer (give location) | | | |
| Tuberculosis | | | |
| Diabetes (adult-onset?) | | | |
| Heart trouble | | | |
| High blood pressure | | | |
| Stroke | | | |
| Convulsions | | | |
| Migraine headaches | | | |
| Alcoholism | | | |
| Ulcer | | | |
| Mental illness | | | |
| Kidney disease | | | |
| Glaucoma | | | |
| Arthritis | | | |
| Sickle cell disease | | | |
| Parkinson's disease | | | |
| Multiple sclerosis | | | |

*Developed by the Medical Historian Department at St. Luke's Hospitals, St. Louis, Missouri. This form is completed by patients prior to their admission, and is used by medical historians when interviewing patients upon their arrival.*

# Nursing Health History

Identify client or informant (if different from client) and include assessment of reliability.
State briefly in client's words why the client is seeking assistance with health needs.

### Assessment of Needs of the Individual

## Physiological Needs

### Oxygenation
Factors that interfere with breathing (position, emotions, weather, smoking, activity):

Smoking history (form of tobacco, amount, number of years):

Presence of:

| | |
|---|---|
| Dyspnea _____ | Bruises _____ |
| Sputum _____ | Exercise intolerance _____ |
| Cough _____ | Temperature/color change of extremities _____ |
| Fatigue _____ | |

Aids to improve oxygenation (drugs, position, elastic support stockings, oxygen, etc.):
Date of last chest x-ray:
Client's health concerns in this area:

### Fluids/Electrolytes
Usual fluid intake:
Preferred liquid choices:
Fluid dislikes and intolerances:
Use of alcoholic beverages:
If yes, describe type, amount, and frequency of use.
Use of salt in cooking and at table:
Use of salt substitute:
Client's health concerns in this area:

### Nutrition
Usual eating habits (number and timing of meals, inclusion of Basic Four Food Groups, preferred foods, restrictions
   and intolerances):
Food allergies:
Appetite:
Recent changes in eating habits and/or appetite:
Height: _____      Present weight: _____
Weight gain/loss pattern:
Perception of weight status:
Use of dietary aids to maintain weight:
Importance of food to well-being:
Symbolic meanings of food (reward, love, punishment, etc.):
Religious dietary restrictions:

Cultural preferences:
Economic restraints:
Geographic constraints:
Person responsible for food preparation in the home:
Use and care of oral prosthetics (braces, dentures, plates, etc.):
Fit of prostheses:
Date of last dental visit:

Presence of:

| | | |
|---|---|---|
| Bad taste in mouth _____ | Belching _____ | Bleeding gums and mucous membranes _____ |
| Difficulty chewing _____ | Nausea _____ | Adequate salivation _____ |
| Difficulty swallowing _____ | Heartburn _____ | Frequent sores on gums and mucous membranes _____ |
| Alterations in taste _____ | Caries _____. | |

Use of drugs or other substances to handle the above:
Client's health concerns in this area:

In addition to the above, when gathering health history on a child, ask about feeding patterns:

## *Elimination*
Usual pattern of bowel elimination (frequency, color, consistency, and amount):
Changes in pattern of elimination:
Incontinence (methods of management):

| | |
|---|---|
| Constipation _____ | Rectal bleeding _____ |
| Diarrhea _____ | Flatulence _____ |

Aids used to manage problems of elimination (laxatives, beverages, foods, positions):
Usual pattern of urination (amount, frequency, color, and odor):
Changes in pattern of urination:
Incontinence (methods of management):
Client's health concerns in this area:

In addition to the above, when gathering health history on a child, ask if the child is toilet-trained:

## *Rest/Sleep*
Usual time of retiring and rising:
Naps:
Changes in sleep pattern:
Bedtime rituals:
Aids to sleep:
Client's health concerns in this area:
Presence of discomfort and/or pain:
Sources of discomfort:
Aids used for relief:
Recent stress at home or on the job:
Current stressful situation:
Usual response to stress/crisis:
Resources used to cope with stress (personal strengths, activities, persons, drugs and/or substances, i. e., tobacco, alcohol):
Client's health concerns in this area:

## *Immunization*

| | Date of Disease | Date of Immunization |
|---|---|---|
| Chickenpox | _____ | _____ |
| Diphtheria | _____ | _____ |
| Influenza | _____ | _____ |
| Mumps | _____ | _____ |
| Pertussis | _____ | _____ |
| Polio | _____ | _____ |
| Rubella | _____ | _____ |
| Rubeola | _____ | _____ |
| Scarlet Fever | _____ | _____ |
| Tetanus | _____ | _____ |
| Tuberculosis | _____ | _____ |

## Sexual Growth

*Female*
Age at menarche _____    Age at menopause _____
Date of last vaginal/rectal examination:
Date of last pap smear:
Date of last breast examination (self and/or health care provider):
Knowledge of sexuality, reproduction, family planning methods, etc.:
Attitudes toward own sexuality:

Obstetrical History
Number of pregnancies:
Number of full-term deliveries:
Number of stillbirths:
Number of abortions:
Complications during pregnancy and/or delivery:
Family planning method used:
Infertility problems:

*Male*
Knowledge of sexuality, reproduction, family planning methods, etc.:
Attitudes toward own sexuality:
Number of natural offspring:
Circumcised:
Date of last rectal examination for prostatic enlargement:
Date of last testicular examination:
Client's health concerns in this area:

*Sexual Activity* (assess only if applicable)
Libido:
Last sexual contact:
Usual frequency of sexual contact:
Satisfaction with sexual performance:
Any concerns related to marital relations:

*Child*
Knowledge of own sexuality:
Sexual activities:
Interest in sexual relations:
Physical development of sex organs:

## Safety/Security Needs

### Physical Safety

*Perception/Coordination*
Sensory status (visual, auditory, olfactory, skin/tactile):
Visual
Date of last eye examination:
Restrictions in vision: R _____    L _____
Prosthesis (glasses, contact lenses, artificial eye):
Use and maintenance, purpose, and effectiveness of prosthesis:
History of problems (including any surgery):

Auditory
Date of last hearing examination:
Restrictions in hearing: R _____    L _____
Cause for restriction: _____
Use and maintenance of prosthesis (hearing aid):
History of problems (including any surgery):

Olfactory
Presence of:
Problems with smelling _____ nosebleeds _____ rhinorrhea _____ sinusitis _____ obstruction of nasal
    passage _____

Skin/Tactile
Use of/intolerance to soaps, lotions, etc.:
Mode and frequency of bathing (tub, shower, sink):
Altered integrity
Rashes, acne, dryness:
Wounds:
Altered sensation:
Excessive perspiration:
Pruritis:

*Mobility*
Usual daily exercise/activity patterns (e.g., ambulation, household chores, personal hygiene, job, planned exercise
   programs):
Activity tolerance (endurance):
Stressors compromising ability to perform ADL (personal hygiene, food preparation):
Fatigue _____   Pain _____
Limitation of range of motion _____
Muscular weakness/paralysis _____
Degree of independence in performing tasks:
Use of aids for ambulation:
Client's health concerns in this area:

**Emotional Safety**
Changes in affect:
Sleep problems (dreams, nightmares):
Frequent crying:
Withdrawal:
Problems with decision making, work, sex:
Suicidal thoughts and/or attempts:
Depression:
Anxiety:
Behavioral response when angry:
Behavioral response when sad:
Use of drugs, substances, or other coping activities:
History of problems in this area, including hospitalizations or outpatient treatment:
Client's health concerns in this area:

**Environmental Safety**
Occupation:

*Employment History*
Present place of employment:
Length of present employment:
Job description:

*Economic Status*
Total family income per week/month/year:
Significance of health status on financial security:
Type of medical insurance coverage:

*Living Situation*
Housing accommodations (apartment, house, duplex, etc.):
With whom shared:
Number of rooms and their description:
Furnishings adequate/inadequate:
Plumbing/heating facilities adequate/inadequate:
Number of stairways involved:
Character of neighborhood/community:
Presence of allergens, pollutants, noise within community:
Availability of community resources (health clinics or crisis centers):
Means of available transportation within community:
Means of personal transportation:

Profile of school (distance from home, means of transportation, type, grade, relationship with teacher, success or difficulties):
Client's health concerns in this area:

In addition to the above, when gathering a health history on a child, ask:

*Play facilities:*
Safety of home structure:
Safety of community environment:

## Love/*Belonging Needs*
Marital status:
Members of family unit (family as perceived by client)—
    Names:
    Birthdates:
    Sexes:
    Relationships to client:
    Household tasks performed by each member:
Autonomy of individual family members:
Allocation of family and personal roles:
Distribution of power and authority:
Achievement of developmental tasks:
Family goals (education, health futures, children):
Sharing of thoughts and feelings among members (amount, type):
Interactions with friends, co-workers, and neighbors:
Means by which family members express kindness and consideration (cards, flowers, gifts, telephone calls):
Care of ill family members:
Geographic distance from extended-family support system:
Type and number of pets:
Membership in any organization or group:
Religious affiliation:
Level of involvement in religious activities:
Cultural group with whom client identifies:
Influences of cultural group on life-style:
Client's health concerns in this area:

## Esteem/Recognition Needs

*Communication*
Dominant language:
Facility with language:
Interferences with communication:

*Motivation*
Motivating forces (money, status, prestige, fulfillment, acknowledgement):
Ability to initiate changes:
Reaction to changes:
Acceptance of present life-style:
Changes desired in life-style:
Accomplishments during life time:

*Perception of self*
Assets or strengths:
Positive traits:
Client's health concerns in this area:

## Self-Actualization Needs
Value system with which client identifies:
Means of coping with changing values:
Moral/ethical code with which client identifies:
Personal philosophy:

Beliefs about health care system:
Attitude about own ability to produce changes:
Degree of goal orientation:
Perception of degree of independence/dependence:
Perception of successes/failures:
Perception of self as creative:
Perceived areas of lack of fulfillment:

# Nutritional Assessment Forms

I. Identifying Data
   - A. Name _____
   - B. Sex _____
   - C. Age _____
   - D. Height _____
   - E. Weight _____

II. Does client complain of
   - Constipation _____
   - Diarrhea _____
   - Food allergens _____
   - Food intolerances _____
   - Nausea _____
   - Vomiting _____
   - Feeling of fullness _____
   - Heartburn _____
   - Choking _____
   - Loss of appetite _____
   - Denture problems _____

   Weight gain or loss (over 5 pounds) over past year _____
   Describe all items checked in terms of onset, frequency, severity, and character as well as client's perception of cause and interference with normal eating patterns.

III. Food Attainment and Preparation
   - A. Food shopping
     1. Who does most of the shopping?
     2. What is the major source of food?
     3. What is the frequency of shopping?
     4. Is transportation a problem?
     5. Are food storage facilities adequate?
   - B. Financial
     1. Is there an economic problem in obtaining adequate food?
     2. Is the client receiving WIC vouchers or food stamps?
   - C. Food preparation
     1. Are cooking facilities adequate?
     2. Who prepares client's meals?
     3. Are food additives used?
     4. Where does the client usually eat meals?
     Describe any areas of concern:

IV. Nutritional Habits
   - A. Gross meal assessment
     What items are most frequently eaten for
     Breakfast _____

     Lunch _____

     Dinner _____

Snacks _____

_____

B. At what hour does the client usually eat:
Breakfast _____
Lunch _____
Dinner _____
C. With whom does the client share meals?
D. Estimate frequency of
Use of soft drinks _____
Use of coffee _____
Use of tea _____
Intake of alcohol _____
Skipped meals _____
E. Are there specific ethnic, cultural, or religious food habits?
F. Food likes, dislikes, intolerances?
Description of any _____
G. Does the client take a dietary supplement?
Type _____
Dose _____
Frequency _____
H. Does the client have unusual dietary practices such as fad diets?
V. Special Diets
If the client has ever been on a special diet, describe:
A. Reason for diet as perceived by client
B. Assigned by whom? (physician, self, or other)
C. Expected and attained results
D. Compliance as perceived by client

346

**FOOD DIARY FORM—A. RECORD ALL FOODS AND DRINKS THAT YOU HAD DURING THE LAST 24 HOURS**

| Meal | Hour | Food and Quantity |
|------|------|-------------------|
| Breakfast | | |
| Snack | | |
| Lunch | | |
| Snack | | |
| Dinner | | |
| Bedtime snack | | |

## B. NUTRITIONAL ANALYSIS

| (1) Basic Food Group | (2) Food and Quantity | (3) RDA= Cal. | (4) RDA= Fat | (5) RDA= CHO Total | (5) RDA= CHO Fiber | (6) RDA= PRO | (7) RDA= Fe | (8) RDA= Ca | (9) RDA= Vit. A | (10) RDA= Vit. C | (11) RDA= Vit. $B_1$ | (12) RDA= Vit. $B_2$ | (13) RDA= Niacin |
|---|---|---|---|---|---|---|---|---|---|---|---|---|---|
| Milk Group RDA___ No. Svgs.___ H, L, A | | | | | | | | | | | | | |
| Meat Group RDA___ No. Svgs.___ H, L, A | | | | | | | | | | | | | |
| Vegetable-Fruit Group RDA___ No. Svgs.___ H, L, A | | | | | | | | | | | | | |
| Bread-Cereal Group RDA___ No. Svgs.___ H, L, A | | | | | | | | | | | | | |
| Miscellaneous | | | | | | | | | | | | | |

Evaluation:
A. Total of each column
B. Compare to RDA; state H, L, A (High, Low, Average)

*Adapted from forms used at SIUE School of Nursing, Edwardsville, Ill., with permission.*

# Life-style and Health Habits Assessment Form

Please place an X before each statement that is true regarding your *present* way of life or personal habits. That is, what you generally do.

## General Competence in Self-care (14)
_____ Take 12–15 deep breaths at least three times daily
_____ Drink 6–8 glasses of water each day in addition to other liquids
_____ Do not smoke
_____ Read articles or books about promoting health
_____ Know my body contours and physical sensations well
_____ Do not take laxative medications
_____ Know what my blood pressure and pulse readings should be
_____ Protect my skin from excessive sun exposure
_____ Know the seven danger signs of cancer
_____ Observe my body monthly for cancer danger signs
_____ Understand how to correctly examine my breasts (women only)
_____ Conduct monthly breast self-examination (women only)
_____ Use soft toothbrush regularly
_____ Dental floss regularly
Total number of items checked _____ Percent checked _____

## Nutritional Practices (16)
_____ Know about the "basic four" food groups
_____ Plan or select meals to meet nutritional needs
_____ Eat breakfast daily
_____ Eat three meals a day
_____ Avoid between-meal snacks
_____ Drink only small amounts (no more than 3 cups/day) of caffeinated beverages (coffees, teas, or colas)
_____ Do not consume alcoholic beverages or do so in very limited amounts
_____ Limit intake of refined sugars (junk foods or desserts)
_____ Frequently use unprocessed foods or foods without preservatives or other additives
_____ Maintain adequate roughage (fiber) in diet (whole grains, raw fruits, raw vegetables)
_____ Read labels for nutrients in packaged food
_____ Eat more poultry and fish than red meats
_____ Chew foods thoroughly and eat slowly
_____ Add little or no salt to my food when cooking or during eating
_____ Keep weight within recommended limits for my height
_____ Avoid frequent consumption of charcoaled foods
Total number of items checked _____ Percent checked _____

## Physical or Recreational Activity (9)

_____ Walk up stairs rather than riding the elevator
_____ Exercise vigorously for 30–40 minutes at least four times per week
_____ Regularly engage in recreational sports (swimming, soccer, bicycling)
_____ Perform stretching exercises at least four times per week to increase flexibility.
_____ Participate in individual sports for the pleasure of movement and physical fitness
_____ Engage in competitive sports primarily for enjoyment rather than competition
_____ Maintain good posture when sitting or standing
_____ Often elevate my legs when sitting
_____ Seldom sit with legs crossed at knees
Total number of items checked _____ Percent checked _____

## Sleep Patterns (9)

_____ Get 7 hours of sleep per night (not 1½ hours less or more)
_____ Wake up feeling fresh and relaxed
_____ Take some time for relaxation each day
_____ Fall asleep easily at night
_____ Sleep soundly
_____ Systematically relax voluntary muscles before sleep
_____ Sleep on a firm mattress
_____ Use a small pillow for sleep that maintains head and neck in a natural position
_____ Allow the thoughts and worries of the day to leave my mind, concentrating on passive but pleasant thoughts at bedtime
Total number of items checked _____ Percent checked _____

## Stress Management (11)

_____ Can laugh at myself
_____ Frequently laugh out loud with others
_____ Maintain adequate vitamin C intake when experiencing high stress
_____ Practice relaxation or meditation for 15–20 minutes daily
_____ Understand the relationship between stress and illness
_____ Create relaxed atmosphere at meal time
_____ Forget my problems and enjoy myself when immediate solutions are not possible
_____ Enjoy spending time in unstructured activities
_____ Consider it acceptable to cry, feel sad, angry, or afraid
_____ Find constructive ways to express my feelings
_____ Have attended training classes or biofeedback sessions to gain relaxation skills
Total number of items checked _____ Percent checked _____

## Self-Actualization (12)

_____ Maintain an enthusiastic and optimistic outlook on life
_____ Enjoy expressing myself in hobbies, the arts, exercise, or play
_____ Like myself and enjoy occasional solitude
_____ Continue to grow and change in positive directions
_____ Am happy most of the time
_____ Am a member of one or more community groups
_____ Feel fulfilled in my work
_____ Aware of personal strengths and weaknesses
_____ Am proud of my body and my personality
_____ Respect my own accomplishments
_____ Find each day interesting and challenging
_____ Look forward to the future
Total number of items checked _____ Percent checked _____

## Sense of Purpose (4)

_____ Aware of what is important to me in life
_____ Have identified short-term and long-term life goals
_____ Am realistic about the goals that I set
_____ Believe that my life has purpose
Total number of items checked _____ Percent checked _____

## Relationships with Others (11)

_____ Have persons close to me with whom I can discuss personal problems and concerns
_____ Perceive myself as being well accepted by others
_____ Maintain meaningful and fulfilling interpersonal relationships

_____ Communicate easily with others
_____ Recognize accomplishments and praise other people easily
_____ Enjoy my neighbors
_____ Have a number of close friends
_____ Thoughtfully consider constructive criticism rather than reacting defensively
_____ Enjoy being touched and touching people close to me
_____ Find it easy to express concern, love, and warmth to others
_____ Enjoy meeting new people and getting to know them
Total number of items checked _____ Percent checked _____

**Environmental Control (6)**
_____ When possible, prevent overwhelming changes in my environment
_____ Avoid purchasing aerosol sprays
_____ Seldom listen to loud rock music
_____ Do not permit smoking in my home or car
_____ Provide resources to meet my own personal needs
_____ Maintain safe living area free from fire or accident hazards
Total number of items checked _____ Percent checked _____

**Use of Health Care System (8)**
_____ Report any unusual signs or symptoms to a physician
_____ Question my physician or seek a second opinion when I do not agree with the recommended
treatment
_____ Expect prompt, helpful, and courteous personalized service from health care personnel
_____ Discuss health care concerns or problems with the health professional most qualified to provide
meaningful assistance
_____ Have breasts examined at least once a year by nurse or physician
_____ Have a pap smear at intervals recommended by my physician
_____ Have a rectal examination at intervals recommended by my physician
_____ Attend educational classes on personal health care provided within the community
Total number of items checked _____ Percent checked _____

*Scoring:* Calculate the percentage of items checked in each category by dividing the number of items that you
checked by the total number of items listed in the category (total number of items in each category is listed in
parentheses by category title). Record below the percentage of items checked from each category.

| Category | Percentage of Items Checked | Rating (see below) |
|---|---|---|
| Competency in self-care | _____ | _____ |
| Nutritional practices | _____ | _____ |
| Physical or recreational activity | _____ | _____ |
| Sleep patterns | _____ | _____ |
| Stress management | _____ | _____ |
| Self-actualization | _____ | _____ |
| Sense of purpose | _____ | _____ |
| Relationships with others | _____ | _____ |
| Environmental control | _____ | _____ |
| Use of health care system | _____ | _____ |

For each category, the following scale may be used to evaluate the extent to which the client's life-style and health
habits maintain or promote personal health.

| Rating | Percentage of Items Checked |
|---|---|
| Excellent | Greater than 85% |
| Good | 75–84% |
| Average | 65–74% |
| Fair | 55–64% |
| Poor | Below 55% |

From Pender, N: *Health Promotion in Nursing Practice.* Norwalk, Conn.: Appleton-Century-Crofts, 1982, with permission.

# Physical Assessment Tool

Client's name: _____
Health care facility: _____
Date of assessment: _____
Reason for seeking health care: _____

I. Social status
   Age:
   Sex:
   Race:
   Marital status:
   Living relatives:

   Religious affiliation:
   Occupation:
   Housing accommodation:
   Financial status:

II. Pertinent information about family history

III. Pertinent information from past medical–surgical history

IV. General behavior
   Apathy:
   Lethargy:
   Hyperirritability:
   Depression:
   Mental sluggishness:
   Apprehension:
   Alertness:

   Hyperactivity:
   Emotional lability:
   Tenseness:
   Restlessness:
   Rapidity of speech:
   Euphoria:
   Anxiety:

V. Whole organism
   A. Growth
      Height:
      Weight:
      Alteration in body proportion and features:
      Nutritional status:
   B. Metabolism
      Metabolic rate—
         Basal metabolic rate:
         Tolerance to cold:
         Tolerance to heat:
         Temperature of skin:

         Body temperature:
         Shivers:
         Tolerance to drugs:

      Metabolism of fats, proteins, and carbohydrates—
         Weakness:
         Muscle wasting:
         Glycosuria:
         Fatigue:

         Hypoglycemia
         Hyperglycemia:
         Trunkal obesity:
         Fat pads:

      Assessment of plasma and/or serum levels—
         Glucose:
         Total protein:

Albumin:
Cholesterol:
Triglycerides:
Assessment of urine levels—
Albumin:
Glucose:
Ketone bodies:
Metabolism of minerals
Serum and plasma levels—
Sodium:
Potassium:
Chloride:
Calcium:
Phosphorus:
Urine levels of minerals—
VI. Organ systems
A. Integumentary system
Characteristics of skin (texture, rashes, color, pigmentation changes, presence of lesions or bruises, etc.):
Characteristics of hair (dry, soft, brittle, alopecia, color, distribution, texture, etc.):
Characteristics of nails (color, brittle, soft, grooved, etc.):
B. Circulatory system
Arterial circulation (color and temperature of extremities, presence or absence of peripheral pulses, characteristics of pulses, etc.):
Venous circulation (presence of peripheral edema, presence of varicosities, etc.):
Characteristics of peripheral arteries and veins:
Blood pressure:
C. Respiratory system
Rate and rhythm of breathing:
Note shape of chest, width of costal angle, use of accessory muscles for breathing, level of diaphragm, presence of retraction, symmetry of respiratory movements, etc.:
D. Musculo-skeletal system
Determine presence or absence of tetany, atrophy, tremors, deformities, limitation of motion, redness of joints or muscles, decreased muscle strength, vertebral tenderness, curvature of the spine, crepitation as joint moves, bony enlargements, subcutaneous nodules around joints, etc.:
E. Lymphatic system
Enlargement, lack of consistency, or tenderness of lymph nodes (check cervical, axillary, epitrochlear, inguinal):
F. Digestive system
Assess abdomen for scars, tenderness, herniations, enlargement of liver or spleen, striae, dilated veins, rashes, lesions, contour, symmetry, presence of peristalsis and pulsations on auscultation, etc.:
Assess rectum for hemorrhoids, fissures, fistulas, presence of tenderness or masses, sphincter tone, etc.:
G. Urinary system
Characteristics of urine (color, odor, specific gravity, RBC, WBC, bacteria):
Determine presence of frequency, urgency, dysuria, nocturia, retention, incontinence, difficulty starting stream, etc.:
Palpate kidneys for tenderness, size, and contour:
H. Reproductive system
Male —
Assess scrotum for nodules, inflammation, masses, ulcers, swelling, etc.:
Assess penis for discharge, tenderness, size, contour, etc.:
Female —
Describe appearance of perineum and external genitalia, vagina, cervix, fundus:
Determine presence of masses, tenderness, bleeding, ulcerations, etc.:
Assess breasts (size, symmetry, contour, thickening of skin, venous pattern, etc.:
Assess nipples (size, shape, color, presence of rashes, ulcerations, discharge, etc.:
I. Nervous system
Assess cranial nerves, motor function, muscle strength, sensory system, reflexes:
VII. Tissues or organs
A. Eyes

       Determine color of conjunctiva and sclera:
       Pupils (size, shape, reaction to light, equality):
       Eyeballs (prominence, motion, tension, position, alignment, etc.):
       Eyelids (presence of ptosis, edema, skin changes, etc.):
       Vision:
  B. Ears
       Determine presence of discharge, mastoid tenderness, etc.:
       Describe appearance of external ear:
       Assess condition of canal and tympanic membranes:
       Bone conduction:
       Air conduction:
       Hearing:
  C. Mouth and throat
       Describe characteristics of tongue, breath, mucous membranes, teeth, tonsils, gums, etc.:
  D. Nose
       Describe appearance of mucosa:
       Determine presence of drainage, sinus tenderness, septal deviation, etc.:
  E. Heart
       Determine heart borders, heart sounds, presence of murmurs, PMI, presence of arrhythmias, etc.:
  F. Lungs
       Determine lung borders, breath sounds, vocal fremitus, presence of fluid, mucus, or obstruction in the air passages, air flow through the tracheobronchial tree, presence of adventitious or abnormal sounds, etc.:
VIII. Cellular level
       Red blood cell count:
       White blood cell count:
  IX. Subcellular level:
       Hemoglobin level:
       Hematocrit level:

A semistructured format is used for this tool. Suggested topics are listed, but the tool is not meant to be inclusive.

# Family System Assessment Tool

| | Points |
|---|---|
| I. Family members relating to one another | |
| A. Individuality and autonomy | |
| 1. a. Each family member demonstrates respect for self | (2) _____ |
| b. Some family members demonstrate respect for self | (1) _____ |
| c. Very few or no family member(s) demonstrate(s) respect for self | (0) _____ |
| 2. a. Each family member demonstrates respect for individuality of every other family member | (2) _____ |
| b. Some family members demonstrate respect for individuality of other family members | (1) _____ |
| c. Very few or no family members show respect for individuality of other family members | (0) _____ |
| 3. a. Each family member is tolerant and responsive to other family members | (2) _____ |
| b. Some family members are tolerant and responsive to other family members | (1) _____ |
| c. Very few or no family members are tolerant and show responsiveness to other family members | (0) _____ |
| 4. a. Each family member feels a sense of freedom to grow | (2) _____ |
| b. Some family members feel a sense of freedom to grow | (1) _____ |
| c. Family members feel constricted in ability to grow | (0) _____ |
| 5. When conflicts arise in the family individual views are | |
| a. Always respected | (2) _____ |
| b. Sometimes respected | (1) _____ |
| c. Scarcely ever or never respected | (0) _____ |
| 6. Individuals in the family are unique and | |
| a. Clearly distinct from one another | (2) _____ |
| b. Fairly distinct from one another | (1) _____ |
| c. Very similar in thoughts, feelings, and actions | (0) _____ |

Total points possible ___12___

Total not applicable _____

Total applicable _____

Total points attained _____

| | |
|---|---|
| B. Communication | |
| 1. Family members communicate with each other | |
| a. Regularly | (2) _____ |
| b. Sometimes | (1) _____ |
| c. Hardly ever | (0) _____ |
| 2. Communication among family members shows | |
| a. Much variety | (2) _____ |
| b. Some variety | (1) _____ |
| c. Very little variety | (0) _____ |
| 3. Communications are | |
| a. Always open and spontaneous | (2) _____ |

      b. Sometimes open and spontaneous                (1) _____

      c. Constricted and rigid                          (0) _____

   4. Communications show humor and wit

      a. Frequently                                  (2) _____

      b. Sometimes                                  (1) _____

      c. Infrequently or hardly ever               (0) _____

   5. Family members discuss

      a. Any matter of interest to the family       (2) _____

      b. Only what certain family members wish to discuss   (1) _____

      c. Very few interests of anyone in the family    (0) _____

   6. Communications occur

      a. Usually in depth                           (2) _____

      b. Sometimes in depth                       (1) _____

      c. Usually superficially                      (0) _____

   7. The emotional tone of the family is one of

      a. Warmth                                 (2) _____

      b. Coolness                               (1) _____

      c. Neutrality—no emotional tone detected     (0) _____

   8. Family members

      a. Frequently express feelings about each other   (2) _____

      b. Sometimes express feelings about each other   (1) _____

      c. Hardly ever or never express feelings about each other  (0) _____

   9. The family permits

      a. Expression of a range of emotions        (2) _____

      b. Expression of only certain emotions      (1) _____

      c. Little to no expression of any emotions    (0) _____

  10. Communications are

      a. Straightforward most of the time        (2) _____

      b. Straightforward some of the time       (1) _____

      c. Usually filled with hidden meanings     (0) _____

  11. Communications are

      a. Clear, spontaneous, with interruptions tolerated   (2) _____

      b. Clear, well-punctuated, with interruptions not tolerated  (1) _____

      c. Unintelligible and frequently misinterpreted   (0) _____

  12. When disagreements arise when communicating, family members

      a. Seldom feel threatened                  (2) _____

      b. Sometimes feel threatened              (1) _____

      c. Usually feel threatened                (0) _____

  13. Family communications show

      a. A high degree of empathy              (2) _____

      b. A moderate degree of empathy        (1) _____

      c. Very little or no empathy             (0) _____

  14. Family members

      a. Usually feel understood               (2) _____

      b. Sometimes feel understood            (1) _____

      c. Seldom or never feel understood       (0) _____

|  |  |
|---|---|
| Total points possible | _28_ |
| Total not applicable | |
| Total applicable | |
| Total points attained | |

C. Bonding

   1. Bonds are evident through relationships among/between

      a. All family members                     (2) _____

      b. Some family members                   (1) _____

      c. No family members                      (0) _____

   2. Family demonstrates

      a. Much capacity for changing bonds over time   (2) _____

      b. Little capacity to change bonds       (1) _____

     c. No capacity for changing bonds     (0) _____
3. Interdependence among family members is demonstrated among
     a. All family members     (2) _____
     b. Some family members     (1) _____
     c. Few family members     (0) _____
4. Each marital partner feels his/her needs are met
     a. Nearly all of the time     (2) _____
     b. Some of the time     (1) _____
     c. Hardly ever or never     (0) _____
5. Marital partners function with
     a. A high degree of complementarity     (2) _____
     b. Some complementarity     (1) _____
     c. Very little complementarity but much separateness     (0) _____
6. Marital partners express affection for each other
     a. Frequently     (2) _____
     b. Sometimes     (1) _____
     c. Seldom or never     (0) _____
7. Marital partners demonstrate
     a. Pride in each other's assets and strengths     (2) _____
     b. Some pride but some indifference in each other's assets and strengths     (1) _____
     c. Hostility, anger, resentment, or jealousy in each other's assets and strengths     (0) _____
8. Marital partners demonstrate
     a. Much cooperation with each other     (2) _____
     b. Some cooperation but some competition with each other     (1) _____
     c. Much competition with each other     (0) _____
9. A feeling of security within the family is experienced by
     a. All family members     (2) _____
     b. Some family members     (1) _____
     c. Few or no family member(s)     (0) _____

    Total points possible     *18*
    Total not applicable _____
    Total applicable _____
    Total points attained _____

II. Family Members Functioning Together
  A. Roles and Role Relationships
    1 Roles within the family are accepted by
     a. All family members     (2) _____
     b. Some family members     (1) _____
     c. Few or no family member(s)     (0) _____
    2. Parents show acceptance of work roles
     a. Most of the time     (2) _____
     b. Some of the time     (1) _____
     c. Hardly ever or never     (0) _____
    3. Parents show acceptance of parental roles
     a. Most of the time     (2) _____
     b. Some of the time     (1) _____
     c. Hardly ever or never     (0) _____
    4. Parents show acceptance of marital roles
     a. Most of the time     (2) _____
     b. Some of the time     (1) _____
     c. Hardly ever or never     (0) _____
    5. Mutual expectations of marital partners are met
     a. Or surpassed     (2) _____
     b. To some degree     (1) _____
     c. To a minimal degree or not at all     (0) _____
    6. Marital partners consider that their physical and emotional needs are met
     a. Consistently and to a high degree     (2) _____
     b. Irregularly or to a moderate degree     (1) _____
     c. Seldom or never or to a minimal degree     (0) _____

7. Parents enjoy their children
   a. Most of the time                                                    (2) _____
   b. Some but not much of the time                                       (1) _____
   c. Seldom or not any of the time                                       (0) _____
8. Parents feel satisfaction in childrearing
   a. Most of the time                                                    (2) _____
   b. Some of the time                                                    (1) _____
   c. Seldom or never                                                     (0) _____
9. Parents use discipline
   a. Usually to guide children                                           (2) _____
   b. Sometimes to guide but often to force or punish children            (1) _____
   c. Usually to force, punish, or constrict children                     (0) _____
10. Roles within the family are
    a. Highly flexible as the situation changes                           (2) _____
    b. Sometimes flexible                                                 (1) _____
    c. Rigidly followed all the time                                      (0) _____
11. Responsibility for discipline of the children is
    a. Shared by both parents                                             (2) _____
    b. Assumed by only one parent                                         (1) _____
    c. Assumed by neither parent                                          (0) _____

                                         Total points possible    ___22___
                                         Total not applicable      _____
                                         Total applicable          _____
                                         Total points attained     _____

B. Division of Tasks and Activities
   1. Performance of tasks is
      a. Highly interchangeable and flexible                             (2) _____
      b. Somewhat interchangeable and flexible                           (1) _____
      c. Always closely adhered to                                       (0) _____
   2. Task roles in the family are determined
      a. Mostly by each individual                                       (2) _____
      b. Sometimes by each individual but also by the leader in the family (1) _____
      c. Mostly by the leader in the family                              (0) _____
   3. Task performance roles are developed according to
      a. Interest and ability of the person                              (2) _____
      b. Sometimes according to interest and ability but also by age and sex (1) _____
      c. Age and sex stereotypes only                                    (0) _____
   4. The organization of family tasks is
      a. Usually flexible                                                (2) _____
      b. Sometimes flexible                                              (1) _____
      c. Usually rigid                                                   (0) _____

                                         Total points possible    ___8___
                                         Total not applicable      _____
                                         Total applicable          _____
                                         Total points attained     _____

C. Governance and Power
   1. Governance in the family is characterized by
      a. Each person being guided by principles of good judgment         (2) _____
      b. Mutual agreement of family members to a set of rules            (1) _____
      c. Each person attempting to achieve his or her ends through threats, coaxing,
         and negativism                                                  (0) _____
   2. Rules in the family are
      a. Agreed on by all members by mutual consent                      (2) _____
      b. Agreed on by some members and forced on others                  (1) _____
      c. Forced on all members by the leader                             (0) _____
   3. Governance is characterized by patterns of
      a. Egalitarianism                                                  (2) _____
      b. Some egalitarianism but also some authoritarianism              (1) _____

       c. Authoritarianism and dominance/submission             (0) _____

  4. Each member of the family is

       a. Usually self-governed                                 (2) _____

       b. Sometimes self-governed but sometimes governed by an authority figure     (1) _____

       c. Governed by some authority figure                      (0) _____

  5. Power in the family is

       a. Shared among family members                           (2) _____

       b. Sometimes shared but sometimes assumed by one person       (1) _____

       c. Usually controlled by one person                       (0) _____

  6. Children are given opportunities for self-determination and self-governance

       a. Frequently according to growth and developmental stages      (2) _____

       b. Sometimes but not often, according to growth and developmental stages   (1) _____

       c. Hardly ever, or never, at any stage of growth and development     (0) _____

  7. Governance by principles is used in

       a. Most decision-making situations                       (2) _____

       b. Some decision-making situations                      (1) _____

       c. Few or no decision-making situations                (0) _____

                                   Total points possible     *14*

                                   Total not applicable   _____

                                     Total applicable   _____

                                   Total points attained   _____

D. Decision Making and Problem Solving

  1. Decision making and problem solving are characterized by

       a. Much creativity                                     (2) _____

       b. Some creativity                                    (1) _____

       c. Little to no creativity                               (0) _____

  2. When an alternative does not work, the family

       a. Usually tries another alternative                       (2) _____

       b. Sometimes tries another alternative but tries to make the first one work   (1) _____

       c. Keeps trying to make the first option work              (0) _____

  3. The family is willing and able to deal with a

       a. Wide range of problems, including emotional ones          (2) _____

       b. Narrow range of problems, but sometimes including emotional ones   (1) _____

       c. Narrow range of problems, not including emotional ones     (0) _____

  4. The family

       a. Tends to all problems in some way                    (2) _____

       b. Tends to some problems, but also avoids dealing with other problems   (1) _____

       c. Avoids dealing with any problems as much as possible     (0) _____

  5. Difficult problems are seen as

       a. Solvable, and therefore are dealt with                 (2) _____

       b. Not usually solvable but attempts are made to try to solve them    (1) _____

       c. Not solvable and therefore are avoided               (0) _____

  6. The family views small problems as

       a. Small problems and not as threatening                 (2) _____

       b. Sometimes small problems but sometimes as very complex    (1) _____

       c. Very complex and threatening                     (0) _____

  7. The family attempts to cope with life's problems

       a. On a daily basis                                  (2) _____

       b. Only when the problem becomes a large one          (1) _____

       c. Seldom or infrequently                         (0) _____

  8. In handling problems and decisions, the family is

       a. Open to new ideas, information, and resources          (2) _____

       b. Not always willing to try new ideas, information, or resources    (1) _____

       c. Resistant to any new ideas, information, or resources     (0) _____

  9. When making decisions, the family involves in the decision-making process

       a. All those who are affected by the decision           (2) _____

       b. Some but not all persons who are affected by the decision    (1) _____

       c. Only the leader in the family                     (0) _____

10. Rules for making decisions are
   a. Highly flexible      (2) _____
   b. Somewhat flexible      (1) _____
   c. Rigid      (0) _____
11. Decision making involves
   a. Little of the family's time      (2) _____
   b. A moderate amount of the family's time      (1) _____
   c. Much of the family's time      (0) _____
12. Skills in decision making are learned by
   a. All family members      (2) _____
   b. Some family members      (1) _____
   c. Few family members      (0) _____
13. When the family is unable to reach a decision
   a. All family members agree on who will make the final selection of alternatives      (2) _____
   b. Some or one family member(s) decide(s) on who will make the final selection of alternatives      (1) _____
   c. The impasse prevails and no decision is reached      (0) _____

Total points possible   26
Total not applicable   _____
Total applicable   _____
Total points attained   _____

E. Leadership and Initiative
1. Leadership is
   a. Usually shared, depending on the situation      (2) _____
   b. Sometimes shared, depending on the situation      (1) _____
   c. Always assumed by one person      (0) _____
2. Leadership is
   a. Usually effective      (2) _____
   b. Sometimes but not always effective      (1) _____
   c. Usually ineffective      (0) _____
3. With regard to leadership in the total family, parents have
   a. Greater influence than children      (2) _____
   b. About the same influence as children      (1) _____
   c. Less influence than children or no influence at all      (0) _____
4. When one parent assumes a more dominant leadership role, the other parent is
   a. Always cooperative and supportive      (2) _____
   b. Sometimes cooperative and supportive      (1) _____
   c. Contradictory and divisive      (0) _____
5. The family's system of leadership is
   a. Mutually respectful of all family members      (2) _____
   b. Sometimes respectful but sometimes authoritarian      (1) _____
   c. Highly authoritarian most of the time      (0) _____
6. In meeting the family's needs, leadership in the family is
   a. Highly effective      (2) _____
   b. Sometimes effective      (1) _____
   c. Usually ineffective      (0) _____
7. Children are encouraged to seek and use opportunities to develop leadership skills
   a. Often      (2) _____
   b. Sometimes      (1) _____
   c. Seldom or never      (0) _____
8. The climate in the family for leadership development in the children is
   a. Always warm and supportive, and tolerant of failure      (2) _____
   b. Sometimes warm and supportive, and tolerant of failure      (1) _____
   c. Apathetic and nonsupportive, and intolerant of failure      (0) _____
9. The family unit as a whole
   a. Frequently shows initiative and actively seeks new experiences      (2) _____
   b. Sometimes shows initiative and sometimes seeks new experiences      (1) _____

      c. Is passive and seldom seeks new experiences       (0) _____

                    Total points possible    *18*

                    Total not applicable    _____

                    Total applicable    _____

                    Total points attained    _____

III. Involvement in Outside Community
    A. Groups and activities external to the family are participated in by
        1. All family members     (2) _____
        2. Some family members     (1) _____
        3. No family members     (0) _____
    B. The family provides input into the larger community
        1. Frequently     (2) _____
        2. Sometimes     (1) _____
        3. Seldom or never     (0) _____
    C. Use of the community's recreational, cultural, or educational resources is
        1. Extensive     (2) _____
        2. Limited     (1) _____
        3. Nonexistent     (0) _____
    D. The family seeks out community resources
        1. Frequently     (2) _____
        2. Sometimes     (1) _____
        3. Seldom or never     (0) _____

                    Total points possible    *8*

                    Total not applicable    _____

                    Total applicable    _____

                    Total points attained    _____

| Assessment Tool Summary | Subtotal Points Possible | Subtotal Not Applicable | Subtotal Applicable | Subtotal Points Attained |
|---|---|---|---|---|
| 1. Family Members Relating to One Another | | | | |
|   A. Individuality and Autonomy | 12 | \_\_\_\_ | \_\_\_\_ | \_\_\_\_ |
|   B. Communication | 28 | \_\_\_\_ | \_\_\_\_ | \_\_\_\_ |
|   C. Bonding | 18 | \_\_\_\_ | \_\_\_\_ | \_\_\_\_ |
| II. Family Members Functioning Together | | | | |
|   A. Roles and Role Relationships | 22 | \_\_\_\_ | \_\_\_\_ | \_\_\_\_ |
|   B. Division of Tasks and Activities | 8 | \_\_\_\_ | \_\_\_\_ | \_\_\_\_ |
|   C. Governance and Power | 14 | \_\_\_\_ | \_\_\_\_ | \_\_\_\_ |
|   D. Decision Making and Problem Solving | 26 | \_\_\_\_ | \_\_\_\_ | \_\_\_\_ |
|   E. Leadership and Initiative | 18 | \_\_\_\_ | \_\_\_\_ | \_\_\_\_ |
| III. Involvement in Outside Community | 8 | \_\_\_\_ | \_\_\_\_ | \_\_\_\_ |

                    Total points possible    *154*

                    Total not applicable    _____

                    Total applicable    _____

                    Total points attained    _____

From Kandzari, J. et al. *The Well Family*. Boston: Little, Brown, 1981, with permission.

# Family Assessment Tool

---

## General Description

Family Composition (family as perceived by client)

| Name | Sex | Birthdate | Place of Birth | Relationship to Client |
|------|-----|-----------|----------------|------------------------|
| | | | | |
| | | | | |
| | | | | |
| | | | | |
| | | | | |

Professional and/or volunteer person/agencies working with family: _____

---

## Assessment of Needs of the Family

### Physiological Needs
Use of tobacco by family members:
Use of alcoholic beverages by family members:
Use of prescribed medications by family members:

### *Usual Eating Habits*
Appearance indicating adequate nutrition (adult and children):*
Number and timing of meals:
Inclusion of Basic Four food groups:
Storage facilities for food:
Frequency of food purchases (daily, biweekly, weekly, or monthly):
Effect of financial restraints on food purchases:
Amount of money spent on food weekly:
Cultural preferences:
Person primarily responsible for food preparation in the home:

*If there is doubt about nutritional state, use complete Nutritional Assessment and Analysis form.

### *Sleeping Patterns of Individual Family Members*
Which family members sleep together:
Which family members sleep alone:
Sleeping accommodations available for family members (beds, bed linens, and pillows):

Room in which family members sleep: Bedroom _____
Living room _____ Basement _____ Family room _____
Usual time of retiring and rising: Adults _____
Children _____
Presence of allergies within family:

### General Impression of Family Relationships*
Relationship of adults with one another:
Relationship of each adult with children:
Relationship of children with one another:
Relationship of each child with adults:

*Information as perceived by each member of the family.

### Stress
Recent family stress:
Current stressful situation for family:
Family's usual response to stress/crisis:
Family resources utilized to cope with stress:

### Family Planning Practices
Consistency of use:
Conflict over method:
Implications for health:

## Safety/Security Needs

### Type of Health Maintenance
Source of family health care (clinics, private physicians, hospital emergency room, Health Maintenance Organizations):
Manner in which care is financed:

### Preventive Health Care Practices*
Date of last chest x-ray:
Date of last TB skin test:
Date of last eye examination:
Date of last hearing examination:
Date of last dental examination:
Date of last physical examination:
Immunizations:
Use of over-the-counter medication:

*Consider for each family member.

Use of prostheses and appliances (glasses, dentures, hearing aids):

### Type of Emergency Medical Plan
Availability of telephone numbers of ambulance, pharmacy, poison control, hospitals, physicians:
Availability of transportation in the event of an emergency:
Availability of support system:
Finances designated for emergency health care use:
Present health concerns of the family:
Usual activities of family members (adults and children):
Type of recreational activities (frequency, group, individual):

### Growth and Development (individual family member)

*Evidence of normal development patterns*
Biological:
Psychological:
Social:
Cognitive:
Moral/Ethical:
Achievement of developmental tasks:
Barriers to achievement:
Growth and development (family unit):

Stage of family development:
Achievement of developmental tasks:
Barriers to achievement:
Concerns related to individual or family development:

*Behavior patterns perceived as detrimental to individual family member(s) or family unit*

### Environmental safety

### Employment history of each family member
Present place of employment:
Length of present employment:
Job description:
Previous employment:
Potential threats to the health of family members related to employment:
Income adequate to meet family expenses:
If inadequate, determine presence of budgeting; amount saved monthly; method of paying expenses (cash or checks):
Total family income per week/month/year:

### Living Situation
Housing accommodations (apartment, house, duplex, etc.)
Rent or own:
Number and description of rooms:
Adequate/inadequate laundry facilities:
Adequate/inadequate furnishings:
Adequate/inadequate plumbing, sewage and heating facilities:
Adequate/inadequate trash collection:

*Presence of hazards in the home*
Poor lighting in halls and stairways:
Poisonous substances within reach of children:
Unsecured floor coverings:
Structural defects (deteriorating wood, broken concrete and brick):
Size and condition of yard for recreational activities:
Yard fenced or unfenced:
Proximity to busy street or alley:
Characteristics of neighborhood and community:
Presence of allergens, pollutants, noise within community:
Means of available transportation within community (bus, taxi service, street cars, car):
Means of personal transportation:
Present concerns of the family related to environmental safety:

### Love and Belonging Needs
Marital status:

### Allocation of family and personal roles
Adults:
Children:
Ability to shift roles to facilitate growth of family unit:
Childrearing practices:
Distribution of power and authority:

### Member Making Decisions Which Affect Family Unit
Adult members:
Children:
Member responsible for family finances:
Adequate/inadequate quality of interactions of family unit:
With—
    Extended family:
    Friends:
    Neighbors:
    Co-workers:
    Social groups:

Church members:
Means by which family unit expresses kindness and consideration:
Religious affiliation:
Level of involvement in religious activities:
Cultural groups with whom family identifies:
Influences of cultural groups on family lifestyles:

## Esteem and Recognition Needs
Dominant language used by family:
Family communication patterns:
Motivation—
    Educational level of each family member:
    Implications of educational levels for health teaching:
    Plans for future education:
    Relationship of educational level to family's socioeconomic goals:
Family's ability to adapt to changes affecting family unit:
Family's willingness to seek assistance when needed:

## Self-Actualization Needs

### Values and Goals of Family Unit
Adults:
Children:
Entire family:

### Ways in which family values are reflected
Neighborhood:
Residence:
Furnishings:
Type of reading material:
Wardrobe:
Health beliefs and practices:
Family's perception of its image:
Norms for social behavior accepted by family unit:
Philosophical and spiritual beliefs:

## Summarization of Family's Assets

# Community Assessment Tool

---

## Identify the Community to be Assessed

Name of community:
Geographical boundaries:
Census tract:
Area in square miles:

## Sources of Community Data

Interviews, census reports, books, newspapers, directories, etc.:

**History of Community**
Historical account of founding:
Developmental growth:
Dates of founding of major hospitals, health institutions, health departments, nongovernmental health agencies, nursing organizations:
Dates of epidemics and disasters:
Dates of court decisions and laws relating to health:

## Assessment of Needs of the Community

**Physiological Needs**
Urban/suburban/rural community:

***Physical description***
Geography:
Climate (temperature range, yearly precipitation, humidity):
Terrain:
Unusual topographical features:
Natural resources:

***Major concerns***
Crime rate:
Substance abuse:
Financial ability:
Poverty level (percentage below):

**Safety/Security Needs**

***Physical safety***
Adequate and Inadequate Protective Services—
    Ambulance:
    Civil defense:

Community nursing:
Educational (ecology, conservation, etc.):
Fire:
Health (immunization, chest x-ray, etc.):
Hospital:
Police:
Social agencies (Visiting Nurses Association, Easter Seals, etc.):
Transportation:
Summary of assets in this area:
Summary of potential health needs in this area:

### Environmental Safety
*Housing*
Types of dwellings (approximate percentage of each)—
    Single-family dwellings:
    Apartment complexes:
    Housing projects:
Condition of dwellings (old, new, substandard):
Median cost of single-family dwelling:
Median monthly rent:

*Water source*
Public:
Private (well):
Method of treatment:

*Sewage disposal methods*
Public:
Private (septic tank, outdoor toilets):
Method of treatment:

*Solid waste disposal methods*
Garbage collection
    Private:
    Public:
Public dump:
Landfill:
Vector control (rodent):

*Food and milk supply*
Approximate number of stores selling food items:
Approximate number of restaurants:

*Surface pollutants*
Presence of toxic substances (dioxin, asbestos, lead, etc.):
Abandoned cars:
Junk yards:
Standing water:

*Vector control methods*
Insects:
Mosquitos:
Rodents:
Others:

*Air pollutants*
Sources of pollution:
Presence of
    Smoke:
    Gases:
    Odors:
    Vapors:
    Pollens:
    Others:

Local restrictions governing industry, burning leaves, car emission, incinerators:

*Noise pollutants*
Sources of pollution (industry, airports, etc.):
Frequency, intensity, and time period involved:
Local restrictions (use of sirens on emergency vehicles, air traffic control, adherence to Environmental Protection Agency mandates, etc.):
Summary of assets in this area:
Summary of potential health needs in this area:

### Health Services

*Primary Health Care*

*Facilities*
    Dental, optical, and audio services:
    School health services:
    Occupational health agencies:
    Community health agencies:
    Health Department Services:
    Health Maintenance Organizations (HMOs):
Staffing pattern for facility (physicians, dentists, nurses, social workers, dietitians, etc.):
Screening programs (blood pressure, diabetes mellitus, stress surveys, etc.):

Health Education Activities
Types of programs and sponsoring agencies:
Speakers bureau for health topics:

*Secondary Health Care*

*Facilities*
    Hospitals (indicate services provided):
    Ambulatory care centers:
    Emergency services:
Staffing pattern for facility (physicians, nurses, radiologists, pathologists, laboratory and x-ray technicians, etc.):

Health Education Activities
Types of programs and sponsoring agencies:

*Tertiary Health Care*

Facilities
    Long-term (nursing home, etc.):
    Extended care:
    Rehabilitation:
    Hospice:
    Respite care:
Staffing pattern for facility (occupational therapists, physical therapists, nurses, rehabilitation specialists, dietitians, psychologists, social workers, etc.):

Health Education Activities
Type of programs and sponsoring agencies:

### Prevalent Health Concerns
*Morbidity/Mortality*
    Maternal:– Morbidity _____     Mortality _____
    Infant:–     Morbidity _____     Mortality _____
    Adult:–     Morbidity _____     Mortality _____
Identify existing patterns of morbidity and mortality (i.e., leading cause of death, types of chronic illness):
Incidence of communicable disease (type and percentage of occurence):

### Available Immunization Programs
Types of programs and sponsoring agencies:
Prevalent social concerns that may affect health:
Venereal disease (note type and prevalence):

Suicide rate:
Divorce rate:
Crime rate:
Other:
Summary of assets in this area:
Summary of potential health needs in this area:

### Economic Status

*Employment Distribution*
    Percent employed/unemployed
    Percent professional/white collar/blue collar:
Major industry and businesses (list and indicate number of employees):
Banks, savings and loan, credit unions (list and indicate number of employees):
Median income of population (compare with state/national median income):
Concerns of the community:

### Educational facilities
Type and number of facilities (indicate if private or public):
Available special educational programs (sensory impaired, mentally and/or physically handicapped, etc.):
Available health manpower facilities (medical, nursing, dental, allied health, etc.):
Libraries, museums, cultural centers:

*Educational Level of Population*
Percentage with
    Grade school education:
    High school education:
    Community college degree:
    Baccalaureate degree:
    Graduate degree:
    Concerns of the community:

### Transportation Facilities
Available major routes and services (buses, trains, taxis, etc.):
Concerns of the community:

### Governance
Form of government (mayor, city manager, etc.):
Key leaders:
Influential groups (NAACP, Jaycees, Community Service League, etc.):
City offices (location, hours, services):
Concerns of the community:

### Welfare Agencies
List resources, location, population served and service provided
    Public:
    Private (voluntary):

## Love/Belonging Needs

### Religion
Facilities and distribution (percentage) by denomination (list):
Religious leaders:
Community programs and services (day-care centers, food distribution, senior-citizen programs, respite programs, etc.):

### Population
Total population:
Number of people per square mile:

*Population composition*
    Sex ratio:
    Age distribution:

Cultural groups represented:
Race distribution:
Existing family structures:
Average number of children per family:
Summarize predominant characteristics of the current population (divorce rate, marriage rate, mobility):
Summarize changes that have occurred in the population in the past ten years:

## Esteem/Recognition Needs

### Communication
Languages spoken within community:

*Sources of communication*
Newspapers (consider frequency and readership):
Radio stations:
Television stations:

### Recreation
Type and number of facilities (indicate if private or public):
Type of other activities frequently used (list):
Leadership/supervision available during recreational hours:
Programs for special population groups (elderly, handicapped, etc.):

## Self Actualization Needs
Priorities of the community:
Attitudes, values, and belief systems projected by community:
Goals of the community for the next 5 years:
Community perception of its image:
Norms for social behavior accepted by community:

## Summarization of Community Assets

# National Conference on Classification of Nursing Diagnoses

Activity intolerance
Activity intolerance, potential
Airway clearance, ineffective
Anxiety
Bowel elimination, alteration in: constipation
Bowel elimination, alteration in: diarrhea
Bowel elimination, alteration in: incontinence
Breathing pattern, ineffective
Cardiac output, alteration in: decreased
Comfort, alteration in: pain
Communication, impaired: verbal
Coping, family: potential for growth
Coping, ineffective family: compromised
Coping, ineffective family: disabling
Coping, ineffective individual
Diversional activity, deficit
Family process, alteration in
Fear
Fluid volume alteration in: excess
Fluid volume deficit, actual
Fluid volume deficit, potential
Gas exchange, impaired
Grieving, anticipatory
Grieving, dysfunctional
Health maintenance, alteration in
Home maintenance management, impaired
Injury, potential for
Knowledge deficit (specify)
Mobility, impaired physical
Noncompliance (specify)
Nutrition, alteration in: less than body requirements
Nutrition, alteration in: more than body requirements
Nutrition, alteration in: potential from more than body requirements
Oral mucous membrane, alteration in
Parenting, alteration in: actual
Parenting, alteration in: potential
Powerlessness
Rape trauma syndrome

Self-care deficit: feeding, bathing/hygiene, dressing/grooming, toileting
Self-concept, disturbance in: body image, self-esteem, role performance, personal identity
Sensory–perceptual alteration: visual, auditory, kinesthetic, gustatory, tactile, olfactory
Sexual dysfunction
Skin integrity, impairment of: actual
Skin integrity, impairment of: potential
Sleep pattern disturbance
Social isolation
Spiritual distress (distress of the human spirit)
Thought processes, alteration in
Tissue perfusion, alteration in: cerebral, cardiopulmonary, renal, gastrointestinal, peripheral
Urinary elimination, alteration in patterns
Violence, potential for: self-directed or directed at others

From Kim, M. J., McFarland, G. & McLane, A. *Classification of Nursing Diagnoses: Proceedings of the Fifth National Conference.* New York: McGraw-Hill, 1984.

# Sample Teaching Plans

Code Number <u>P-4.1</u>
Date of Origin <u>July, 1979</u>
Revision Date _____

**Policy Heading:** Breast Self-Examination Teaching

**Policy Statement:** Female patients 20 years of age and older demonstrating need for breast self-examination teaching or reinforcement of prior teaching are to be taught following approved breast self-examination teaching plan.

---

**Patient Teaching Plan—Female Breast Self-Examination**

---

**Purpose:** To teach the patient breast self-examination.
To emphasize the need for monthly breast self-examination.
To emphasize the need for prompt medical attention for any breast lump or other changes.

| Content | Content Delivered *Date and Name* | Content Reinforced *Date and Name* |
|---|---|---|
| I. Discussion of need for monthly breast self-examination | _____ | _____ |
| II. Discussion of normal breast changes | _____ | _____ |
| III. Factors which influence development of breast cancer | _____ | _____ |
| IV. What to look for during breast self-examination | _____ | _____ |
| V. When to examine breasts | _____ | _____ |
| VI. Procedure for breast self-examination: | | |
| A. In the shower or tub | _____ | _____ |
| B. Before a mirror | _____ | _____ |
| C. Lying down | _____ | _____ |
| VII. Review of take-home literature | _____ | _____ |

**Learner Objectives Met:**

*Date and Name*

_____

**Learner Objectives**

I. Patient states breast cancer prevalence in women and explains that the best hope for cure is through early detection and treatment     _____

II. Patient discusses the following breast changes which may normally occur:

   A. Changes before and after the menstrual period     _____

   B. When wrinkling might normally appear     _____

   C. Changes in the areola during pregnancy     _____

 III. Patient marks her risks in hand-out, "Breast Cancer . . . What is your risk?" and evaluates her score according to directions in pamphlet     _____

 IV. Patient states she will check for any lumps, thickening, changes in contour, puckering, dimpling, swelling, persistent skin irritation, redness, pain, tenderness, scaliness, inversion of nipple or nipple discharge and will report any of these changes to her physician     _____

 V. Patient states she will examine her breasts at the following times:

   A. Approximately one week following her monthly menstrual period     _____

   B. On the first day of each month if she is post-menopausal     _____

 VI. Patient states steps of breast self-examination:

   A. In the shower or tub     _____

   B. Before a mirror     _____

   C. Lying down

   Patient uses anatomical breast model to demonstrate the procedure as if she were:

   A. In the shower     _____

   B. Before a mirror     _____

   C. Lying down     _____

 VII. Patient has take-home literature on breast self-examination     _____

**Evaluation and Comments:**

**Total Learner Objectives Met:**
**Total Possible Points:**

## Patient Teaching Guidelines—Female Breast Self-Examination

  I. Patient states breast cancer prevalence in women and explains that the best hope for cure is through early detection and treatment. Cancer of the breast causes more deaths in women than any other type of cancer; however, breast cancers which are found early and treated promptly have excellent chances for cure. Monthly breast self-examination is the first line of defense against breast cancer. *Emphasize to the patient the importance of making breast self-examination a monthly lifetime habit. Emphasize also that if a woman finds a breast lump or other change, she should see her physician as soon as possible.* Finding a breast lump is frightening, but it helps to remember that four out of five breast lumps are benign. If a lump is malignant, delay allows the opportunity for spread from the site of origin. Biopsy with microscopic examination is the most accurate method of diagnosis.

 II. Patient discusses the following breast changes which may normally occur:

   A. Changes before and after the menstrual period.

   B. When wrinkling might normally appear.

   C. Changes in the areola during pregnancy.

   The female breast is composed of glandular, fibrous, and fatty tissue. Lobes of glandular tissue are arranged like the spokes of a wheel and are drained by ducts which open on the surface of the nipple. The glandular tissue is supported by fibrous tissue which may feel lumpy or stringy. Premenstrual tenderness, fullness and nodularity commonly occur but should decrease or disappear during the week following the menstrual period because of lower hormonal levels. The skin of the breast is usually smooth, but increasing age or weight loss may cause wrinkling. The areola or circular area around the nipple may enlarge and darken in color during pregnancy.

 III. Patient marks her risks in hand-out, "Breast Cancer . . . What is your risk?" and evaluates her score according to directions in pamphlet. The following factors influence the development of breast cancer:

   *Late Menopause:* Incidence of breast cancer increases with age. Seventy-five percent of new cases occur after age forty. However, after menopause the incidence decreases. Therefore, women who have late menopause are considered high risk.

*Family History:* Women whose sisters or mothers have had breast cancer have increased risk for development of breast cancer.

*Race:* Caucasian women are at higher risk for breast cancer than Blacks or Orientals.

*Cancer of the Opposite Breast:* Women who have had breast cancer in one breast have a higher risk for developing primary or secondary cancer in the other breast.

*Marital Status:* Single women have a higher incidence of breast cancer than married women.

*Pregnancy after 20:* Women whose first pregnancies occurred after age twenty and women who have never been pregnant are at higher risk for breast cancer than those having teenage pregnancies.

*Breast Feeding:* Women who have not breast fed are at higher risk than those who have breast fed.

IV. Patient states she will check for any lumps, thickening, changes in contour, puckering, dimpling, swelling, persistent skin irritation, redness, pain, tenderness, scaliness, inversion of nipple or nipple discharge and will report any of these changes to her physician. Carcinoma may develop anywhere in the breast or nipple but is frequently found in the upper outer quadrant. It usually occurs as a painless lump or thickening. Puckering, dimpling, swelling, persistent skin irritation, redness, pain or tenderness are other changes which should be brought to the physician's attention. On the nipple and around the areolae look for whitish scale, distorted shape, inverted nipple or nipple discharge.

V. Patient states she will examine her breasts at the following time:
  A. Approximately one week following her monthly menstrual period. In the week following the menstrual period, the breasts are usually not tender or swollen. A woman's breasts rarely match exactly, but regular inspection will let her know what is normal for her so that abnormalities can be detected early.
  B. On the first day of each month if she is post-menopausal. Changes are best noted by examination at the same time each month. The choice of a certain day each month makes remembering easier.

VI. Patient states and demonstrates steps of breast self-examination:
  A. In the shower or tub—Examine breasts during bath or shower. Hands glide easier over wet skin. With fingers flat, move gently over every part of each breast. Use right hand to examine left breast and left hand to examine right breast. Check for any lump, hard knot, or thickening.
  B. Before a mirror—Inspect breasts with arms at sides. Next, raise arms high overhead. Look for any changes in contour of each breast, a swelling, dimpling of skin, or changes in the nipple. Then rest palms on hips and press down firmly to flex the chest muscles. The breasts will not match exactly, but regular inspection will show what is normal for each individual.
  C. Lying down—To examine the right breast, place a pillow or folded towel under the right shoulder. Place right hand behind head—this distributes breast tissue more evenly on the chest. With left hand, fingers flat, press gently in small circular motions around an imaginary clock face. Begin at outermost top of right breast at 12 o'clock, then move to 1 o'clock, and on around the circle to 12 o'clock. A ridge of firm tissue in the lower curve of each breast is normal. Then move in an inch, toward the nipple and repeat. Keep circling to examine every part of the breast including nipple. This requires at least three more circles. Also check the tail of breast, the tissue extending from the breast upward toward axilla. Then slowly repeat procedure on left breast with a pillow under left shoulder and left hand behind head. Finally, in sitting position, squeeze the nipple of each breast gently between thumb and index finger. Any discharge, clear or bloody, should be reported to the physician immediately.

A woman who has had a mastectomy should include several additional steps in her regular breast self-examination:
  1. Watch for a brown spot or blister on the involved arm near the armpit. This may indicate a rare inflammatory cancer.
  2. Be aware of any pain in shoulder, hip, lower back, or pelvis, which are possible symptoms of bone involvement. Other symptoms are weakness, constipation, and confusion.
  3. Note any unusual breast ache or pain that does not come and go regularly with the menstrual cycle. Cancer is not usually painful, but one rare kind (generalized) does cause pain and soreness—but no lump or thickening. (A breast cancer patient should report any new pain any place in her body to her physician.)

**Take-Home Literature:**
American Cancer Society, "Breast Cancer . . . What is your risk?"
American Cancer Society, "How to examine your breasts."

**REFERENCES**
American Cancer Society, "Breast Cancer . . . What is your risk?"
American Cancer Society, "How to examine your breasts."
American Cancer Society, "Facts on Breast Cancer," 1978.
Bates, B. *A Guide to Physical Examination.* Philadelphia. Lippincott, 1974, 145–157.
Tully, J. P., & Wagner, B. "Breast Cancer . . . Helping the mastectomy patient live life fully," *Nursing,* January 1978, *78,* 18–25.

## Breast Palpation Simulator

**Purpose:** How to obtain breast model for breast self-examination demonstration and prevent cross contamination.

**Equipment Needed:** Breast model
Bath towel
Wash cloth
Teaching plan for breast self-examination

## Essential Steps:

1. Call Nursing Service for availability of breast models.
2. Obtain model from Nursing Service and sign log book.
3. Use model in conjunction with breast self-examination teaching plan.
4. Instruct patient to wash hands thoroughly with soap and water before handling model.
5. Place clean dry bath towel between patient and model at all times. If model is held upright, place towel lengthwise across chest; if held on lap or bed, place towel under model.
6. Wash front of model with soap and water using clean wash cloth between each patient demonstration and before returning to Nursing Service, taking care not to wet back part of model.
7. Return model to Nursing Service at close of teaching session(s) and sign log to indicate return.

*Note:* Not to be used with infectious patients, elevated temperatures, draining wounds or isolations.

**Documentation:** Complete breast self-examination teaching plan.

From Saint Elizabeth's Medical Center, Granite City, Illinois.

# Glossary

**Affective domain.** A classification of learning objectives that is concerned with emotional development and is related to interests, attitudes, values, and goals.

**Analysis.** The act of isolating and examining separately each component of the whole in order to better understand the whole and to provide a basis for arriving at some type of judgment or conclusion.

**Assessing.** The act of gathering, verifying, and communicating data in a comprehensive and systematic manner for the purpose of accurately identifying the health needs and problems of individuals, families, and communities.

**Auditing.** A method of evaluating the quality of care received by the client by examining or verifying the data in the client's health records.

**Behavioral objective.** Statement containing observable behaviors that describe the change that should be evident in the person.

**Care plan.** Written source of client information that serves as a guide to client-centered nursing care.

**Cerebral specialization.** The tendency to rely more heavily on one hemisphere than the other when processing information.

> **Left.** The language-processing, sequential, if-then (hypothetical) brain that mediates input in a "sorting out" way, processing information systematically to find the best solution.

> **Right.** The global view, visual-spatial brain that functions on multiple image inputs, experiences, emotions, and a wide assortment of mental operations in a way that encourages invention.

**Change agent.** One who assists members of a social system to modify their own behavior or that of the system.

**Change, planned.** A deliberate action that has as its goal the modification of the present structure and process of a social system.

**Change, unplanned.** Unpredictable and unintentional change that takes place without being wanted.

**Changing phase—identification.** The time when the target population learns of the desired behavior changes from a resource person.

**Changing phase—internalization.** The time when the environment is changed in ways that require the target population to use the new behaviors to function effectively.

**Client.** Individual, family, or community that the nurse serves.

**Cognitive domain.** A classification of learning objectives that is concerned with the intellectual abilities and the development of thought processes.

**Cognitive style.** The characteristic way of thinking that is exhibited in the activities of a person.

**Communication.** A transactional process which allows for the generation and transmission of information.

**Community.** Specific population living in the same locality and under the same government; a social group that has common values, interests, and needs.

**Concept.** An abstract idea of universal significance; an organized group of ideas about phenomena that have identifiable characteristics.

**Conceptual model.** A group of interrelated concepts that provide the means for categorizing patterns of observations.

**Counseling.** Interaction process used to facilitate understanding of self and environment.

**Cue.** A perceived signal for action that produces a conditional response.

**Data.** Information that has been gathered and organized for analysis and for use as the basis for decisions.

> **Objective.** Information that can be determined by the nurse through observing, listening, feeling, smelling, or measuring.

> **Subjective.** Information provided by the client and that cannot be described or verified by another person.

**Decision making.** A deliberate and systematic analysis used to select a particular course of action.

> **Deliberation phase.** Phase in which inductive and deductive reasoning are used for the purpose of organizing and interpreting isolated assessment data.

> **Discrimination phase.** Phase in which the nursing diagnosis is formulated, and then given a priority following validation.

**Deductions.** Conclusions that are reached by logically proceeding from a clarification of definitions.

**Deductive thinking.** The act of moving from a conclusion or generalization to specific data using prescribed rules of logic.

**Diagnostic conclusions.** Generalizations or summary statements that reflect the client's (individual, family, community) health status and the locus of decision making in the nurse–client interaction.

**Diagnostic label.** Specific statement that represents the conclusions concerning the client's (individual, family, community) health status.

**Diagnostic medical examination.** An examination which seeks to identify the health problem of an apparently ill person so that appropriate treatment may be initiated.

**Directional hypothesis.** Refers to the direction of the expected results.

**Directive change cycle.** Change that is imposed on a target population by an external force.

**Distribution, frequency.** A systematic arrangement of individual measurements from lowest to highest.

**Empathy.** Ability to recognize and share the thoughts and feelings of another, and to understand the meaning and significance of that individual's behavior.

**Evaluating.** The process of assessing the client's progress toward the attainment of the established goals and objectives.

**Evaluation, retrospective.** Evaluation that occurs after the client is no longer receiving care from a particular agency.

**Experiential readiness.** Refers to whether or not a person has had experiences that allow learning what is desired.

**Family.** A unit of interdependent people.

**Field dependence.** The tendency to accept a background as it is; to adhere to the existing structure without any attempt to restructure.

**Field independence.** The tendency to mentally separate embedded figures from contextual backgrounds.

**Field perception.** The tendency toward perceiving events in one mode versus another.

**Formal family roles.** Explicit roles which each family role structure contains. These roles represent a cluster of more or less homogeneous behaviors.

**Goal.** Broad statement of what is to be accomplished; the outcome, end state, or point to be achieved.

**Goal-setting behavior.** The act of making a judgment concerning the desired outcome of a particular situation.

**Health history.** Written record of specific subjective data from the client.

**Help-seeking behavior.** The act of obtaining assistance from another.

**Hypothesis.** A tentative proposition suggested as explanation of abstract phenomena or a solution to a problem.

**Implementing.** Involves the initiation and completion of the actions necessary to accomplish defined goals and objectives and to resolve or support the nursing diagnosis.

**Inductive thinking.** A cognitive process used to gather together isolated pieces of unassociated information.

**Informal family roles.** Implicit roles which are maintained to meet the emotional needs of individuals or to maintain family equilibrium.

**Information-seeking behavior.** The act of using questioning and examining methods to obtain information.

**Interpersonal skills.** Techniques used to enhance the meaning of a transaction between two or more individuals.

**Intervention.** Action that prevents harm from occurring to a client or that maintains or improves the mental, physical, or psychological function of a client; actions, therapies, and/or strategies.

    **Dependent.** Action needed to implement the medical order.

    **Independent.** Action described in the nursing order or the action needed to implement the order.

    **Interdependent.** Action which the nurse performs in collaboration with multidisciplinary health team members.

**Interview.** An exchange of verbal and nonverbal communication by two people for the purpose of sharing information and data pertinent to a particular subject.

**Leadership.** Interpersonal process of influencing a person, group, family, or community toward goal-setting and goal achievement.

**Learning.** The process whereby clients change their behavior as a result of experience.

**Management.** Process whereby human and physical resources are manipulated in order to accomplish specific predetermined results.

**Mastery.** The act of gaining a full command of knowledge of a particular subject.

**Medical examination.** Diagnostic evaluation of the client's health status.

**Medical health history.** Written record of subjective data from the client that concentrates on the disease process—symptoms, contributing factors, and progression of the disease. It seeks to identify information that will aid in the diagnosis and treatment of the client's disease process.

**Model.** Patterns or word descriptions that depict a concept in shortened form.

**Nondirectional hypothesis.** Refers to the nonspecification of direction that expected differences or relationships may take.

**Null hypothesis.** Statement that conveys there is no relationship between the variables of the problem.

**Nurse–client relationship.** Helpful, purposeful interaction between the care-giver and the recipient of the care.

**Nursing.** The act of diagnosing and managing human responses to potential or actual changes in health status; care is provided to maintain health, restore life and well-being, and prevent illness and injury.

**Nursing diagnosis.** Primary statement that reflects the client's healthy/unhealthy response(s) or potentially unhealthy response(s) and the sustaining factor(s) for each response.

**Nursing health history.** A written record of subjective data that deals with the client's responses, physically and psychologically, to the health status.

**Nursing order.** Written description of the actions needed to implement independent behavior of the nurse.

**Nursing process.** An organized systematic method of examining the client's needs and determining appropriate solutions to meet these needs. The nursing process uses the steps of assessing, diagnosing, planning, implementing, and evaluating.

**Nursing prognosis.** Prediction or forecast of the probable course of events or outcome with a particular nursing diagnosis.

**Operational definition.** Defines a variable in terms of the procedures necessary to measure that variable.

**Outcome criteria.** Standards used to determine the responses to or the results of nursing interventions.

**Participative change cycle.** Change that is initiated when new information is made available to the target population and that population makes a decision to accept the information, determine behaviors in need of change, and decide ways to change the behaviors.

**Perception.** Mental process that is used to select, categorize, and interpret data; recognition and interpretation of sensory stimuli through unconscious associations.

**Periodic health appraisal.** Examination done to rule out any health problems, detect disease in an early more treatable stage, or supply the physician or nurse with clues regarding future health problems.

**Physical assessment/examination.** Evaluation of the client's health status through the use of the examiner's special senses of sight, hearing, touch, and smell.

**Planned change—changing phase.** Second phase of planned change; consists of identification and internalization

**Planned change—refreezing phase.** The time when the new behavior is incorporated into one's life-style.

**Planned change—unfreezing phase.** Target population becomes motivated to accept proposed change; a desired readiness implying that the target population sees the need to change and is ready to change.

**Planning.** Nursing strategy or scheme designed to assure goal-directed care for the client.

**Principle of parsimony.** Refers to the simplicity of language (for stating hypotheses) used to convey the intended meaning.

**Priorities.** Preferential ratings in order of importance or urgency.

**Problem.** A question in need of a solution or an answer.

**Problem solving.** The process used to find the answer to a question raised for solution.

**Process.** The act of continuously moving forward, proceeding from one point to another on the way to a goal: a method used to produce, accomplish, or attain a specific result.

**Prognosis.** A prediction or forecast of the probable course of events or outcome associated with a particular nursing diagnosis.

**Psychomotor domain.** A classification of learning objectives that is concerned with motor activities and skills.

**Rapport.** Sense of mutuality and understanding; feeling of harmony, accord, confidence, and respect that underlies a relationship between two individuals.

**Reliability.** The extent to which a measuring device is consistent in what it is measuring.

**Research design.** Refers to the specified plan and structure of the research.

**Research hypothesis.** A simple, clear statement of the specific relationship between two variables.

**Research method.** Refers to the way in which one collects data.

**Restructuring problem.** A problem that can only be solved by changing the initial perception of the problem.

**Role transition.** Changes in role relationships, expectations, and abilities which occur throughout a person's life-cycle and the cycle of the family unit.

**Scientific approach.** A process in which one moves inductively from observations to hypotheses and then deductively from hypotheses to logical implications of the hypotheses.

**Selective attention.** A person can pay attention to only a limited number of stimuli at one time, blocking out some stimuli in order to receive others.

**Selective exposure.** Persons choose messages that expose them to ideas and attitudes that reaffirm those already held.

**Selective perception.** Interpretation of data usually coincides with preconceptions held about the data or idea represented.

**Selective retention.** Individuals remember only those things they want to remember.

**Statistics, descriptive.** The procedures used to describe and summarize observations.

**Statistics, inferential.** Procedures used to infer that what was observed in part will be observed in the whole.

**Straightforward problem.** A problem that does not require a change in perception.

**Strategies.** Plans of actions that bring about unfreezing, changing, and refreezing within planned change. These strategies are comprised of tactics.

**Subsystems.** Component parts of a system that are interrelated and interdependent.

**Sustaining factors.** Contributory elements that cause or perpetuate the response(s) designated by the diagnostic label.

**Synthesis.** The linking of data to a specific problem and bringing them into meaningful relationships; the ability to tie together concepts, data, methods, and ideas from one source with those available from other sources.

**System, content of.** Refers to the sum of the discrete parts that are organized to accomplish a particular goal.

**Systems.** A set of interacting and interdependent parts.

    **Feedback.** The return to the input of a part of the output of a system.

    **Inputs.** Information entering a system from the environment.

    **Outputs.** The energy and waste products that go to other subsystems and out into the environment.

    **Throughputs.** The process that converts inputs into outputs.

**Tactics.** Activities aimed at implementing the different parts of the overall plan.

**Target population.** The persons about whom one wants to learn.

**Teaching.** Any activity by which one person helps another person to learn; an interpersonal act directed at changing the way a person behaves; an intentionally structured communication that is sequenced to produce learning.

**Theory.** A systematic set of interrelated concepts, definitions, and deductions that describe, explain, or predict certain phenomena.

**Trust.** Belief in the dependability, credibility, and reliability of another individual.

**Validity.** The extent to which an instrument measures what it is supposed to measure.

**Variable.** A concept or collection of ideas expressed by a single word that is also operationally defined.

    **Dependent.** The outcome or behavior resulting from the action of an independent variable or treatment.

    **Independent.** The cause, stimulus, or treatment that one manipulates in order to study its effect on the dependent variable.

# Index

(Italicized numbers refer to illustrations and tables.)